EMS Safety and Risk Management

Jeffrey T. Lindsey, PhD, PM, EFO, CFO

*Distance Education Coordinator
for the Fire and Emergency Services Programs*

University of Florida

Gainesville, Florida

EMS Management Series

SERIES EDITOR, *Jeffrey T. Lindsey, PhD, PM, EFO, CFO*

PEARSON

Boston   Columbus   Indianapolis   New York   San Francisco   Upper Saddle River
Amsterdam   Cape Town   Dubai   London   Madrid   Milan   Munich   Paris   Montreal   Toronto
Delhi   Mexico City   São Paulo   Sydney   Hong Kong   Seoul   Singapore   Taipei   Tokyo

Publisher: Julie Levin Alexander	**Project Manager:** Julie Boddorf
Publisher's Assistant: Regina Bruno	**Full-Service Project Manager:**
Editor-in-Chief: Marlene McHugh Pratt	Munesh Kumar, Aptara®, Inc.
Product Manager: Sladjana Repic	**Editorial Media Manager:** Amy Peltier
Program Manager: Monica Moosang	**Media Project Manager:** Ellen Martino
Development Editor: Jo Cepeda	**Creative Director:** Jayne Conte
Editorial Assistant: Kelly Clark	**Cover Designer:** Suzanne Behnke
Director of Marketing: David Gesell	**Cover Image:** Shutterstock/B Calkins
Executive Marketing Manager: Brian Hoehl	**Composition:** Aptara®, Inc.
Marketing Specialist: Michael Sirinides	**Text Font:** Times Ten LT Std
Project Management Lead: Cynthia Zonneveld	

Credits and acknowledgments borrowed from other sources and reproduced, with permission, in this textbook appear on the appropriate pages within text.

Copyright © 2015 by Pearson Education, Inc. All rights reserved. Manufactured in the United States of America. This publication is protected by Copyright, and permission should be obtained from the publisher prior to any prohibited reproduction, storage in a retrieval system, or transmission in any form or by any means, electronic, mechanical, photocopying, recording, or likewise. To obtain permission(s) to use material from this work, please submit a written request to Pearson Education, Inc., Permissions Department, One Lake Street, Upper Saddle River, New Jersey 07458, or you may fax your request to 201-236-3290.

Notice: The authors and the publisher of this volume have taken care that the information and technical recommendations contained herein are based on research and expert consultation, and are accurate and compatible with the standards generally accepted at the time of publication. Nevertheless, as new information becomes available, changes in clinical and technical practices become necessary. The reader is advised to carefully consult manufacturers' instructions and information material for all supplies and equipment before use, and to consult with a health care professional as necessary. This advice is especially important when using new supplies or equipment for clinical purposes. The authors and publisher disclaim all responsibility for any liability, loss, injury, or damage incurred as a consequence, directly or indirectly, of the use and application of any of the contents of this volume.

Many of the designations by manufacturers and sellers to distinguish their products are claimed as trademarks. Where those designations appear in this book, and the publisher was aware of a trademark claim, the designations have been printed in initial caps or all caps.

Library of Congress Cataloging-in-Publication Data
Lindsey, Jeffrey.
  Safety and risk management / Jeffrey Lindsey, Ph.D., EMT-P, CHS IV, EFO, CFO, St. Petersburg College, St. Petersburg, Florida.—1 [edition].
    pages cm
    ISBN-13: 978-0-13-502472-0
    ISBN-10: 0-13-502472-2
  1. Emergency medical services. 2. Emergency medical technicians. 3. Health facilities—Risk management—United States. I. Title.
  RA645.5.L563 2015
  362.18—dc23
                                        2012033080

PEARSON

ISBN 13: 978-0-13 502472-0
ISBN 10:   0-13-502472-2

Dedication

I want to dedicate this book to the three best kids in the world—Natasha, Melissa, and Matthew Lindsey—who have always supported me, and in memory of their mother Kandace. I also acknowledge and thank my stepson, Austin Wolfangel, and hope his career ambitions in fire and EMS come true. I also dedicate this to my wife, Sue Wolfangel-Lindsey, with gratitude for her love and understanding. And in gratitude to my parents, Thomas and Janet Lindsey, for always encouraging me in everything I do, I also dedicate this work.

Contents

Preface ix
About the Author xii
About FESHE xiii

Chapter 1

Introduction to Risk and Safety 1
Objectives 1
Overview 1
Key Terms 1
What Would You Do? 2
Introduction 2
Accreditation Agencies 2
EMS Safety and Risk Managers 3
A High-Risk Profession 3
Risk Management vs. Loss Control 5
Safety 6
Chapter Review 7
Summary 7
What Would You Do? Reflection 7
Review Questions 7
References 7
Key Terms 8

Chapter 2

The EMS Safety Officer 9
Objectives 9
Overview 9
Key Terms 9
What Would You Do? 10
Introduction 10
Role of the EMS Safety Officer 10
   Incident Safety Officer 11
   EMS Safety Officer 12
Basic Duties and Responsibilities 14
   Knowledge of Duties 14
   Role Model 14
   Incidents 14
   Minimum Requirements for an EMS Safety Officer 15
Characteristics of an Effective EMS Safety Officer 16
Chapter Review 17
Summary 17
What Would You Do? Reflection 17
Review Questions 18
References 18
Key Terms 18

Chapter 3

Safety Program Management 19
Objectives 19
Overview 19
Key Terms 19
What Would You Do? 20
Introduction 20
Management 21
   Areas of Improvement 21
   Overview of System Components 22
   Leadership in Safety and Health 22
   Safety-and-Health Policy 23
   Visible Top Management Leadership 24
   Program Evaluation 25
Strategic Map for Change and Improvement 25
Hazards 29
   Job Hazard Analysis 29
   Identifying Workplace Hazards 31
   Correcting or Preventing Hazards 33
Financial Aspects 34
Insurance Concerns 35
   A Brief History of Insurance 35
   Insurance Today 38
   Insurance Is Not the Answer to All 42

Chapter Review 43
Summary 43
What Would You Do? Reflection 44
Review Questions 44
References 44
Key Terms 45

Chapter 4

Developing a Safety Program 47
Objectives 47
Overview 47
Key Terms 47
What Would You Do? 48
Introduction 48
The Hierarchy of Controls 48
   Engineering Controls 49
   Administrative Controls 49
   Personal Protective Equipment 51
   Interim Measures 51
Safety Program 52
   Designating Responsibility 52
   Ask for Help 53
   Facts About Your Situation 53
   Safety-and-Health Program 55
The Safety Culture 61
   Building a Safety Culture 62
   Improving Management
      Processes 63
Safety Committee 63
   Roles and Responsibilities 63
   The Committee's Purpose 64
   Starting the Safety Committee 65
   Safety Committee Training 72
   Safety Meetings 73
Hazard Identification and Control 74
   Hazard Analysis 74
   Hazard Classifications 76
   Principles of Hazard Identification
      and Control 76
   Processes to Identify Hazards 76
   Catching Hazards 78
   Hazardous Materials 79
   Hazardous Equipment 79

   Systems to Track Hazard Corrections 80
   Preventive Maintenance Systems 80
Chapter Review 82
Summary 82
What Would You Do? Reflection 83
Review Questions 83
References 83
Key Terms 85

Chapter 5

Risk Management Process 86
Objectives 86
Overview 86
Key Terms 86
What Would You Do? 87
Introduction 87
Risk 88
   Risk Assessment 88
   Risk Management 88
The Risk Management Process 90
   Identifying and Analyzing Loss
      Exposures 90
   Feasibility of Alternative Risk Management
      Techniques 91
   Selecting the Best Risk Management
      Techniques 94
   Implementing the Techniques 95
   Monitoring the Program 98
Loss Control 98
   Finance 99
   Customer Service 99
   Leadership and Supervision 100
Safety and Prevention 100
   Safety Inspections 100
   Legal Responsibility 101
   Acceptance of Risk 102
   Consensus Standards 102
Chapter Review 103
Summary 103
What Would You Do? Reflection 103
Review Questions 104
References 104
Key Terms 104

Chapter 6

Vehicle Driving and Fleet Maintenance   106
Objectives   106
Overview   106
Key Terms   106
What Would You Do?   107
Introduction   107
Crash Injury and Fatalities   107
   The Research   107
   Human Factors   108
The Safe Driver   109
   Driver Selection   110
   Driver Training   112
   Driver Proficiency   119
Maintenance   125
   Tires   127
   Support Equipment   131
   Vehicle Inspection   131
   Inspection Schedule   131
   Refusing to Drive an Unsafe Vehicle   135
   Comprehensive Maintenance Programs   135
Chapter Review   138
Summary   138
What Would You Do? Reflection   139
Review Questions   139
References   139
Key Terms   141

Chapter 7

Scene Operations   143
Objectives   143
Overview   143
Key Terms   143
What Would You Do?   144
Introduction   144
Streets and Roadway Scenes   144
   Manual on Uniform Traffic Control Devices for Streets and Highways   144
   The Challenge   145
   Safety   145
   Command and Control   146
   Personnel Functions   147
   Limited Access Highway Operations   147
   Traffic Cones   148
   Personal Protective Equipment   149
   Scene Lighting   149
   Emergency Vehicle Markings   151
Building Fires   151
   Forecasting Tools   152
   Functioning at Building Fires   154
Wildland Fires Operations   154
Infectious Disease   155
   Exposure Control Plan   155
   Information and Training   160
Patient Handling   161
   Causes of Patient Drops   162
   Improper Maintenance   164
   Injury Prevention   165
   Proper Lifting Dynamics   166
Violent Situations   167
   Violence to EMS   167
   Uniforms   169
   Highway Safety   169
   Residences   171
   Violent Groups and Situations   172
   Clandestine Drug Labs   173
   Domestic Violence   174
   Other Tactics   174
   EMS at Crime Scenes   176
Hazmat Scenes   176
Air Operations   177
   Background   178
   FAA Oversight   178
Chapter Review   180
Summary   180
What Would You Do? Reflection   181
Review Questions   181
References   182
Key Terms   185

Chapter 8

Station, Office, and Facility Safety   186
Objectives   186
Overview   186

Key Terms   186
What Would You Do?   187
Introduction   187
Organize the Workplace   187
   Self-Inspection Scope   188
   Required Postings   189
Office, Station, and Facility   189
   Safety and Health   200
Vehicle Maintenance Areas   211
   Eye Protection and Protective
      Clothing   211
   Work Clothing   211
   Housekeeping   212
   Lifting Devices   212
   Flammables   212
Towing and Changing Tires   212
Compressed Gases   212
Chapter Review   214
Summary   214
What Would You Do? Reflection   214
Review Questions   214
References   215
Key Terms   215

Chapter 9

Accident Investigation   217
Objectives   217
Overview   217
Key Terms   217
What Would You Do?   218
Introduction   218
The Accident/Incident Investigation   219
   Near Misses   219
   The Investigator   220
   Accident Investigations   220
   Purpose of an Investigation   221
   Effective Investigation Planning   222
   Initiating the Process   223
   Accident Investigator's Kit   224
   Methods to Document the
      Accident   224
Analyze the Accident Process   229
   Accident Causation Theories   229
Determining the Sequence of Events   232

Determining Surface and Root Causes   233
   Management Perceptions   234
   Analyze for Cause   234
Developing Recommendations   236
   Effective Recommendations   236
   Hierarchy of Controls   236
   Recommend System Improvements   237
Writing the Report   241
   The Accident Report Form   241
   Recommendations   246
   Accident Summary   247
   Review and Follow-up Actions   247
   Attachment   247
Chapter Review   248
Summary   248
What Would You Do? Reflection   248
Review Questions   248
References   249
Key Terms   249

Chapter 10

Recordkeeping   251
Objectives   251
Overview   251
Key Terms   251
What Would You Do?   252
Introduction   252
Recordkeeping   252
   Documenting Your Activities   253
   Safety and Health Recordkeeping   253
   Injury/Illness Records   253
   Injury Reports   254
   Infectious Diseases   256
   Privacy Issues   258
   Tuberculosis Cases   258
   Respirator Fit Testing   259
Training   260
Safety Audits   261
Accident Reports   261
   Benefits of Recordkeeping   261
Safety Meetings   262
Vehicle and Equipment Maintenance   262
   Vehicles   262
   Equipment   265

Recordkeeping Checklist 267
Chapter Review 267
Summary 267
What Would You Do? Reflection 268
Review Questions 268
References 268
Key Terms 269

Chapter 11

EMS Provider Health and Wellness 270
Objectives 270
Overview 270
Key Terms 270
What Would You Do? 271
Introduction 271
High Risk Factors 272
   Lack of Physical Fitness 272
   Lack of Pre-employment Physical Ability Testing 272
   History of Illness 272
   Medications 273
   Use of Tobacco 274
   Hearing Loss 274
   Back Injuries 275
   Cancer 275

Wellness Programs 276
   Annual Medical Evaluations 276
   Infection Control 277
   Employee Assistance Program 278
   Physical Fitness Program 278
   Incident Rehabilitation 280
   Return to Work 284
   Stress and Mental Health 288
Chapter Review 289
Summary 289
What Would You Do? Reflection 289
Review Questions 289
References 290
Key Terms 291

Appendix I Occupational Safety and Health Administration (OSHA) 293

Appendix II Federal Resources 302

Appendix III Associations 304

Appendix IV Other Resources 306

Glossary 307

Index 312

Preface

This book on EMS safety and risk management has been written to assist EMS providers in the reduction of line-of-duty injuries, illnesses, and fatalities. It provides a framework for developing programs that will create an appropriate margin of health and safety during the performance of EMS duties.

ORGANIZATION OF TEXT

The chapters of this text are designed to give you a strong foundation in the realms of safety and health. The book concentrates heavily on safety principles and foundations. Chapter 1 introduces you to the concept of risk and safety. Chapter 2 gets into the role of a safety officer at the scene of incidents. Chapter 3 discusses establishing the safety program, emphasizes the administrative side of the safety program, and covers the management viewpoint, financial impact, and insurance perspective.

Chapter 4 addresses the application of a well-defined safety program by discussing the various components. It describes the position of the safety officer within the safety program, gets into safety program components, and describes the safety culture of an organization. It reviews the required postings for organizations and gives a detailed review of a safety committee.

Chapter 5 discusses and describes the risk management process, and Chapter 6 provides an overview of emergency vehicle operations as related to the safety officer.

Chapter 7 focuses on the operational side. It gets into the various operation scenes in which the safety officer may be called to function.

Chapter 8 describes station safety, and Chapter 9 gives a detailed description of conducting an accident/incident investigation.

Chapter 10 discusses recordkeeping for the safety officer. Chapter 11 concludes the text with a discussion on EMS provider wellness. The four appendices provide additional resources on OSHA, federal resources, associations, and additional resources as it pertains to risk and safety.

FEATURES

Chapter Objectives: Objectives are identified at the beginning of each chapter and outline the material the reader should understand upon completion of the chapter.

Key Terms: Key terms are listed at the beginning of each chapter and are bold upon introduction in the chapter. Each chapter's terms are defined at the end of the chapter, and all terms are included in the comprehensive glossary at the end of the book.

What Would You Do? Case Study: Every chapter starts with an EMS manager tackling some issue related to public information and education that is related to the content of the chapter. How he resolved the issue based on information in the chapter is presented in the What Would You Do? Reflection feature at the end of the chapter.

Best Practice: Every chapter includes a real-world example that illustrates information from the chapter having been used successfully by an EMS agency.

Sidebars: This feature relates interesting information that corresponds very closely to text discussion.

Review Questions: Students are required to draw on the knowledge presented in the chapter to answer the questions.

References: A list of bibliographical references appears at the end of each chapter.

ROADMAP/HOW TO USE THIS TEXT

This text does not focus solely on the incident scene. Responding to incident scenes comprises most of what EMS personnel do; however, accidents happen in the station, and they too must be addressed as an administrative component of the safety program. Safety is much more than understanding the inherent risks at incident scenes; it is understanding of the entire system.

As you read the text, you will notice that it addresses all types of agencies. EMS is very diverse; there are volunteer agencies, career agencies, third service, fire department, hospital, and various other types of services. It is difficult to write a text that fits every variation; however, the information contained in this text can be applied to virtually every organization.

Terminology was considered, so when you read "personnel," this refers to EMS personnel in general. Whether paid or volunteer, all personnel are considered members of the organization. Likewise, "managers" and "supervisors" refer to the leadership in your organization, as does "chief." In this text, "management" refers in most instances to the upper management team and supervisors, who are typically referred to as your "shift supervisor" and "street supervisors."

This text is devoted to giving the reader a strong foundation and global perspective on health and safety for EMS providers. EMS personnel have a high risk of injury, and as a safety officer it is your job to reduce the incidence of injury.

TEACHING AND LEARNING RESOURCES

For information on instructor resources, including PowerPoint presentations and assessment tools, please contact your Brady sales representative.

ACKNOWLEDGMENTS

To the wonderful staff at Brady: Marlene Pratt and Monica Moosang.

To the developmental editor: Jo Cepeda.

To all the reviewers for their feedback and encouragement to make this a great text!

To all those who read this text, thanks for taking the time. It is my desire that your efforts make an impact in the EMS profession for the betterment of all.

REVIEWERS

Chief Andy Baillis, OFE, FF/EMT-P, EMS-I
Rittman EMS
Rittman, Ohio

Larry J. Hill, EMT-P/FF/SAFETY SPECIALIST
Bloomingdale, GA

Jeffrey L. Huber
Interim Chair Public Service Careers
Lansing Community College
Lansing, MI

Kurt Krumperman
Clinical Assistant Professor, Emergency Health Services, UMBC
Baltimore, MD

Kevin S. Walker, JD, MBA
Eastern Oregon University
Fire Service Administration

Ryan Watson
Public Safety Director
Oregon City Schools & Adult Education

Jason J. Zigmont, MA, NREMT-P
Executive Director
The Center for Public Safety Education
East Berlin, CT

About the Author

JEFFREY T. LINDSEY, PH.D., PM, EFO, CFO

Dr. Jeffrey Lindsey has served in a variety of roles in the fire and EMS arena for the past 30 years. He has held positions of firefighter, paramedic, dispatcher, educator, coordinator, deputy chief, and chief. He started his career in Carlisle, Pennsylvania, as a volunteer firefighter/EMT. In 1985 Dr. Lindsey pioneered the first advanced life support service in Cumberland County, Pennsylvania. He is retired as the Fire/EMS Chief for Estero Fire Rescue, where he served as the South Division Incident Commander during major events. He was also part of the Area Command for Lee County EOC. Currently he is the Distance Education Coordinator for the Fire and Emergency Services Programs at the University of Florida.

He has served as an inaugural member on the National EMS Advisory Council, representing fire-based EMS, and is a past member of the State of Florida EMS Advisory Council, where he served as the firefighter/paramedic representative. He currently serves as representative to the Fire and Emergency Services Higher Education EMS degree committee. He has been active in the IAFC, serving as liaison to ACEP and attending various meetings representing fire-based EMS, and as the inaugural chair of the Community Paramedic committee, and he is an associate member of the Prehospital Research Forum.

He was a monthly columnist on product reviews for 3 years for *The Journal of Emergency Medical Services (JEMS)*, a national EMS journal. He is a columnist for Firerehab.com and has authored numerous fire and EMS texts for Brady/Pearson. He is currently the Chief Learning Officer for the Health and Safety Institute, which produces *24-7 EMS* and *24-7 Fire* videos. He also was an EMS professor for St. Petersburg College (Florida).

Dr. Lindsey has been involved in a number of large events and has served within the incident command system at the upper level, including during a number of wildland fires and Hurricane Charley. He has also been involved in the preparations for a number of other hurricanes and tropical storms.

He holds an associate's degree in paramedicine from Harrisburg Area Community College, a bachelor's degree in Fire and Safety from the University of Cincinnati, a master's degree in Instructional Technology from the University of South Florida, and a Ph.D. in Instructional Technology/Adult Education from the University of South Florida.

In addition, Dr. Lindsey has completed the Executive Fire Officer Program at the, National Fire Academy. He has designed and developed various courses in fire and EMS. Dr. Lindsey is accredited with the Chief Fire Officer Designation. He also is a certified Fire Officer II, Fire Instructor III, and paramedic in the state of Florida; holds a paramedic certificate for the state of Pennsylvania; and is a certified instructor in these and a variety of other courses.

Dr. Lindsey has an innate interest in alternative health. He is a certified nutritional counselor, a master herbalist, and a holistic health practitioner.

About FESHE

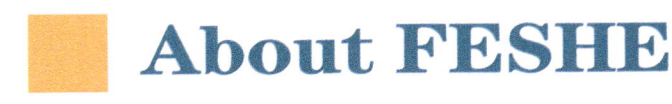

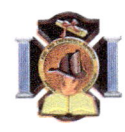

FESHE (Fire and Emergency Services Higher Education) is a dedicated group of individuals from around the country. It is hosted by the United States Fire Administration through the National Fire Academy. The mission of this group is to develop a uniform model curriculum for associate's, bachelor's, and master's degrees. In December 2006, a group of EMS educators convened as the inaugural EMS committee for FESHE. The mission was to develop a model curriculum in EMS management at the bachelor's level. It was the consensus of the leaders across the United States that the committee focus on the management issues of EMS. The clinical portion of the industry is addressed through the National EMS Education Standards and is mainly focused at the associate's level.

This text is written to meet the needs of the national model curriculum for EMS management at the bachelor's level. The EMS management curriculum includes six core courses and seven elective courses. Following are titles in Brady's *EMS Management Series*, designed to meet the FESHE curriculum.

CORE

- Foundations of EMS Systems
- Management of EMS
- EMS Community Risk Reduction
- EMS Quality Management and Research
- Legal, Political and Regulatory Environment in EMS
- EMS Safety and Risk Management

ELECTIVE

- Management of Ambulance Services
- Foundations for the Practice of EMS Education
- EMS Special Operations
- EMS Public Information and Community Relations
- EMS Communications and Information Technology
- EMS Finance
- Analytical Approaches to EMS

Introduction to Risk and Safety

CHAPTER 1

Objectives

After reading this chapter, the student should be able to:

1.1 Explain the need for effective risk management research, planning, and action in an EMS agency.
1.2 Define the terms *risk management*, *loss control*, and *safety*.

Overview

This title on EMS safety and risk management has been written to assist EMS providers in the reduction of line-of-duty injuries, illnesses, and fatalities. It provides a framework for developing programs that will create an appropriate margin of health and safety for providers during the performance of EMS duties.

Key Terms

EMS safety officer **risk management**
loss control **safety**

WHAT WOULD YOU DO?

You have just been named EMS safety officer. It is a brand new position in the department, and your chief really does not know what he expects of you at this point. As your first assignment, you are to describe the difference between risk management and loss control. He is preparing to go in front of the organization's board of directors, who have asked him to be able to define the difference because they see the two areas as the same. You are not sure where to begin, but you know that there must be a difference. You set out to determine what that difference is.

1. Who can you contact to find the difference between *risk management* and *loss control*?
2. What other sources could help you prepare to present the difference between risk management and loss control?
3. What is one way you can present your findings to the chief?

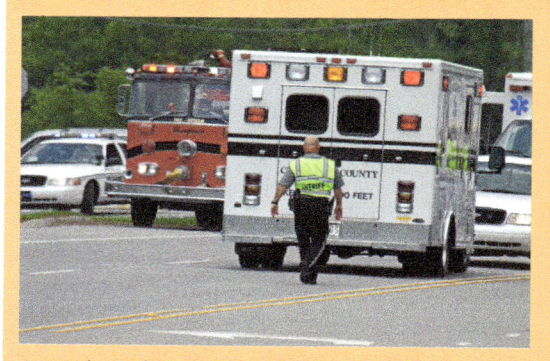

A number of resources are available to the EMS safety officer. *Source:* Fotolia/© Sir_Eagle.

INTRODUCTION

The hazards of hostile or unknown environments, communicable diseases, violence, hazardous materials, and critical-incident stress are, unfortunately, on the rise and affect emergency responders in EMS systems across the United States. Additional hazards such as those associated with driving, lifting and moving, and overexertion also affect the morbidity of those providing EMS services.

ACCREDITATION AGENCIES

Three major standards bodies are applicable to EMS services. They are the Commission on Accreditation of Ambulance Services (CAAS), Commission on Accreditation of Medical Transport Systems (CAMTS), and Commission on Fire Accreditation International (CFAI). Each of these accreditation bodies strives to meet its individual standards in order to achieve the level of service set forth by the agency. Safety is an integral part of the efforts of each of these accreditation bodies.

- **Commission on Accreditation of Ambulance Services (CAAS).** CAAS has identified a number of criteria that should be met in order to gain accreditation. Section 202 of the manual provides the standards for an organization that is seeking accreditation for its service on safe operations and managing risk. The purpose of fulfilling this requirement is to provide a comprehensive safety standard to ensure that patients, employees, and the organization are protected from unnecessary risk.
- **Commission on Accreditation of Medical Transport Systems (CAMTS).** CAMTS is dedicated to improving the quality of patient care and safety of the transport environment for services providing rotor-wing, fixed-wing, and

ground-transport systems. The organization's standards incorporate safety throughout.

- **Commission on Fire Accreditation International (CFAI).** CFAI is committed to assisting and improving fire and emergency service agencies around the world in achieving organizational and professional excellence through its strategic self-assessment model and accreditation process to provide continuous quality improvement and enhancement of service delivery to the community and the world at large. As part of that effort, safety is incorporated into the standards.

Each of the accrediting agencies listed above has a website where you can access additional information on the accreditation process and the standards as they relate to safety in EMS. You can find the Internet addresses at the end of this chapter.

EMS SAFETY AND RISK MANAGERS

This book is intended to be used for the implementation of programs that identify and describe the hazards and risks faced by EMS providers and the ways in which safety and risk managers can and should deal with those risks. However, all EMS providers should address the issue of occupational safety and health programs, not just safety and risk managers.

EMS is a diverse profession around the world. The terms and systems are not always the same. A safety and risk manager may be referred to as a *safety officer* in one organization and in another as the *health officer*. Regardless of the title, the person who is in charge of the health and safety of the organization provides a crucial role to the well-being of the organization's personnel. The term **EMS safety officer** (Figure 1.1) will be used in this text. The EMS safety officer is the person responsible for the safety, health, and well-being of the EMS provider.

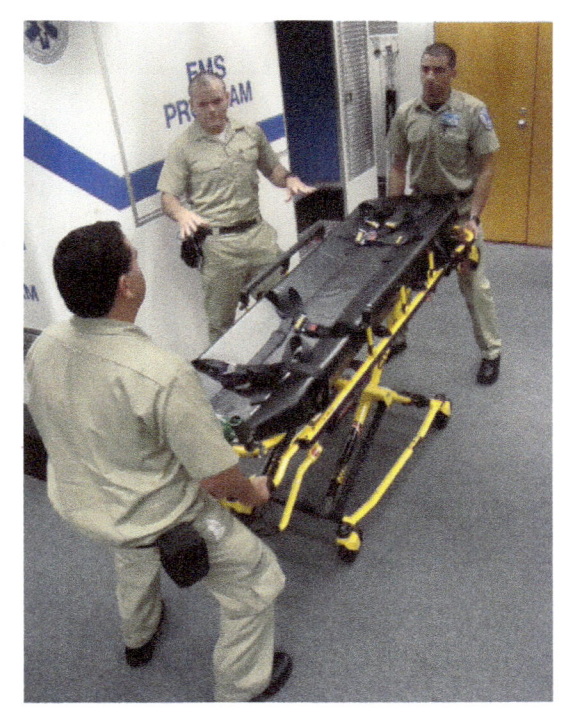

FIGURE 1.1 ■ The EMS safety officer is tasked with the responsibility of ensuring the health and safety of the providers of the EMS organization. *Courtesy of Jeffrey T. Lindsey, Ph.D.*

In addition, a properly protected, trained, and staffed EMS response will provide a greater margin of safety to its members, and it will also enhance service to the citizens that EMS responders are sworn to protect. With a positive approach to these issues, EMS personnel will better understand and, most important, prevent the injuries and fatalities that plague the occupation.

A HIGH-RISK PROFESSION

The Science Daily published a report (Ohio State University, 2008) that almost 10% of the EMTs in the United States missed work because of injuries or illnesses they suffered on the job. In comparison, the rate of injuries

Best Practices

In its October 2007 newsletter, Contra Costa EMS reported on a new system it was implementing on patient safety. It illustrates a great model that can be implemented for provider safety:

EMS Event Reporting: New Patient Safety

Reporting & Provider Recognition Program EMS Event Reporting replaces the old Unusual Event Report Policy (#32) and has undergone major redesign. Over the last eight months, EMS has been working with all of our fire and transport agencies to develop a best practices patient safety and provider recognition program. The new program called "EMS Event Reporting" is focused on patient and provider safety and builds in mechanisms to acknowledge exemplary care in the field. The program uses a consistent process to report, review, analyze, and track patient safety and exemplary care. It is a program that promotes accountability throughout the EMS system.

In the April 2007 Best Practices, we talked about what happens when things don't go according to plan. The new EMS Event reporting program is geared to focus on the root causes of these issues while giving provider agency leadership tools and information to understand "why" things happen. Experts agree that patient safety reporting systems that punish people for making "honest mistakes" do little to improve overall system safety. Leaders in this area know that most safety events can be prevented through training, positive corrections, and understanding the frequency and type of problems people face while trying to deliver patient care. As an EMS agency we are interested in the "what" and "why" behind patient and provider safety events. In a recent review we found that communication was a factor in 61% of our patient safety events. The implications . . . just imagine how many patient safety events could be reduced by improving communication skills in our system. What are we doing with this information? We are in the process of defining the complex communication issues involved and will be redesigning our patient handoff reporting and base contact communication standards to reduce these events. We understand that patient safety reports only capture a small portion of the safety events out there. This new program is designed to encourage better reporting and better problem-solving.

Another innovative aspect of the EMS Event reporting program is that it acknowledges exemplary care in the field. Most of what happens in EMS goes right and we should never forget that. So we want to make sure that we have a way to consistently capture field excellence. Prehospital personnel can also be recognized for "great catches." These are near miss events that are caught before doing harm. Our plan for this program is that EMS event reporting will become an important backbone to our Quality Improvement Program at Contra Costa EMS. As we roll out this new program, we are interested in your comments and experiences with it. If you have questions contact your agency QI coordinator or Pat Frost, EMS QI coordinator, at *pfrost@hsd.cccounty.us*.

Source: Contra Costa Emergency Medical Services. (2007). "EMS Event Reporting: New Patient Safety Reporting & Provider Recognition Program." *EMS Best Practices* 5, 2. (See the organization website.)

---

requiring work absence among EMS personnel far exceeds the national average of 1.3 per 100 lost-work injury cases reported in 2006. This makes the EMS profession a high-risk occupation compared to other occupations in the United States.

The Ohio State University study (2008) to which the *Science Daily* article refers cites two common characteristics associated with an increase in EMS personnel injuries: high call volume (40 or more calls per week) and preexisting back problems. In addition, the study determined that there is a risk of injury in any system serving a population of 25,000 or more. This does not mean that those who work in a low-volume system or in an area with a population of fewer than 25,000 will not sustain an injury; it just means that there is proportionally less chance of an injury.

The need to concentrate on reducing injuries and illnesses is paramount in EMS. As the EMS safety officer, you will be expected to help in the reduction of injuries and illnesses by investigating incidents and by looking for ways to improve the health and safety of personnel in your organization. (The role of the EMS safety officer will be discussed in greater depth in Chapter 10.)

■ RISK MANAGEMENT VS. LOSS CONTROL

Taking risks is an unavoidable practice undertaken every day by individuals from all walks of life, but emergency services have a greater incidence of being exposed to risks. Although there are similarities in both the nature of the work and risk for all of the emergency services, this text will focus on the EMS community.

As an EMS safety officer, you will need to increase your own awareness and understanding of risk management and how it can posi-

> **Side Bar**
>
> According to a study done by Ohio State University (2008), almost 10% of the EMTs in the United States miss work because of injuries or illnesses they suffered on the job. In comparison, the rate of injuries requiring work absence among EMS personnel far exceeds the national average of 1.3 per 100 lost-work injury cases reported in 2006. EMS personnel have almost eight times the rate of injuries or illnesses as any other worker in the United States.

tively affect your EMS organization. So, when researching, look to multiple sources, including information from the insurance and EMS industries. It also is important to realize that risk management is neither costly nor burdensome. A good risk management plan will assist you in coordinating your organization's activities, whether it is daily activities or at major events.

The terms *risk management* and *loss control* sometimes are used interchangeably, but in fact are two separate functions. **Risk management** encompasses all management activities directed at the prevention, reduction, or elimination of the pure risks of business. It can be described as the concept by which an organization deters loss from occurring. Risk management can be accomplished by means of evaluation of the workplace environment, job performance, practices, and coordinated efforts to reduce lost work hours, property, and supplies.

In contrast, **loss control** is a function of management that occurs after an incident. For example, if a person hurts his or her back at work, loss control recognizes the financial loss to the organization and attempts to control the financial consequences. This is done by way of selecting a physician who understands the EMS organization's business, who works with both the patient and the business to get the employee back to work in a normal functional state, and who does both as quickly as possible without expending more dollars than necessary. Another option for loss control is for the organization to have a return-to-work program that will help to reduce the financial payout to the injured employee, who is sitting at home (nonproductive time) collecting workers' compensation instead of being at work helping in some productive manner. In other words, loss control is the process of controlling the loss.

Both risk management and loss control for EMS are rather new ideas. For example, for years risk management was a concept that was fairly exclusive to the insurance and commercial industries. With an openly litigious society and the increasing need to operate EMS services as a business, risk management has become an invaluable tool. An effective and proactive risk management program is essential for maintaining and improving a company's financial success, customer service, management, employee morale, and equipment serviceability.

SAFETY

Safety is a term that is used frequently to mean being "free from risk, injury, or danger." The EMS safety officer is tasked with creating a safe environment for EMS personnel. Sometimes that can be difficult, because the environment in which EMS personnel function is by no means a safe one.

Current research on the problem of occupational injury and illness among EMS personnel presents cause for concern, but offers only a limited understanding of the problem. Maguire, Smith, Hunting, and Guidotti (2005) state that in the year 2000, the occupational injury rate was highest for EMS personnel compared to other industries. An earlier study by Maguire, Levick, Hunting, and Smith (2002) found that the occupational fatality rate for EMS personnel was more than twice that of the national average.

Compared to information on EMS occupational injury, our depth and scope of knowledge regarding EMS workforce occupational illness is severely lacking. Even in the limited areas where EMS workforce illness is better understood, there is still a large reliance on analyses of infectious disease reports mandated by law and studies of the respiratory illness that has plagued World Trade Center rescuers.

A limited understanding of the size of the EMS workforce contributes to the difficulty of conducting adequate surveillance of occupational injury and illness in this population. EMS providers function within a number of different types of organizations, including career and volunteer fire departments, commercial ambulance services, third-service public utilities, rescue squads, and others, thus further obscuring the true dimensions of the EMS workforce. Maguire and Walz (2004) estimated that the total number of EMS providers in the United States is around 900,000. Of these, the U.S. Bureau of Labor Statistics estimates that approximately 192,000 paramedics and emergency medical technicians (EMTs) work in full-time paid positions. Other data suggest that the size of the EMS workforce may be larger.

The National Highway Traffic Safety Administration (NHTSA) funded a work group—the EMS Steering Committee—to develop a document entitled "Feasibility for an EMS Workforce Safety and Health Surveillance System" in order to better understand occupational injuries and illnesses among EMS personnel (Becker and Spicer, 2007). The panel concluded that no single data system exists in the United States today that alone can serve as an effective surveillance data source for EMS workforce illness and injury. Systems that do exist include the National Electronic Injury Surveillance System (NEISS), Census of Fatal Occupational Injuries (CFOI), and Fatality Analysis Reporting System (FARS). A comprehensive surveillance program should rely on an integration of data systems, and those who manage data systems should consider sharing them. Data owners and other data providers should be encouraged to explore new approaches to data aggregation to address EMS issues. EMS stakeholders should work together with data holders/owners to encourage analysis and dissemination of information on EMS workforce illness and injury. A national injury and illness surveillance program should be established for this workforce, spanning surveillance to prevention because, ultimately, the goal of the program is to improve the health and safety of EMS workers.

CHAPTER REVIEW

Summary

EMS safety is still in its infancy stage. A concerted effort needs to be made to improve the safety and well-being of EMS providers. As the EMS safety officer, it is important for you to be able to implement programs and create an environment that will reduce the injuries and enhance the safety of your organization. More research and studies are needed in the area of EMS safety. After reading through this text, you will be better prepared to be part of the solution for a safer EMS work environment.

WHAT WOULD YOU DO? Reflection

There is a difference between *risk management* and *loss control*. You can contact your insurance carrier and speak to the risk management services department to get a better understanding. There also is informative literature available that can enable you to distinguish between the two terms. After some study, you feel you understand. "Chief," you report, "I am ready to explain the difference between risk management and loss control. Let me put it to you this way: You can pay me now, or you can pay me later. Risk management is paying me now. It is the programs and precautions you put into place to avoid potential injuries and property loss. Loss control happens after an incident occurs and involves the programs and procedures that help to reduce the financial losses, damages, and personal recovery after an incident occurs."

The chief thanks you for your response. He is ready to respond to the questions of the board of directors.

Review Questions

1. Define *loss control*, *risk management*, and *safety*.
2. Compare and contrast loss control and risk management.
3. Describe your organization's risk management program.
4. Describe the current status of research in EMS regarding safety issues.

References

Becker, L. R., and R. Spicer. (2007, June). "Feasibility for an EMS Workforce Safety and Health Surveillance System." DOT HS 810 756. Washington, DC: National Highway Traffic Safety Administration.

Bureau of Labor Statistics. (2006). *Occupational Outlook Handbook.* Washington, DC: U.S. Department of Labor. (See the organization website.)

Contra Costa Emergency Medical Services. (2007, October). "EMS Event Reporting: New Patient Safety Reporting and Provider Recognition Program." *EMS Best Practices 5*, 2. (See the organization website.)

Maguire, B. J., N. R. Levick, K. L. Hunting, and G. S. Smith. (2002). "Occupational Fatalities in Emergency Medical Services: A Hidden Crisis." *Annals of Emergency Medicine 40*(6), 625–632.

Maguire, B. J., G. S. Smith, K. L. Hunting, and T. L. Guidotti. (2005). "Occupational Injuries Among Emergency Medical Services Personnel." *Prehospital Emergency Care 9*(4), 405–411.

Maguire, B. J., and B. Waltz. (2004). "Current Emergency Medical Services Workforce Issues in the United States." *Journal of Emergency Management 2*(3), 17–26.

Ohio State University. (2008, January 8). "Emergency Responders at High Risk to Miss Work Because of Injuries." *ScienceDaily*. (See the organization website.)

Key Terms

EMS safety officer The person responsible for the safety, health, and well-being of the EMS provider.

loss control A function of management that occurs after an incident.

risk management Encompasses all management activities directed at the prevention, reduction, or elimination of the pure risks of providing emergency medical services.

safety Being free from risk, injury, or danger.

The EMS Safety Officer

CHAPTER 2

Objectives

After reading this chapter, the student should be able to:

2.1 Identify the role of EMS personnel in risk management and safety.
2.2 Describe the role of the EMS safety officer.
2.3 Explain the duties of a EMS safety officer.

Overview

This title on EMS safety and risk management has been written to assist EMS providers in the reduction of line-of-duty injuries, illnesses, and fatalities. It provides a framework for developing programs that will create an appropriate margin of health and safety for providers during the performance of EMS duties.

Key Terms

EMS Safety Officer
incident action plan
incident command system
incident safety officer
medical plan
unit log

CHAPTER 2 The EMS Safety Officer

WHAT WOULD YOU DO?

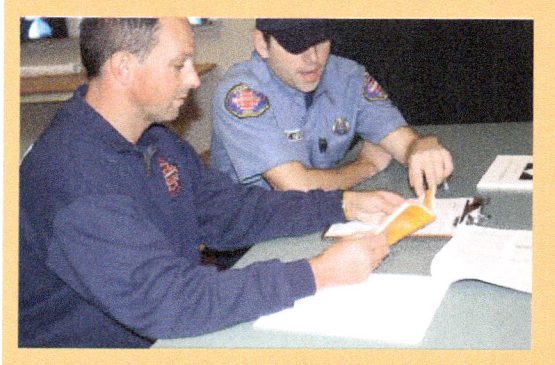

You may be called upon to answer a variety of questions regarding the safety program. It is important that you understand the importance of each aspect of the program and the positions.
Courtesy of 24-7 EMS®, a member of the HSI family of brands.

You are called into the office of the chief. He has been reading about the benefits of having a safety program and he wants to start one. He is unclear about whether he needs to have an incident safety officer or an EMS safety officer. So he would like you to tell him the difference between the two titles. He also would like you to make a recommendation about which position to implement in the organization. What is the difference between the two titles? What would be your recommendation of which position to implement? How could you have multiple safety officers?

INTRODUCTION

The EMS safety officer is by no means the individual solely responsible for the safety of the personnel in an organization. The safety officer is the person charged with overseeing the safety program of the organization. The leadership of the organization must be committed to the safety program and the safety officer. This chapter examines specifically at the EMS safety officer. The following chapters will discuss the safety and risk program, and the EMS safety officer's role.

The fire service has recognized the safety officer role for many years. However, EMS has not developed any programs or criteria for a safety officer in general. A number of years ago a text was written by Gordon Sachs entitled *The Fire and EMS Department Safety Officer* (Sachs, 2001). Sachs (p. 3) writes in the very first chapter that there is little guidance available on the EMS-related responsibilities of the safety officer. The National Fire Academy has three courses targeted for EMS safety officers. These courses are limited for attendance.

The fire service uses NFPA 1500, "Standard on Fire Department Occupational Safety and Health Program" (NFPA, 2007), and NFPA 1521, "Standard for Fire Department Safety Officer" (NFPA, 2008), as the guideline for its safety officers. EMS has not traditionally followed NFPA standards unless except for a fire-based system. However, there has been an effort to involve non-fire based EMS services in the NFPA standard process.

ROLE OF THE EMS SAFETY OFFICER

The appointment of an **EMS safety officer** does not diminish the particular responsibilities of supervisors or the primary responsibility of every

Best Practices

Advanced Safety Operations and Management (R154)

This is a 6-day course that focuses on applying the risk management model to health and safety aspects of emergency services operations, including program management, day-to-day operations, and incident safety. Content areas include firefighters and emergency services fatality and injury problems; the risk management process; safety responsibilities of department members; regulations, standards, and policies affecting emergency services safety; and appropriate documentation and recordkeeping pertaining to firefighter and emergency services health and safety.

Student Selection Criteria

Company-level officers, chief officers, and civilian managers who have department-level health and safety responsibilities (such as program planning and implementation), who may serve as an incident safety officer (ISO).

Incident Safety Officer (F729)

This 2-day course examines the safety officer's role at emergency responses. A specific focus on operations within an **Incident Command System** (ICS) as a safety officer is a main theme. Response to all-hazards types of situations will be emphasized.

Student Selection Criteria

Individuals who have a safety officer responsibility at emergency operation situations. Persons attending this course should have a working knowledge of the ICS, as taught by NFA, building construction principles, hazardous materials management, applicable National Fire Protection Association (NFPA) guidelines, and federal regulations.

Health and Safety Officer (F730)

This 2-day course examines the health and safety officer's role in identifying, evaluating, and implementing policy and procedures that affect health and safety aspects for emergency responders. Risk analysis, wellness, and other occupational safety issues will be the main emphasis of this course.

Student Selection Criteria

Individuals who have department-level health and safety responsibilities. Persons attending this course should have a working knowledge of the ICS, as taught by NFA, applicable NFPA and Occupational Safety and Health Administration (OSHA) requirements and recommendations, and responsibility for setting policy for the department on such issues.

Source: United States Fire Administration. (2009). "MD Emergency Medical Services and Health and Safety Training Programs FA-322." Emmitsburg, MD: Author. (See the organization website.)

---

individual for maintaining occupational health and safety standards. The EMS safety officer role may actually be divided into two separate roles, depending on the size of the organization. There may be an **Incident safety officer**, and/or a safety officer, and both will be discussed in this chapter; however, the term *EMS safety officer* will be used exclusively throughout the text.

INCIDENT SAFETY OFFICER

The Incident safety officer is the individual who is responsible and accountable for safety at the scene of incidents. This person may be the EMS safety officer of the organization or a separate individual in the organization; in larger incidents, it may be an individual from another department or agency. Like most public safety organizations in the United States, the titles may be different but the duties are the same.

The focus or role of the incident safety officer is to ensure scene safety at an incident. He should not be involved with any other aspect of the incident and must have the power and authority to cease or mitigate any unsafe operation. The bottom line is for all personnel to be kept safe. The EMS incident safety officer also is responsible for the following:

- Responding to or having a designated individual respond to major incidents or those that involve or may involve unusual safety hazards
- Community and responder safety impacts to life, property, and the economy
- Managing potentially hazardous materials
- Considering weather and other environmental influences
- Predicting the likelihood of cascading events
- Preparing for potential crime scenes, including terrorism
- Assessing personnel at incident scenes, especially those of prolonged duration, to determine who needs on-site rehabilitation
- Attending post-incident analyses, adding positive and negative reviews of the safety angle, where appropriate
- Developing or implementing a safety action plan at incident scenes
- Ensuring that hazards and risks are identified and adequately monitored for the duration of the incident
- Sharing the action plan with the incident commander and incident staff and revising it as necessary
- Correcting any incident hazards and risks and including them in the safety action plan, safety messages, and/or safety briefings, as appropriate
- Coordinating elements of the safety action plan with the **incident action plan** (IAP)
- Inspecting incident facilities, as appropriate
- Conducting a general inspection of the base and camp facilities soon after they become operational and following up on a periodic basis throughout the incident for compliance to all health and safety standards, such as for a disaster medical assistance team (DMAT) facility at a major incident
- Identifying and documenting all unsafe conditions and providing this information to the incident commander or the base/camp manager, such as at a DMAT facility

EMS SAFETY OFFICER

The role of an EMS safety officer can be more administrative, such as coordinating the safety and wellness aspects of the organization and guiding the organization's policy as it applies to occupational safety practices and personnel welfare issues. The EMS safety officer is responsible for knowing and understanding all rules, regulations, and standards and their applications to safety and health issues in the emergency services. Examples include bloodborne and airborne pathogen regulations; hazardous materials training requirements, for both field and hazardous communication; personal protective equipment; confined space rescue training; patient lifting and moving; and protocols for civil unrest and violent situations.

To carry out their jobs, the incident safety officer and the EMS safety officer need the support of upper management in the organization. Creating and maintaining a culture of safety in an organization can further support these roles. If upper management is not committed to the safety program and the safety officers, the program will not succeed. In addition, both of these officers, if they are not the same person, need to work together. Both positions will have an impact on a number of areas, and each will be able to assist the other individual to ensure safety for personnel.

Side Bar

According to the Occupational Safety and Health Administration (OSHA, www.osha.org), the main role of an EMS safety officer at EMS scenes is to act as a focal point for all health and safety matters (Figure 2.1). Carrying out the role involves the following:

- Facilitating health and safety awareness
- Providing advice on health and safety problems or obtaining advice on unfamiliar problems
- Informing personnel of health and safety hazards specific to their role or function in the organization
- Alerting the appropriate individual in the chain of command about hazards and risk
- Investigating and reporting on incidents, injuries, and health problems, and notifying OSHA of incidents and hazards
- Actively coordinating with health and safety experts on health and safety activities
- Handling the health and safety issues of the organization
- Maintaining inspection and service records on equipment, vehicles, and facilities
- Knowing what records the vehicle maintenance department is keeping and whether or not these records are thorough and accurate
- Keeping records of situations that pose potential liability to the organization, including threats to sue, actual lawsuits, and other service complaints

Source: Based on Federal Emergency Management Agency (2012), "Safety Officer Position Checklist." (See the organization website.)

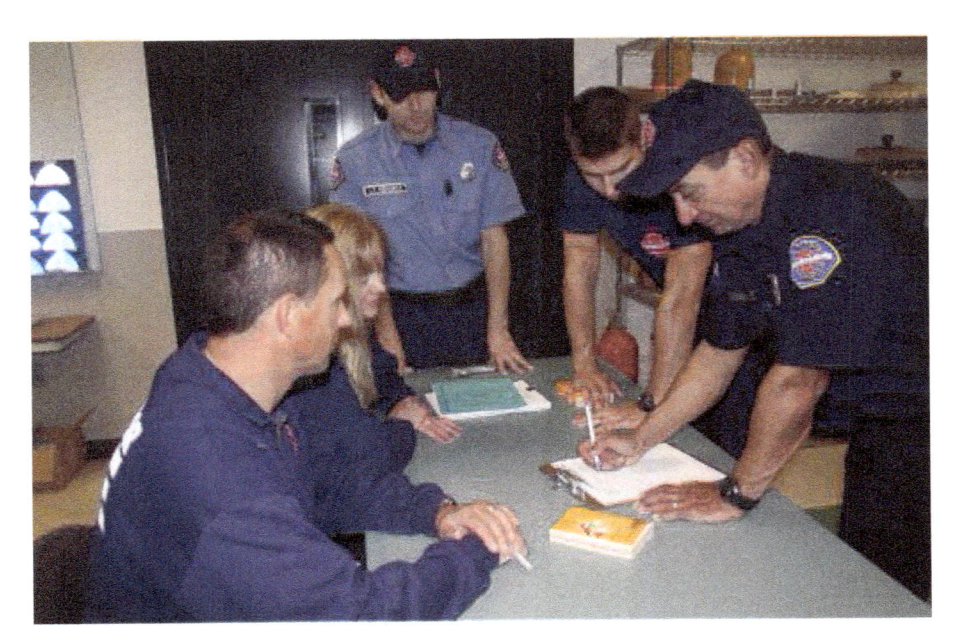

FIGURE 2.1 ■ The safety officer has a variety of roles and duties. *Courtesy of 24-7 EMS ®, a member of the HSI family of brands.*

BASIC DUTIES AND RESPONSIBILITIES

The duties and responsibilities of the EMS safety officer will depend on the organization and its defined role for the EMS safety officer. The following is an overview of some of the basic functions of the EMS safety officer.

KNOWLEDGE OF DUTIES

The EMS safety officer needs to have an understanding of the incident command system (ICS). This includes completing the ICS 100, 200, 300, 400, and 700 courses. In addition, the EMS safety officer needs to fully understand how the safety officer position fits into the ICS and the function of the position within the ICS (Figure 2.2).

The EMS safety officer should have a thorough understanding of the organization's standard operating procedures, medical protocols, and operations. This way the EMS safety officer will be better able to recognize and correct unsafe operations. In addition, he or she needs to know and understand any applicable laws, standards, or regulations.

In general, the EMS safety officer is responsible for knowing current local, state, and federal laws; industry standards; and best practices pertaining to occupational safety and health that apply to EMS. He should also understand the factors related to physical and mental fitness and basic health and should know how to properly and effectively manage a program designated for safety and health.

ROLE MODEL

Being a role model is one of the most important responsibilities for an EMS safety officer. When on the scene of an incident, EMS safety officers must wear the appropriate personal protective equipment (PPE). When traveling in a vehicle, they must be buckled up and not distracted by cell phones or radios. Regardless of the situation, they must consistently set the example. They will lose credibility by requiring personnel to do one thing while doing it completely differently. Safety begins with an attitude that translates into forming a safety culture. It starts with the EMS safety officer.

INCIDENTS

The EMS safety officer is expected to respond to various incidents. With that expectation comes the additional expectation that the individual will exhibit a certain level of knowledge

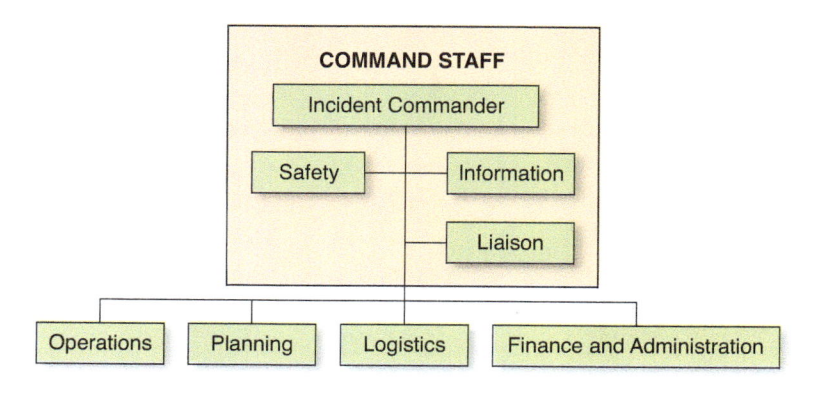

FIGURE 2.2 ■ EMS safety officers need to understand the ICS structure and where they fit into it.

at an incident scene. This knowledge should include the following:

Fireground
- Building construction
- Fire behavior
- Flame spread
- Limits to PPE
- Wildland fire operations

EMS Responses
- Infection control procedures
- Scene security measures
- Wearing of PPE as required or needed
- Critical incident stress indicators and management
- Lifting and moving of patients

Highway and Street Operations
- Appropriate PPE
- Traffic control
- Vehicle positioning
- Traffic cone placement

Special Operations
- Safety lines, vests, and helmets staffed at water rescues
- Proper shoring at a ditch cave-in and collapse, including gas monitoring
- Approved lifelines at a high-angle rescue: rigging, anchors, ropes, knots, PPE
- For hazmat incidents: product identification, PPE, and safety zones
- Use of technical experts
- Medical helicopter safety

MINIMUM REQUIREMENTS FOR AN EMS SAFETY OFFICER

The following minimum requirements for the position of an EMS safety officer can be used as a checklist. Note that some of the tasks are one-time actions; others are ongoing or repetitive for the duration of the incident.

1. Obtain briefing from incident commander and/or from initial on-scene safety officer.
2. Identify hazardous situations associated with the incident. Ensure adequate levels of protective equipment are available, and being used.
3. Staff and organize function, as appropriate.
   - In multidiscipline incidents, consider the use of an assistant safety officer from each discipline.
   - Multiple high-risk operations also may require an assistant safety officer at each site.
   - Request additional staff through incident chain of command.
4. Identify potentially unsafe acts.
5. Identify corrective actions and ensure implementation. Coordinate corrective action with command and operations.
6. Ensure adequate sanitation and safety in food preparation.
7. Debrief assistant safety officers prior to planning meetings.
8. Prepare Incident Action Plan Safety and Risk Analysis using USFA ICS Form 215A. (National Incident Management System [NIMS], 2009)
9. Participate in planning and tactics meetings.
   - Listen to tactical options being considered. If potentially unsafe, assist in identifying options, protective actions, or alternate tactics.
   - Discuss accidents/injuries to date. Make recommendations on preventative or corrective actions.
10. Attend planning meetings (Table 2.1).
11. Participate in the development of the Incident Action Plan (IAP):
    - Review and approve **Medical Plan** (ICS Form 206). (NIMS, 2009)
    - Provide Safety Message (ICS Form 202) and/or approved document. (NIMS, 2009)
    - Assist in the development of the "Special Instructions" block of ICS Form 204, as requested by the Planning Section. (NIMS, 2009)
12. Investigate accidents that have occurred within incident areas:
    - Ensure accident scene is preserved for investigation.
    - Ensure accident is properly documented.

TABLE 2.1 ■ Sample Planning Meeting Agenda

Agenda Item	Responsible Party
1. Conduct a briefing on situation/resource status.	Planning/operations section chiefs
2. Discuss safety issues.	Safety officer
3. Set/confirm incident objectives.	Incident commander
4. Plot control lines and division boundaries.	Operations section chief
5. Specify tactics for each division/group.	Operations section chief
6. Specify resources needed for each division/group.	Operations/planning section chiefs
7. Specify facilities and reporting locations.	Operations/planning/logistics section chiefs
8. Develop resource order.	Logistics section chief
9. Consider communications/medical/transportation plans.	Logistics/planning section chiefs
10. Provide financial update.	Finance/administration section chief
11. Discuss interagency liaison issues.	Liaison officer
12. Discuss information issues.	Public information officer
13. Finalize/approve/implement plan.	Incident commander/All

- Coordinate with incident compensation and claims unit leader, agency risk manager, and Occupational Safety and Health Administration (OSHA).
- Prepare accident report according to agency policy, procedures, and direction.
- Recommend corrective actions to incident commander and agency.

13. Coordinate critical incident stress, hazardous materials, and other debriefings, as necessary.
14. Document all activity on **Unit Log (ICS Form 214)**. (NIMS, 2009)

CHARACTERISTICS OF AN EFFECTIVE EMS SAFETY OFFICER

An EMS safety officer should possess a number of characteristics. A key characteristic is effective communication. Part of effective communication, and in some cases the most important element, is active listening. The EMS safety officer needs to be able to listen to the activity on the scene via radio, listen to personnel, and be able to interpret what he hears. In the same competent manner, the EMS safety officer must convey messages to the incident commander and personnel on the scene. In some instances, these communications may mean life or death. Messages should be clear and concise and delivered in a manner that anyone can understand.

Some personnel have been doing the job for many years and doing it the same way for all those years. Suddenly someone new shows up and begins to tell them what to do. This is where it is important that the organization recognizes and promotes the EMS safety officer to a rank with authority, and that the EMS safety officer delivers communicates in an effective manner.

An effective EMS safety officer has a genuine concern for safety. The emphasis cannot be stressed enough that the organization needs to buy into the safety program and the EMS safety officer.

The incident scenes that require an EMS safety officer tend to be complex or major incidents. The EMS safety officer should not become involved in the tactical operations nor should they fill any other role on the incident. The EMS safety officer's focus should center completely on the safety of the personnel. Safety should be the highest priority on any scene and in the work environment. The EMS safety officer should focus on making sure the scene and work environment are safe and not be distracted by other events or duties. The EMS safety officer should be a very knowledgeable person and have an understanding of what is happening on the scene. He or she does not have to be the person who has been with the organization the longest but must know how to implement the tactics and strategies needed at incidents. The individual should also be level headed and able to deal with the mental and physical stress of the position. In many instances, especially when a situation starts to go awry, the stress level and confusion on the scene tend to increase.

The EMS safety officer must not be intimidated or afraid to react. He or she must be able to halt operations at any incident if conditions become unsafe, even if personnel do not agree with that decision. Safety must be the top priority at the scene of any incident.

CHAPTER REVIEW

Summary

This chapter describes the fundamentals of establishing a recognized EMS safety officer in an EMS organization. The most important asset in any organization is the personnel. It should be everyone's goal to promote safety on every incident and at all times whether in the station, office, or on a serious incident.

WHAT WOULD YOU DO? Reflection

You explain to the chief that the incident safety officer and the EMS safety officer are two separate and important positions within the organization. The incident safety officer responds to and ensures safety at incidents. The EMS safety officer is action oriented and ensures that the organization has the appropriate safety protocols and procedures in place. You know that staffing is limited, and explain to the chief that one person could fill both roles for now. You also state that you can train multiple individuals to fill the role of the incident safety officer, but that whoever serves on the scene in that position will be unavailable for other assignments, including patient care. You also emphasize the most important aspect of the safety program: Everybody, including the incident safety officer, needs to be 100 percent supportive and committed to the program and the position for it to be successful.

Review Questions

1. Describe the difference between the incident safety officer and the EMS safety officer.
2. Describe at least five things an incident safety officer is responsible for in the organization.
3. Describe at least five roles the EMS safety officer is involved with in the organization.
4. List the tasks that the EMS safety officer should ensure happens at the scene of an incident.
5. What is the most important characteristic of an EMS safety officer?

References

National Fire Protection Association. (2007). "NFPA 1500: Standard on Fire Department Occupational Safety and Health Program." Quincy, MA: Author. (See the organization website.)

National Fire Protection Association. (2008). "NFPA 1521: Standard for Fire Department Safety Officer." Quincy, MA: Author. (See the organization website.)

National Incident Management System (NIMS) Incident Command System. (2009). "ICS Forms Booklet FEMA 502-2." Washington, DC: Author.

Occupational Safety and Health Administration. (n.d.) "Safety Officer." (See the organization website.)

Sachs, G. (2001). *The Fire and EMS Department Safety Officer.* Upper Saddle River, NJ: Prentice Hall Publishing.

Key Terms

EMS safety officer An officer who serves in an administrative role, overseeing health and safety issues within the organization.

incident action plan An oral or written plan that contains objectives reflecting the overall incident strategy and specific tactical actions and supporting information for the next operational period.

incident command system A standardized on-scene emergency management concept specifically designed to allow its users to adopt an integrated organizational structure equal to the complexity and demands of single or multiple incidents, without being hindered by jurisdictional boundaries.

incident safety officer An officer who ensures safety on the scene of an incident.

medical plan A plan that provides information on incident medical aid stations, transportation services, hospitals, and medical emergency procedures.

unit Log (ICS 214) A type of log used to record details of unit activity, including strike team activity. These logs provide the basic reference from which to extract information for inclusion in any after-action report.

Safety Program Management

3 CHAPTER

Objectives

After reading this chapter, the student should be able to:

3.1 Articulate the concepts of a safety program.
3.2 Recognize the importance of a safety program.
3.3 Describe the key components of an insurance program.
3.4 Describe the process and conduct a job hazard analysis.

Overview

This title on EMS safety and risk management has been written to assist EMS providers in the reduction of line-of-duty injuries, illnesses, and fatalities. It provides a framework for developing programs that will create an appropriate margin of health and safety for providers during the performance of EMS duties.

Key Terms

adverse selection	**indirect costs**	**loss exposure**
change process	**insurance**	**peril**
commercial lines	**job hazard analysis**	**personal lines**
direct costs	**liability loss exposure**	**property**
hazard	**loss consequences**	**strategic map**

CHAPTER 3 Safety Program Management

WHAT WOULD YOU DO?

Your phone rings in the middle of night. The dispatcher sounds frantic as she describes the unthinkable event. A unit in your organization was just involved in a fatal crash at the intersection of Main and High Streets. You race to get dressed and drive to the scene. You know how to handle the injured—after all, you are an EMS professional. However, you are faced with the uncertainty of what is going to happen afterward. What insurance coverage is provided for this occurrence? What will the impact be on the organization? How is the community going to respond? So many questions, so few answers. If you could only have been more aware of the insurance policies and the ramifications associated with such an occurrence before it happened, maybe you could have avoided all the problems you are facing now. Not in your wildest dreams did you think this could happen to your organization.

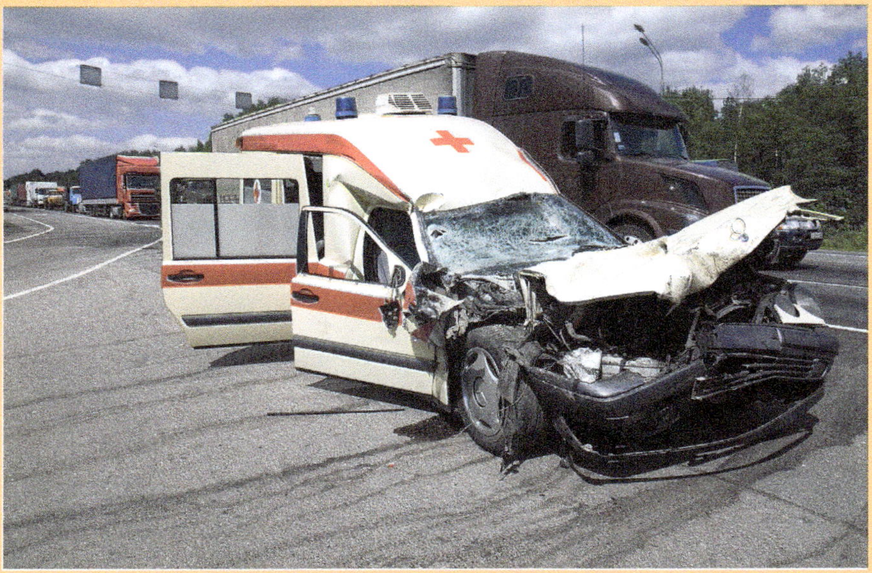

An ambulance crash can have detrimental effects on the agency, personnel, and the community. *Source:* Fotolia/© Alexander Sayganov

INTRODUCTION

As an EMS safety officer, your goals should be to reduce accidents, injuries, illnesses, and their related costs to your organization. You must get everyone to place as much emphasis on safety-and-health issues as they place on other core management issues, such as EMS training and patient care. To be most effective, safety and health must be balanced with and incorporated into the other core processes of your

EMS organization. This chapter describes the necessary components of an effective safety-and-health program.

"Safety first" may sound right, but in reality safety should not be considered in isolation. Rather, it must be integrated into the basic values of your organization. "Safety first" would be better expressed as "Safe procedures are our only standard," which puts emphasis on the idea that it is fine to work as hard and as fast as possible, as long as it can be done safely.

To get an idea of where safety and health fit into your organization, consider the following statements:

- Safety and health are an integral part of our operations.

    True   False   Don't Know

- Teamwork is apparent in all parts of the organization.

    True   False   Don't Know

- Managers and supervisors are out on the scene frequently and always follow the organization's safety and health rules.

    True   False   Don't Know

- Personnel are encouraged to identify safety-and-health hazards and correct them on their own.

    True   False   Don't Know

- Personnel have full and open access to all the tools and equipment they need to do their job safely.

    True   False   Don't Know

If you were able to respond to each statement as true, you are well on your way to developing an active safety-and-health culture. However, if you want to do better, actively work on improving that culture in your organization.

In the final section of this chapter, you will find a description of the means to financially cover your organization when safety fails. It will give you information on how to identify the various means by which you can position your organization to sustain a financial impact from injuries, death, property damage, and bad management decisions.

MANAGEMENT

The role of management and how it fits into the safety program are important considerations in the safety process for an organization. For safety to be integrated into the organization's priorities, it is essential for the EMS safety officer to establish a relationship with management and to be seen as the leader in the safety field for the organization.

AREAS OF IMPROVEMENT

Management processes that are typically ripe for improvement include the following:

- Defining safety responsibilities for all levels of the organization—for example, "Safety is a line management function."
- Developing "upstream measures." These are measures that will let you and your organization learn from the past, such as requiring reports of hazards that were on the scene of an emergency with suggestions for handling them better in the future.
- Aligning management and supervisors by establishing a shared vision of safety-and-health goals and objectives.
- Implementing a process that holds managers and supervisors accountable for visibly being involved, setting the proper example, and leading for improved safety and health.
- Evaluating and rebuilding any incentives and disciplinary systems for safety and health as necessary.
- Ensuring that the safety committee is functioning appropriately. Consider membership, responsibilities/functions, authority, and meeting-management skills.

- Providing multiple paths for personnel to bring forward suggestions, concerns, or problems. One path should be the chain of command.
- Holding supervisors and middle managers accountable for being responsive to subordinates.
- Developing a system that tracks and ensures timeliness in hazard correction. Many sites have been successful in building this in with an already existing work order system.
- Preparing management for an initial increase in incidents and a rise in rates. This will occur if underreporting or an inefficient/poorly organized/poorly disciplined reporting system exists in the organization. It will level off, and then decline, as system changes take hold.
- Evaluating and rebuilding the incident investigation system is necessary to ensure that investigations are timely, complete, and effective. Management should get to the root causes and avoid blaming workers. (OSHA, n.d.–a)

OVERVIEW OF SYSTEM COMPONENTS

A safety-and-health management system and its components should have the following characteristics: It should be an established arrangement of components that work together to attain a certain objective and, in this case, to prevent injuries and illnesses in the workplace. It also should have all its parts interconnected, each one affecting the other. A flaw in one piece probably will impact all the other pieces, and therefore the system as a whole. Specifically:

- Management leadership and personnel involvement are tied together because one is not effective without the other. A shift supervisor can be totally committed, but if EMS personnel follow blindly or are not involved, problems will be solved only temporarily.
- Management must provide the resources and authority so all personnel can identify hazards and, once found, eliminate or control those hazards.
- Training is the backbone of the system. For management to lead, for personnel to analyze the incident for hazards, and for hazards to be eliminated or controlled, everyone involved must be trained.
- No part of this system exists independently. An effective and functioning program is the sum of all its parts. (OSHA, n.d.–b)

LEADERSHIP IN SAFETY AND HEALTH

Management demonstrates leadership by providing the resources, motivation, priorities, and accountability for ensuring the safety and health of its workforce. This leadership involves setting up systems to ensure continuous improvement and maintaining a health and safety focus while attending to patient treatment and emergency mitigation concerns (Figure 3.1).

Enlightened managers understand the value of creating and fostering a strong safety culture within their organization. EMS managers should ensure that safety is elevated in priority within the organization. Safety needs to be seen as a value to the organization as to merely something that must be done or accomplished. Integrating safety-and-health concerns into the everyday management of the organization allows for a proactive approach to accident prevention and demonstrates the importance of working safety into the entire organization.

The importance of leadership in safety and health for EMS is clear. It can increase personnel protection, cut costs, and improve member morale. Industrial worksites participating in OSHA's Voluntary Protection Programs (VPP) have reported OSHA-verified lost-workday cases at rates of 60% to 80% lower than average. For every $1 saved on **direct costs**, such as medical or insurance compensation, an additional $5 to $50 more is saved on **indirect costs**, such as repair to equipment and retraining new workers. The details of this program may not be of value to EMS organizations; however, the overall goal of the program is applicable.

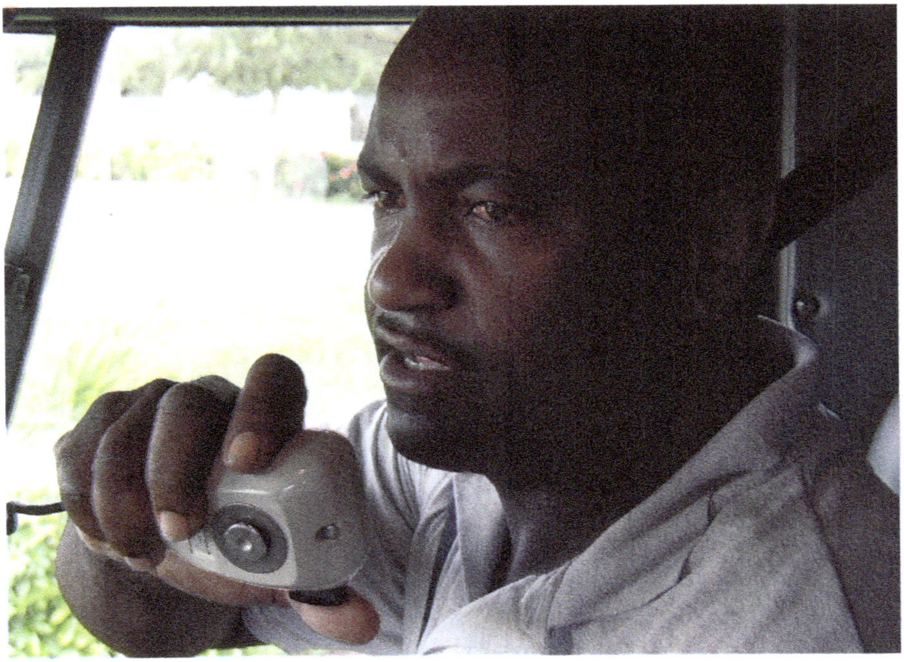

FIGURE 3.1 ■ The incident commander not only commands the strategy and tactics at the scene of an incident, but also takes into consideration the safety of all present. *Courtesy of Jeffrey T. Lindsey, Ph.D.*

During 3 years in OSHA's VPPs a Ford plant noted a 13% increase in productivity and a 16% decrease in scrapped product that had to be reworked. Bottom line: Safety does pay off! Losses prevented go straight to the profit of an organization. EMS is not different from business and industry; loss control should be every manager's concern. Even so, few EMS agencies have been involved in such a program.

Based on the lessons learned from OSHA's VPPs, it is clear that leadership in EMS safety and health begins with management acting on the following:

- Provide visible top management leadership and involvement.
- Establish goals and objectives.
- Establish a safety-and-health policy.
- Provide adequate authority and responsibility.
- Ensure assignment of responsibility.
- Ensure personnel involvement.
- Ensure accountability for management, supervisors, and rank-and-file personnel.

SAFETY-AND-HEALTH POLICY

By developing a clear statement of management policy, you help everyone involved with the worksite to understand the importance of safety-and-health protection in relation to other organizational values. A safety-and-health policy provides an overall direction or vision while setting a framework within which goals and objectives can be developed.

Make goals and objectives realistic and attainable, aiming at specific areas of performance that can be measured or verified (e.g., weekly inspections, hazard correction within 24 hours, training all personnel about the hazards of their jobs and specific safe behaviors before beginning work).

VISIBLE TOP MANAGEMENT LEADERSHIP

Values, goals, objectives, and visions of top management in an organization tend to get emulated and accomplished. If personnel see the emphasis and, equally important, the actions that top management puts on safety and health, they are more likely to emphasize it in their own activities. Besides following set safety rules, managers also can become visible by participating in organization-wide safety-and-health inspections, personally stopping activities or conditions that are hazardous until the hazards are corrected, assigning specific responsibilities, participating in or helping to provide training, and tracking safety-and-health performance.

Assignment of Responsibility

Safety and health are not the sole responsibility of the safety-and-health officer. Rather, they are everyone's responsibility; the safety-and-health officer should be a resource (Figure 3.2). Clear assignments help avoid overlaps or gaps in accomplishing activities. The safety officer should receive initial and ongoing specialized training in *all* aspects of safety (programs, investigation, safety society memberships, human motivation/psychology pertaining to safety, etc.).

Provision of Authority

Any realistic assignment of responsibility must be accompanied by the needed authority and

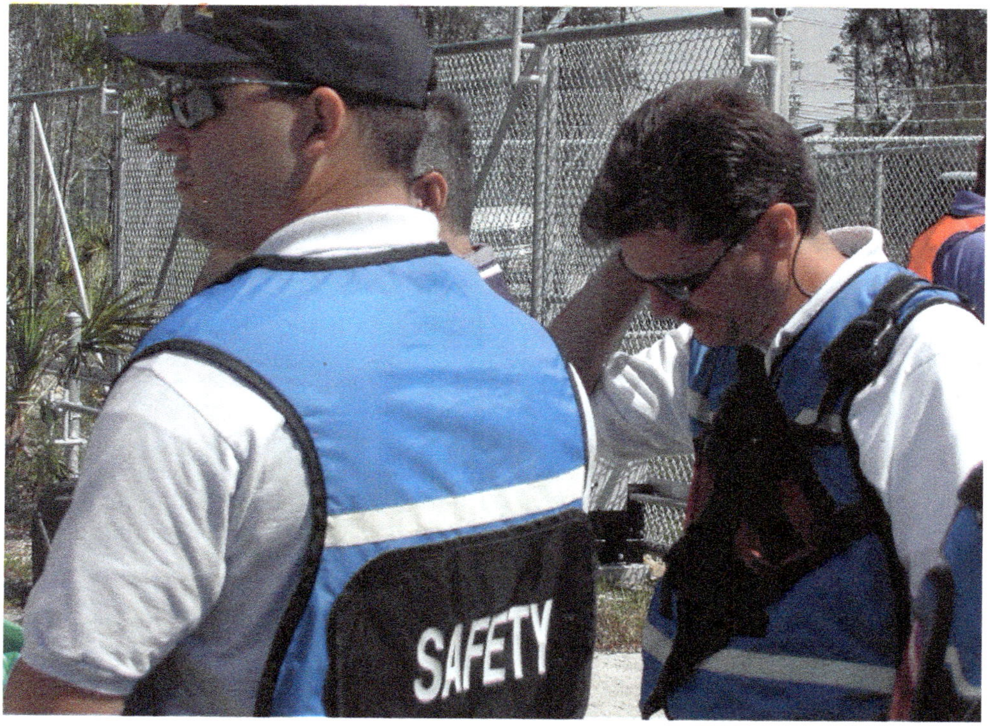

FIGURE 3.2 ■ The safety-and-health officer is the primary individual responsible for the safety of personnel at the scene of an incident; however, it is everyone's responsibility to look out for the safety of all. *Courtesy of Estero Fire Rescue.*

adequate resources. This includes appropriately trained and equipped personnel as well as sufficient operational and capital funding.

Accountability

Accountability is crucial to helping managers, supervisors, and personnel understand that they are responsible for their own performance. Progress should be rewarded and negative consequences enforced when appropriate. Supervisors are motivated to do their best when management measures their performance—what gets measured is what gets done. Take care to ensure that measures accurately depict accomplishments, and do not encourage negative behaviors such as not reporting accidents or near misses. Accountability can be established in safety through a variety of methods, including charge backs, safety goals, and safety activities.

Charge Backs. Charge accident costs back to the department, or prorate insurance premiums. Some organizations have policies that require personnel to pay the deductible of the insurance claim when at fault.

Safety Goals. Set safety goals for management and supervision (e.g., accident rates, accident costs, and loss ratios).

Safety Activities. Conduct safety activities to achieve goals (e.g., hazard hunts, training sessions, safety fairs, and so on that are typically developed from needs based on accident history and safety program deficiencies).

PROGRAM EVALUATION

Once your safety-and-health program is up and running, you will want to ensure its quality, just as you would for any other aspect of your organization's operation. Each program goal and objective should be evaluated in addition to each of the program elements (e.g., management leadership, member involvement, worksite analysis, accident reporting, investigations, surveys, pre-use analysis, hazard analysis, and so on), hazard prevention and control, and training. The evaluation should not only identify accomplishments and the strong points of the safety-and-health program, but it should also identify weaknesses and areas where improvements can be made. Be as objective as you can and identify true weaknesses. The audit then can become a blueprint for improvements and a starting point for the next year's goals and objectives.

Tables 3.1 and 3.2 list obstacles and ways to overcome them in a successful safety-and-health program.

■ STRATEGIC MAP FOR CHANGE AND IMPROVEMENT

A **strategic map** gives an overview of an organization's strategies. The following strategic map describes major processes and milestones that need to be implemented to successfully implement a **change process** for safety and health. This strategy is intended to help you focus on the process rather than on individual tasks, such as training everyone on a particular concern or topic or implementing a new procedure for incident investigations. EMS organizations that maintain their focus on the larger process are far more successful. They can see the forest *and* the trees, and thus can make midcourse adjustments as needed. They never lose sight of their intended goals, and tend not to get distracted or allow obstacles to interfere with their mission. The process itself will take care of task implementation and ensure that the appropriate resources are provided and priorities are set.

The process implementation of the strategic map consists of several steps, which are described below.

TABLE 3.1 ■ Supervisor Identified Obstacles

Obstacles	Solutions
Fear of losing my job	Trust in the system, do the right things, and maintain integrity.
No money for needed changes	Management must support.
Risk in spending money for safety	I must trust and support management.
"What's in it for me" attitude	I must take personal responsibility.
Many people want change but are afraid to take responsibility for it.	I must stop worrying, and instead trust and risk.
No support from upper management	Management must support.
No time or follow-through from upper management	Management must support and provide time and resources.
Competing priorities	Management must balance priorities.
Overwhelmed with workload	Management must provide resources and balance competing pressures.
Turnover too high	Trust that turnover will decrease as culture and work atmosphere improve.
Double standards	Everyone must play by the same rules.
Lack of trust; poor ethics within organization	I must take personal responsibility, stop worrying, trust, and risk.
Lack of open communication and listening	I must be vulnerable and trusting.

Source: OSHA, n.d.–a.

Obtain Top Management Buy-In

Make this the very first step of this process. Top managers must be on board. If they are not, safety and health will compete against other issues. Management needs to understand the need for change and be willing to support it. Showing the costs to the organization in terms of dollars that are being lost (direct and indirect costs of accidents) and the organizational costs (fear, lack of trust, feeling used, and so on) can be compelling reasons for doing something different. Because losses due to accidents are bottom-line costs to the organization, controlling these will more than pay for the needed changes. In addition, as you are successful, you will eliminate organizational barriers such as fear and lack of trust, issues that typically get in the way of all of the organization's goals.

A safety-and-health change process can drive change and bring an organization together very effectively, due to the ability to get buy-in from all levels. This stems from the fact that most people place a high personal value on their own safety. They view change efforts as truly being done for them.

Continue Building Buy-In on a Larger Scale

Build an alliance or partnership among all the personnel of management, your union (if one exists), and employees. A compelling reason

TABLE 3.2 ■ Personnel-Identified Obstacles

Obstacles	Solutions
Fear and lack of trust	Trust in the system, do the right things, and maintain integrity.
Supervisor not willing to listen and support	Supervisors must support and be open, while I must stop worrying and instead trust and risk.
One-way communication (top-down)	Supervisors must risk being vulnerable and open up, while I must not wait to take personal responsibility for my actions.
Organization not aligned on safety	Management must support and provide time and resources.
Supervisors not willing to hear problems and receive feedback	Supervisors must risk being vulnerable and open up, while I must not wait to take personal responsibility for my actions.
Intimidation tactics	If pressures are balanced and I stop worrying, trust, and risk, my supervisor will respond more effectively.
People not willing to take personal responsibility; too easy to shift blame	I must take personal responsibility and operate within guidelines, and must also hold my supervisor and peers accountable.
Lack of consistency and follow through; past efforts fade away	Management must realize this is a long-term effort and commit to it. Excellence is a never-ending journey. I must always be willing to examine myself, receive feedback, and be willing to improve through change.
Them vs. us attitude; win–lose	I take responsibility for myself, and operate from win-win.

Source: OSHA, n.d.–a.

for the change must be spelled out to everyone. People have to understand why they are being asked to change what they normally do and what it will look like when they are successful. This needs to be done up front. If people get wind of something and have not been formally told anything, they will tend to resist and opt out.

Identify key personnel to champion and articulate the reasons for change. These people must be visible. Reasons need to be compelling and motivational. People frequently respond when they realize how many of their co-workers or subordinates are being injured and that they may be next. Management and supervisors also respond when they see money being lost due to accidents, and they realize that their actions toward safety truly influence and define the personnel safety culture.

Build Trust

Trust is a critical part of accepting change, and management needs to know that this is the bigger picture, outside of all the details. Trust will occur as different levels within the organization work together and begin to see success.

Conduct Self-Assessments and Benchmarking

In order to get where you want to go, it is essential to know where you are starting. You can use a variety of self-audit mechanisms to compare your site processes with other recognized models of excellence. VFIS, a division of the Glatfelter Insurance Group, has a number of safety audit forms designed for emergency service organizations.

Use perception surveys to measure the strengths and weaknesses of your safety culture. These surveys can give you data from various viewpoints within the organization. For instance, you can measure differences in personnel and manager perceptions on various issues. This is an excellent way to determine whether or not alignment issues exist and, if so, what they are. One example is the "Safety and Health Program Check-Up" available through OSHA.

At this stage, it is important to look at issues that surface as symptoms of larger system failures. For example, ask what major system failed to detect the defect on the stretcher, or why the system failed to notice that incident investigations are not being performed on time, or if workers are being blamed for the failures. Your greatest level of success will come when these larger system failures are recognized and addressed.

Begin Training

Initial training of management-supervisory staff, union leadership (if present), safety-and-health committee members, and a representative number of members should begin. This may include safety-and-health training and any needed management, team building, hazard recognition, or communication training, which will provide your organization with a core group of people to draw upon as resources. It also gets key personnel on board with needed changes.

Establish a Steering Committee

A steering committee should be made up of management, personnel, union (if present), and safety staff. This group's purpose is to facilitate, support, and direct the change process. Committee members will provide overall guidance and direction and avoid duplication of efforts. To be effective, the group must have the authority to get things done.

Develop Policies

Policies should include a safety vision, goals, measures, and strategic and operational plans. These policies provide guidance and serve as a check-in that can be used to ask yourself if the decision you are about to make supports or detracts from your intended safety-and-health improvement process.

Align the Organization

Establish a shared vision of safety-and-health goals and objectives. Upper management must be willing to provide support by making resources (time) available and holding managers and supervisors accountable for doing the same. The entire management and supervisory staff needs to set the example and lead the change. It is more about leadership than management.

Define Specific Roles and Responsibilities

At all levels of the organization, safety and health must be viewed as everyone's responsibility. Clearly spell out how the organization deals with competing pressures and priorities (e.g., running a high volume of calls versus safety and health).

Develop a System of Accountability

At all levels of the organization, everyone must play by the same rules and be held accountable for their areas of responsibility. The sign of a strong culture is when individuals hold themselves accountable.

Develop an Ongoing Measurement-and-Feedback System

Drive the system with upstream activity measures that encourage positive change. Examples include the number of hazards reported or corrected, number of inspections, number of equipment checks, number of pre-startup reviews conducted, job hazard analysis (JHA), and so on. While it is always nice to know what the bottom-line performance is (e.g., accident rates), overemphasis on rates and using them to drive the system typically only drives accident reporting under the table. It is all too easy to manipulate accident rates, which only results in risk issues remaining unresolved and a probability for future, more serious events to occur.

Create Ways to Reward Participation

Recognition, incentives, and ceremonies for personnel who are doing the right things encourage participation in the upstream activities. Continually reevaluate reward policies for effectiveness and to ensure that they do not become entitlement programs.

Provide Awareness Training for All Personnel

It is not enough for only part of the organization to be involved and know about the change effort. The entire organization must know and be involved in some manner. A kickoff celebration can be used to announce "It's a new day" and seek buy-in for any new procedures and programs.

Implement Process Changes

Involve management, union (if one is present), and personnel using a plan-to-act process such as total quality management (TQM). TQM includes a set of principles, tools, and procedures that provide guidance in the practical applications of running an EMS organization. TQM involves all personnel of the organization in controlling and continuously improving how work is done.

Continually Measure Performance, Communicate Results, and Celebrate Success

Publicizing results is very important to sustaining efforts and keeping everyone motivated. Everyone needs to be updated throughout the process. Sharing progress reports during normal shift meetings (allowing time for comments back to the steering committee) opens communications, but also allows for input. Everyone needs to have a voice; otherwise, they will be reluctant to buy in. A system can be as simple as using current meetings, a bulletin board, or a comment box.

Provide Ongoing Support

That includes reinforcement, feedback, reassessment, midcourse corrections, and ongoing training, which are vital to sustaining continuous improvement.

HAZARDS

A **hazard** is a potential for harm (Figure 3.3). In practical terms, a hazard often is associated with a condition or activity that, if left uncontrolled, can result in an injury or illness. Identifying hazards and eliminating or controlling them as early as possible will help prevent injuries and illnesses.

JOB HAZARD ANALYSIS

A **job hazard analysis** is a technique that focuses on job tasks as a way to identify hazards before they occur. It focuses on the relationship between personnel, the task, the tools, and the work environment. Ideally, after you identify uncontrolled hazards, you will

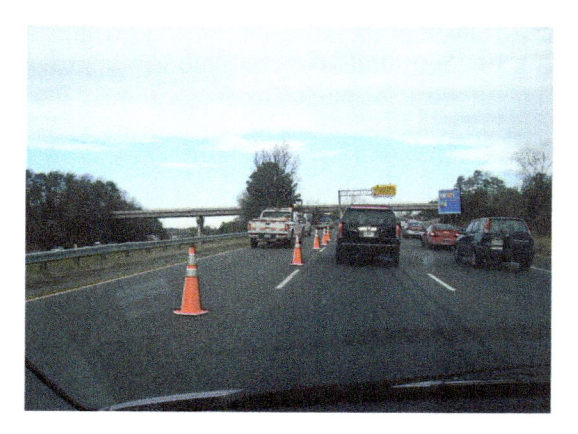

FIGURE 3.3 ■ It is important to identify all of the potential hazards at the scene of an incident. *Courtesy of Jeffrey T. Lindsey, Ph.D.*

take steps to eliminate or reduce them to an acceptable risk level.

EMS personnel are injured and killed at an unacceptable rate in the United States. Safety and health can add value to your organization, your job as an EMS provider, and your life. You can help prevent injuries and illnesses by looking at your workplace operations, establishing proper job procedures, and ensuring that all personnel are trained properly. One of the best ways to do this is by conducting a job hazard analysis, which is one component of the larger commitment of a safety-and-health management system. Supervisors can use the findings of a job hazard analysis to help eliminate and prevent hazards in the work environment, whether at the station or on the scene of an incident. This is likely to result in fewer personnel injuries and illnesses; safer, more effective procedure methods; and reduced worker compensation costs. The analysis also can be a valuable tool for training new personnel in the steps required to perform their jobs safely.

For a job hazard analysis to be effective, management must demonstrate its commitment to safety and health and follow through to correct any uncontrolled hazards that are identified. Otherwise, management will lose credibility and personnel may hesitate to go to management when dangerous conditions threaten them.

To conduct a job hazard analysis, you must involve your personnel, review your accident history, conduct a preliminary job review, list, rank and set priorities for hazardous jobs, and outline the steps or tasks.

Involve Your Personnel

It is very important to involve your personnel in the hazard analysis process. They have a unique understanding of the job, and this knowledge is invaluable for finding hazards. Involving personnel will help minimize oversights, ensure a quality analysis, and get personnel to buy in to the solutions because they will share ownership in their safety-and-health program.

Review Your Accident History

With your personnel, review your organization's history of accidents and occupational illnesses that needed treatment, losses that required repair or replacement, and any near misses, which are events in which an accident or loss did not occur but could have. All of those events are indicators that the existing hazard controls (if any) may not be adequate and deserve more scrutiny.

Conduct a Preliminary Job Review

Discuss with your personnel the hazards they know exist in their current lines of work. Brainstorm with them for ideas to eliminate or control those hazards. If any hazards exist that pose an immediate danger to a individual's life or health, take immediate action to protect him or her. Any problems that can be corrected easily should be corrected as soon as possible. Do not wait to complete your job hazard analysis. Prompt action will demonstrate your commitment to safety and health and enable you to focus on the hazards and jobs that need more study because of their complexity. For those hazards determined to present unacceptable risks, evaluate types of hazard controls.

List, Rank, and Set Priorities for Hazardous Jobs

List jobs with hazards that present unacceptable risks, based on those most likely to occur and with the most severe consequences. These jobs should be your first priority for analysis.

Outline the Steps or Tasks

Nearly every job can be divided into job tasks or steps. When beginning a job hazard analysis, watch the individual perform the job and list each step taken. Be sure to include basic steps, and then record enough information to describe each job action without getting overly detailed. You may find it valuable to get input from other personnel who have performed the same job. Later, review the job steps with the individual to make sure you have not omitted something. Point out that you are evaluating the job itself, not the member's job performance. Include the individual in all phases of the analysis from reviewing the steps and procedures of the job to discussing uncontrolled hazards and recommended solutions.

Sometimes, in conducting a job hazard analysis, it may be helpful to photograph or videotape the individual performing the job. These visual records can be handy references when doing a more detailed analysis of the work.

IDENTIFYING WORKPLACE HAZARDS

A job hazard analysis is an exercise in detective work. Your goal is to discover the following:

- What can go wrong?
- What are the consequences?
- How could it arise?
- What are the contributing factors?
- How likely is it to occur?

To make your job hazard analysis useful, document the answers to those questions in a consistent manner. Describing a hazard in this way helps to ensure that your efforts to eliminate the hazard and implement hazard controls help target the most important contributors to the hazard. This can be difficult as the work environment constantly changes. However, an EMS provider encounters a number of similar scenes. For those hazard scenes, look for answers to these questions:

- Where is it happening (environment)?
- Who or what is it happening to (exposure)?
- What precipitates the hazard (trigger)?
- What will be the outcome should a hazardous incident occur (consequence)?
- What are all the other contributing factors?

Rarely is a hazard a simple case of a single cause resulting in a single effect. More frequently, many contributing factors tend to line up in a certain way to create the hazard. The following is an example of a hazard scenario (Figure 3.4):

> At the scene of a vehicle accident (environment), while assessing a patient (trigger), a member's hand (exposure) comes into contact with broken glass. She brushes against the broken glass and sustains multiple lacerations (consequences).

To perform a job hazard analysis on the preceding scenario, you would ask the following:

What can go wrong?

The EMS provider's hand could come into contact with broken glass.

What are the consequences?

The provider could receive a severe injury and suffer multiple cuts.

How could it happen?

The accident could happen as a result of the provider trying to treat a patient during operations or as part of extrication. Obviously, this hazard

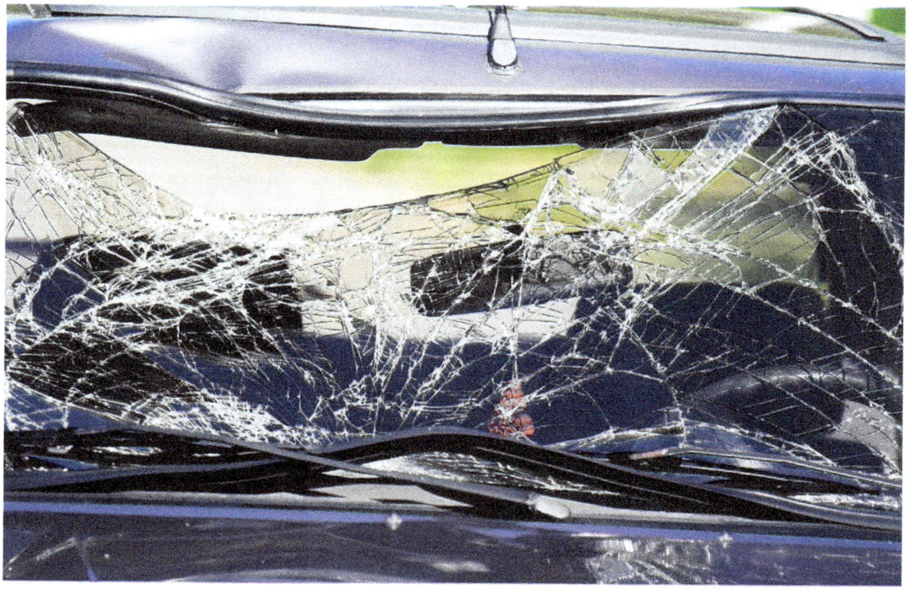

32 CHAPTER 3 *Safety Program Management*

FIGURE 3.4 ■ A motor-vehicle crash has many hazards, broken glass being a typical one. *Source: Fotolia/©drx.*

scenario could not occur if he or she was wearing proper personal protective equipment (PPE).

What are the contributing factors?

This hazard can cause an injury very quickly. It does not give the EMS provider much opportunity to avoid it or recover once her arm comes into contact with the broken glass. This is an important factor, because it helps you determine the severity and likelihood of an accident when selecting appropriate hazard controls. Unfortunately, experience has shown that training is not very effective in hazard control when triggering events happen quickly because human reaction time may not be its equal.

How likely is it that the hazard will occur?

This determination requires some judgment. If there have been near-misses or actual incidents, then the likelihood of a recurrence would be considered high. In the preceding scenario, the likelihood that the hazard will occur is high because the environment is hazardous and uncontrollable, and the treatment is performed without the ability to control the hazard effectively.

See Figure 3.5 for an example of how the steps of an activity can be organized for a job hazard analysis and Figure 3.6 for an example of how the analysis is used to identify the existing or potential hazards in moving a patient down a flight of stairs.

Steps in Moving a Patient Down Stairs

1. Place the patient onto a stair chair.
2. Secure the patient on the stair chair.
3. Wheel the patient to the edge of the steps.
4. Coordinate lifting the patient with a partner.
5. Take one step at a time while moving the patient down the stairs.
6. Set the patient down at the bottom of the stairs.

FIGURE 3.5 ■ Example of how to organize the steps in a patient move.

Job Hazard Analysis Form		
Job Location: Stairway	**Analyst:** Joe Safety	**Date:** January 13, 2013

Task Description: Moving a patient from one level to the next using the stairway.

Hazard Description: The patient could fall. The crew could lose their balance. Potential for a back injury.

Hazard Controls:

1. Properly secure patient to a stair chair.

2. Communicate with partner.

3. Use a spotter or backup person on the foot end.

4. Use proper lifting techniques.

FIGURE 3.6 ■ A sample job analysis form.

CORRECTING OR PREVENTING HAZARDS

After reviewing your job hazard analysis with the EMS provider, consider what control methods will eliminate or reduce each hazard identified on your list. The most effective controls are engineering controls that physically change a machine or work environment to prevent exposure to hazards. The more reliable a hazard control is, the less likely it is that it will be circumvented. If an engineering control is not feasible, administrative controls may be appropriate. This may involve changing how providers do their jobs.

Discuss your recommendations with all EMS providers who perform the job, and consider their responses carefully (Figure 3.7). If you plan to introduce new or modified job procedures, be sure everybody concerned understands the reasons for the changes and what they are required to do.

Periodically review your job hazard analyses to ensure that they remain current and continue to help reduce workplace accidents and injuries. Even if a job has not changed, it is possible that during the review process, you will identify hazards that were not identified in an initial analysis.

It is particularly important to review a job hazard analysis if an illness or injury occurs during a specific incident. Based on the circumstances, the safety officer may determine that the job procedure needs to be changed to prevent similar incidents in the future. If a provider's failure to follow proper job procedures results in a "close call," discuss the situation with all personnel and remind them of proper procedures.

Any time you revise a job hazard analysis, it is important to train all personnel affected by the changes in the new job methods, procedures, or protective measures adopted.

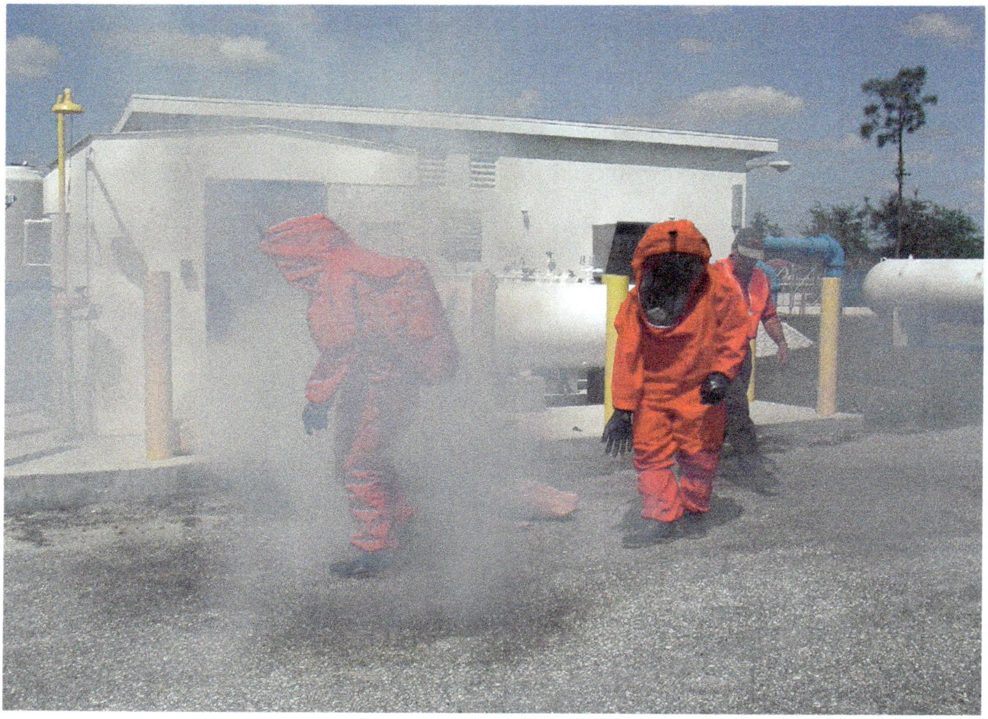

FIGURE 3.7 ■ The safety-and-health officer should provide the appropriate training to personnel to assist them in performing their job safely. *Courtesy of Estero Fire Rescue.*

■ FINANCIAL ASPECTS

> **Side Bar**
>
> Did you know that the average cost of an eye injury is $1,463, when you consider all the hidden costs?
>
> *Source: OSHA, December 13, 2007.*

Accidents (unintentional injuries) are more expensive than most people realize because of hidden costs. Direct costs are obvious—for example, workers' compensation for medical costs and indemnity payments for injured providers. But what about the costs to train and compensate replacement personnel, to repair damaged property, to investigate an accident and implement corrective action, and to maintain insurance coverage? Even less apparent are the costs related to added administrative time, lower morale, increased absenteeism, and poor customer relations both internally and externally. These are the indirect costs—costs that are not so obvious until a closer look is taken.

Here is a quick way to estimate the annual cost of accidents in your workplace: Studies show that the ratio of indirect costs to direct costs varies widely, from a high of 20 indirect:1 direct to a low of 1 indirect:1 direct. OSHA says that the lower the direct costs of an accident, the higher the ratio of indirect to direct costs (Figure 3.8). The more accidents that occur in a workplace, the higher the costs, both

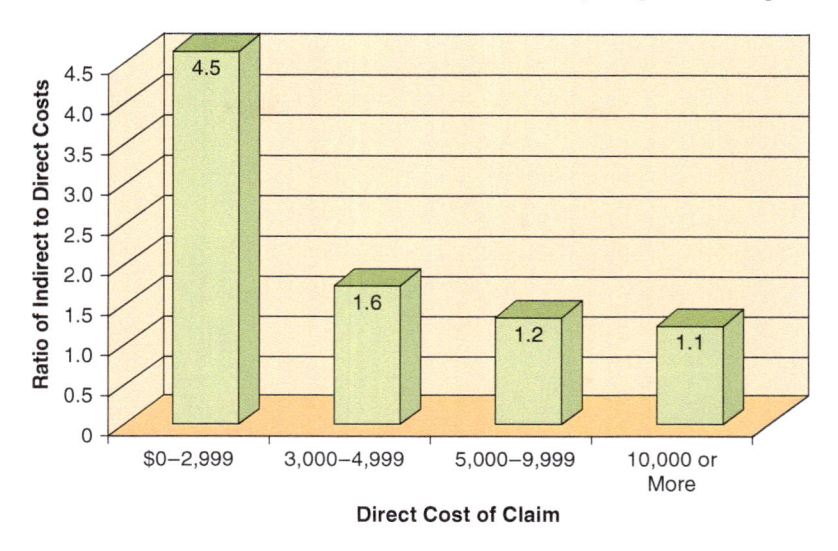

FIGURE 3.8 ■ *OSHA's ratio of indirect to direct costs. Source: Business Roundtable, Improving Construction Safety Performance: A Construction Industry Cost Effectiveness Project Report, Report A-3, January, 1982.*

in increased insurance premiums and greater indirect costs.

To help assess the impact of occupational injuries and illnesses on your organization's profitability, try OSHA's "Safety Pays." It uses a company's profit margin, the average cost of an injury or illness, and the indirect cost multiplier to project the budget you would need to cover costs.

■ INSURANCE CONCERNS

The most common way to transfer the cost of the organization's risk is by purchasing **insurance**. In addition, a large number of companies retain a portion or all of the risk with self-insurance as part of their risk management program. It is your responsibility as the safety officer or risk manager of your organization to oversee the insurance coverage of the entire organization.

A BRIEF HISTORY OF INSURANCE

Insurance is a complex and highly regulated business. When most people hear the word *insurance*, they would rather turn and run the other way. Insurance is a means to pay for your risks; if a loss occurs, you will not be faced with the large dollars to pay for it.

Insurance has been around almost since the beginning of time. Its origins can be found in the form of family, friends, and communities coming together to rebuild structures that were destroyed by nature or otherwise (Figure 3.9). Crops were distributed so that all were not stored at one given location. If a loss should occur, it would affect only some, not all. A variety of these models still exist today. One example is the Amish, members of an Anabaptist Christian denomination with a significant presence in Pennsylvania and Ohio. They pool resources when one of their own is in need. For example, when a barn is destroyed by fire or a natural event, the members of the community designate a day to meet to erect a new barn. It is not uncommon for the Amish to erect a barn in a single day by pooling their resources, including their time, to accomplish such a feat (Figure 3.10). A number of insurance companies were born from religious

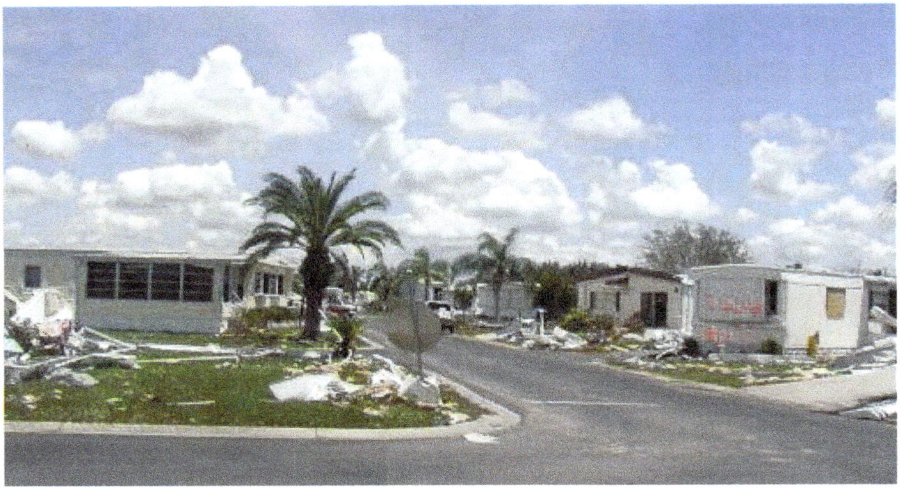

FIGURE 3.9 ■ After a structure is damaged by some event, natural or otherwise, it either will be repaired or torn down and a new structure built in its place. *Courtesy of Jeffrey T. Lindsey, Ph.D.*

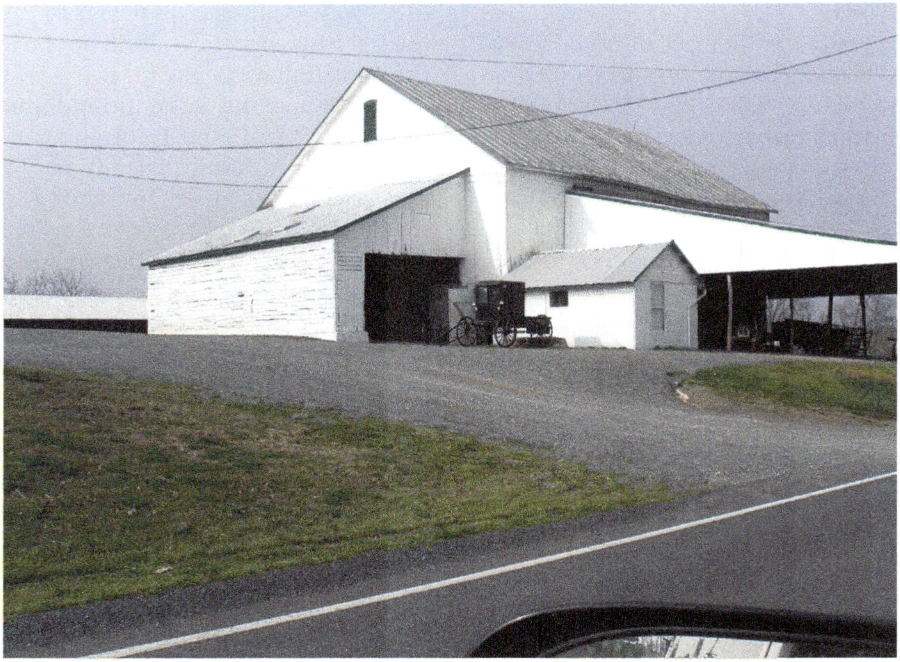

FIGURE 3.10 ■ The Amish are known for raising a barn in a day to replace one destroyed by wind or fire. *Courtesy of Jeffrey T. Lindsey, Ph.D.*

communities; the Lutheran Brotherhood is another example.

In the early days of commerce, Chinese merchants were faced with the treacherous waterways of the Yangtze River. It was not unusual for the mighty river to destroy both the cargo and the vessel. The Chinese merchants knew this and would divide their cargo among the ships so as not to put all their risk on one ship. Thus, if the river destroyed a vessel and its cargo, the merchants would not lose their entire investment.

Insurance has continued to develop since those early days. As the British colonies in America merged into a new country, the insurance conditions birthed new forms that corresponded to the new face and social climate of the country. Today, insurance takes a variety of forms, serving a wide spectrum of needs, from the self-insured to those who purchase every policy available.

The Friendly Society for the Mutual Insuring of Houses Against Fires organization in Charleston, South Carolina, was the earliest known fire insurer, dating back to around 1735. The members of the community gave 1 percent of the value of their home into a pool of monies and agreed to cover any outstanding dollars of others in the event of a loss. After a conflagration that claimed over 300 homes, the company had to go out of business. The members could not pool enough of their monetary resources to withstand the large loss.

Philadelphia was a large city in the New World (Figure 3.11). The design of city blocks by William Penn was aimed to reduce the potential fire threat to the residents of the city. Benjamin Franklin was a well-known Philadelphia resident who had a keen interest in the prevention of fire. His famous saying "An ounce of prevention is worth a pound of cure" was directed to the prevention of fire. In 1736, Franklin also was known for the establishment of the Union Fire Company in the City of Brotherly Love, a volunteer force established to fight fires. By 1750, the fire company organized a mutual insurance company to assist those whose residences were destroyed by fire. Franklin also was instrumental in making the city more fire resistant through the construction of brick buildings, and Philadelphia still reflects that effect today.

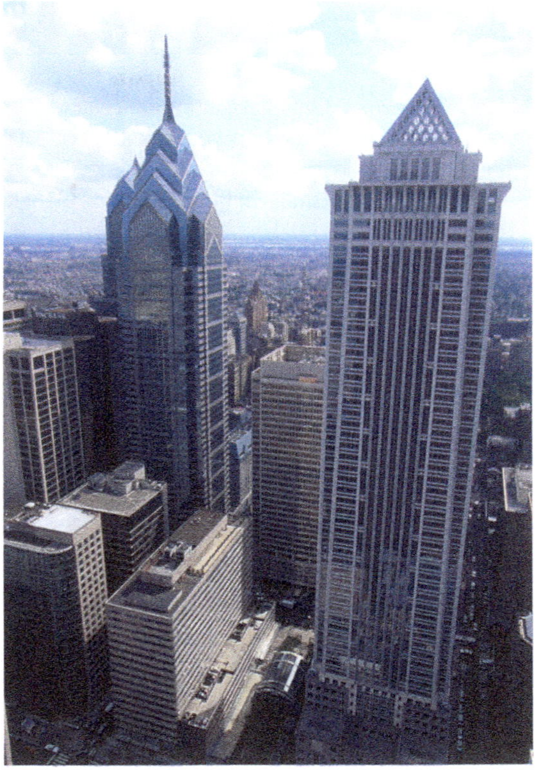

FIGURE 3.11 ■ The city of Philadelphia is best known in the fire service for Ben Franklin's forward thinking regarding fire prevention. *Source: Demetrio Carrasco © Dorling Kindersley.*

As time passed, building construction improved, insurance carriers emerged, and certain trends began to appear. Insurance companies started to establish boundaries regarding what type of businesses they would and would not insure. This holds true today,

Best Practices

In 1969 Arthur J. Glatfelter, an insurance agent, was sent to deliver a check to a young widow of a firefighter who had lost his life. The woman met Glatfelter at her door with a small child in her arms. Glatfelter felt helpless because all he had to offer was a $10,000 check, which was meant to assist her and her child after the loss of her husband. The nation's first insurance company specializing in insuring the emergency service industry emerged as a result of this incident. Volunteer Fireman's Insurance Services (VFIS) was founded by Arthur J. Glatfelter and is still very involved in the emergency services industry today and specializes in insuring it. Today a number of other insurance agencies specialize in insuring emergency service organizations; they include Thomco, ESIP, Fireman's Fund, Provident, and others.

---

with insurance carriers who specialize in catering to those with special needs and risk. EMS is in that category; a number of insurance carriers specialize in insurance for EMS organizations.

INSURANCE TODAY

NOTE: This section provides an overview of insurance and does not serve as a recommendation for or consultation on the insurance policies of your EMS organization.

Insurance is a social device in which a group of individuals transfers the potential cost of their risk in order to combine experience, which permits mathematical prediction of losses and provides for payment of losses from funds contributed by all individuals who transferred risk. Those who transfer risk are called *insureds*. Those whom assume risk are called *insurers*.

An organization may obtain a variety of insurance policies to cover virtually any aspect of business. **Personal lines** are those policies that cover a person's home, auto, and life. **Commercial lines** insure businesses against losses including errors and omissions, theft, vehicle, and liability.

As a consumer, choosing an insurance agent or broker is very important. The agent or broker you use for your personal lines of insurance, such as homeowner's or automobile insurance, may not be the same as your organization's insurance agent. For an EMS organization, the first step toward obtaining insurance is to find an insurance agent or broker who understands the business of EMS. It is imperative that the agent or broker is licensed and reputable. When you purchase coverage, it becomes very difficult to compare apples to apples since the coverage that most companies offer differs to varying degree. This is why it is extremely important that the premium alone is not the sole basis for the selection of insurance coverage. The limitations and exclusions of the policy must be reviewed and discussed to determine what the policy actually covers.

Coverage will vary based on the underwriting capabilities and policies of the insurance company selected. Coverage will include variances on deductibles and coverage limits. The limitation of what the policy actually covers must be considered. A reputable broker or insurance agent who can guide the insurance selection process and explain the ins and outs of any policy is strongly recommended.

When considering insurance, the possibility of self-insuring or self-funding is an option. Self-insuring means the organization establishes an account to lay aside enough funds to cover any event that may occur. For example, if the organization means to self-fund its vehicle coverage, it must put money in reserve to pay for any damages that might occur as a result of a collision. To what extent it can self-fund will depend on the amount of money in reserve.

Self-insuring requires a number of considerations. There are regulations that need to be considered prior to being able to self-insure or self-fund. Most organizations do not have the required cash reserves to be able to do so. The personnel and time required also must be considered when contemplating self-insuring your organization.

Self-insurance is typically seen in large municipalities or large corporations. The majority of small to medium-size organizations cannot consider self-insurance as an option. Still, it is possible to retain a certain amount of risk by self-insuring a portion of the risk.

The insurance deductible is a familiar concept, and acts much like self-insurance does in that the insured decides how much risk he or she wants to assume. The more risk an insured keeps—or the higher the deductible—the less the premium will cost.

The majority of EMS organizations opt to insure through an insurance company. A variety of appropriate insurance policies are available. Property, vehicle, portable equipment, liability, medical malpractice, and errors and omissions all are among the more common policies.

Loss Exposure

To understand why an insurance policy is needed, you must first establish that there is a potential for a financial loss. A **loss exposure** is any condition or situation that presents a possibility of financial loss, whether or not an actual loss ever occurs.

A few particular potential exposures are faced by an EMS organization. A fire, a windstorm, an earthquake, or some other natural peril could damage a station owned by the organization; the organization would not have the capacity to meet the needs the current facility offers—from housing of personnel to the billing office operations and dispatch center. A visitor to the station might be injured while on the premises; a potential liability might be associated with the injury. A medication error or a treatment error may occur; for example, intubations have become one of the most costly errors in patient treatment liability scenarios, ranging from the low millions upward. An EMS provider may be held legally liable for the errors committed by both commission and omission. A vehicle collision involving an EMS unit responding to an incident will in most instances be held legally liable. Emergency service vehicle operators have gone to jail for incidents such as speeding, going through a red light or negative right of way, and deaths occurring as a result of the vehicle being in a collision.

A property loss exists because some party depends on the property to accomplish certain objectives. A property loss exposure has three elements: the **property** that is subject to loss damage or destruction; **peril**, which might lead to loss, damage, or destruction of property; and **loss consequences**, which are the financial results of peril causing property loss, damage, or destruction. Another potential loss for EMS providers and organizations is a liability loss. A **liability loss exposure** is a set of circumstances that presents the possibility that one must spend time and money for the investigation, negotiation, settlement, defense, and/or payment of a claim or suit that arises out of a real or alleged failure to fulfill an obligation or duty imposed by law. A liability claim may be based on an obligation or duty that is imposed by one of four potential areas: common law, statutes, contracts, or contract law. This loss typically is seen in a medical practice claim, a professional liability claim, or a product liability claim in EMS. A workers' compensation claim will fall under this category.

A newly emerging claim that is getting more attention in the EMS arena is employer practice liability. The prevalence of this type of claim is seen in more cases as volunteer organizations begin paying staff. Not knowing and understanding the laws and statutes governing the administration of employees can have a negative impact on an organization, resulting in a claim. It is imperative that the leadership of the organization knows and understands the laws and statutes governing employees and volunteer personnel.

Insurance operates on the law of large numbers. That is, insurance companies compile statistics over many years and then are able to predict with a high level of accuracy the potential for a loss. The potential for the losses then can be spread among a large number of organizations, rather than just one.

For an insurance company to be successful, it depends on losses to affect some but not very many insureds simultaneously. A large number of simultaneous losses has been catastrophic for many insurance companies in the past—from the first fire insurer in the United States going bust from a large conflagration to the most recent hurricanes that caused upheaval in the insurance and building industries. When purchasing insurance, it is imperative to realize and recognize the perils that are covered and those that are not. For example, many insurers do not provide coverage for flood insurance (Figure 3.12) or earthquake insurance; however, such cover-

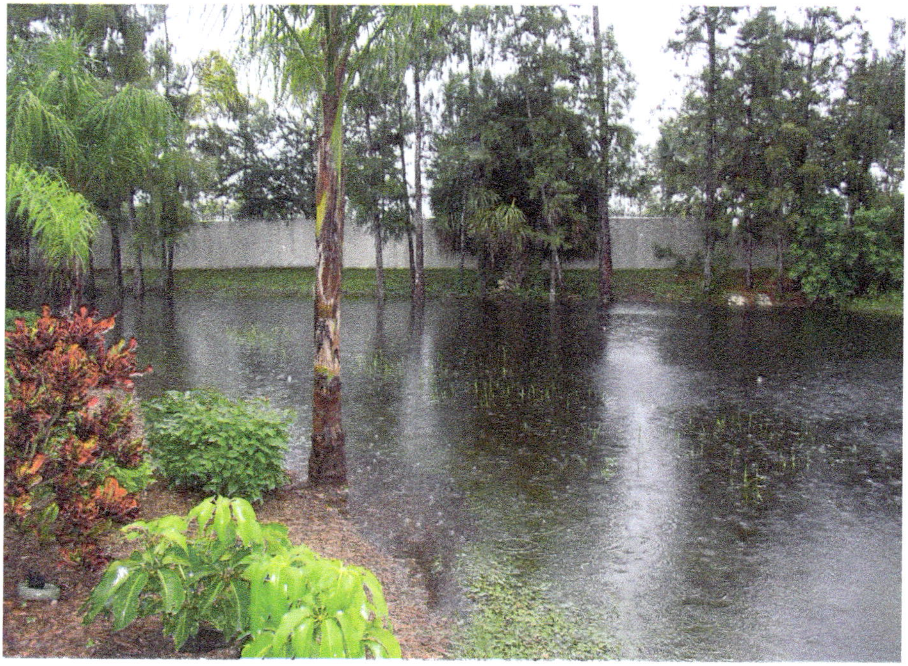

FIGURE 3.12 There are many perils that cause disaster and destruction. Flooding is one that typically requires additional insurance coverage. *Courtesy of Jeffrey T. Lindsey, Ph.D.*

age may be purchased through a separate insurer.

Economic feasibility is another area of consideration when selecting insurance. Insurance companies provide insurance to consumers who purchase policies only if the premium is economically feasible. Two extremes may contribute to the lack of economic feasibility: high frequency and low frequency. If the loss potential is too high, the economic feasibility of the insurer providing such coverage may be prohibitive. If the frequency is too small, there may not be enough of a demand for the protection.

Benefits of Insurance

When describing the benefits of insurance, one immediately thinks of an unfortunate incident for which the insurance company provided payment to remedy the situation. In the overall scheme of things, this is essentially the basics of insurance. But there are other benefits provided by insurance companies.

Insurance companies have an interest in the insured's operation as much as the insured. After all, they have an investment interest in the organization, which is that if the insured has a loss, the insurer will be paying. Insurance companies have handled many claims over the years and compiled statistical evidence and information to determine the cause of a variety of losses. In fact, insurers offer risk management services for the benefit of the insured, which in turn benefits the insurer by making the insured a better risk to insure.

Risk management services include a survey of the premises and operations to evaluate the potential risks and exposures the insured presents. The insurer generates a report, and based upon the findings will send the insured a letter with recommendations for the insured to remedy. These remedies will hopefully make the operations a safer and better risk. The risk management services are provided at no cost to the insured; however, they may be purchased for evaluation purposes when the insured's policy carrier does not provide such services. Risk management is a tool to aid both parties in reducing the potential loss exposures.

A claims service is also provided by some insurance companies. There is more to claims service than just paying claims. The claims service is accustomed to dealing with losses and is more apt to uncover potential fraud and cases where the insured's policy should not be paying. EMS is a specialty business and is unique in the services it provides. For example, the claims service will tap their network of experts in the field, seeking the representation of attorneys who are familiar with and specialize in EMS litigation, something that EMS managers may not be able to do effectively. In addition, some insurance companies offer education services that aid in the reduction of loss potential as a result of a risk management survey or past loss history.

When you are looking for or reevaluating your organization's insurer, pay special attention to the services it provides. An insurer who specializes in EMS is more apt to provide services you need than is an insurer who sells business policies not specific to EMS. So when you pay your premiums, it is not just for the policy, but also for the services the insurer provides. Ask a lot of questions.

Drawbacks to Insurance

There are drawbacks to insurance just as there are benefits. They include the cost of extra services and the cost of the administration of the policy itself. Those costs may be added to your premium. So, when you are considering the purchase of insurance or reevaluating your current policy, ask for and take into account what those costs are and how they affect your organization.

Another drawback is **adverse selection**. Premiums are reflective of claims. The more claims an insurer pays out, the higher the premium has the potential to be. If there are organizations in the insurance pool that have a high incidence of claims, then they may have an adverse effect on all policies, forcing other insureds to look elsewhere for lower premiums.

Moral and morale hazards also are considered a drawback. Some individuals believe insurance is purchased to cover any mishaps that occur, and they do not take personal responsibility for their actions. A number of organizations resolve this issue by creating a pool of dollars they spend on deductions and other costs associated with mishaps. They make a monetary bonus available based on the past dollars paid in claims to their personnel. The personnel must operate in a safe environment without mishaps or claims to be rewarded this money.

INSURANCE IS NOT THE ANSWER TO ALL

Insurance is not the answer to all the problems encountered in EMS. There are a number of issues to take into consideration. When considering any type of loss, there are four areas to look at. These areas are described below.

Injury, Damages, or Death in the Organization

Insurance is purchased to cover the associated expenses incurred when someone is involved in an incident where an injury or death occurs. Life insurance, workers' compensation, accidents, and sickness are a few of the policies that can be purchased to meet immediate needs. However, ongoing costs are also associated with those incidents. Does insurance cover all those costs as well?

In most cases the answer is no. Insurance is designed to cover up to and including the limitations contracted by the policy. However, what are the limitations? Depending on whether or not the EMS provider is a volunteer, career, or on-call paid member, policies may differ. Expectations and contractual obligations within the policy may not be what an individual expects; therefore, it is imperative that the membership and employees of your organization know well in advance any limitations of the organization's insurance policy. They also must determine what their personal insurance will cover should a loss occur, because some personal policies require notifying the insurance agent of any risk-taking activities such as EMS.

Organizations already are operating with limited personnel. What effects would a disabling injury or long-term injury have on the organization or, in a worse-case scenario, if a member or employee was killed? Think of the experience and qualifications of each individual in the organization and what effects it could cause by losing that person. Experience is hard to replace. Recruiting and training are costly for any organization. If a person is injured, who and how will the organization cover the void created until the person can return to full operation with the organization? Insurance cannot cover a number of situations, but it is available to assist the organization in recovering from an incident.

Injury, Damages, or Death to Civilians

Most EMS personnel say they are in the business because they want to help other people. Unfortunately, responders sometimes make mistakes resulting in a patient being injured. The EMS system's insurance will provide monetary assistance in these cases, but patient lawsuits often go far beyond what insurance covers, as does negative publicity, resulting in an EMS system literally being shut down. So, it is imperative for all EMS organizations to implement risk control programs that lower the incidence of life-threatening errors while reducing the organization's potential liability.

The EMS industry changed in the late 1980s when a paramedic was sent to prison for fatally injuring a young woman in her twenties. The paramedic was responding to an incident and collided with this young lady at an intersection. He was found guilty of homicide by vehicle and spent 9 months in prison. He also lost his job, and suffered many times over in his personal life.

A number of other EMS providers have experienced the same misfortunes as that paramedic, including an ambulance company operator from Georgia, who fatally injured a young lady, went to jail, and lost the ambulance service he owned; and a young EMT who killed a pregnant 18-year-old after which the company he worked for filed for bankruptcy. Insurance cannot provide for all the potential factors associated with the losses that occur.

Long-Term Effects

The long-term effects of events can have an everlasting effect on the organization. Future insurance premiums, along with the insurability of the organization, are affected by what happens to the organization today. How will recruiting be affected? It has been recognized that organizations that suffer a severe incident, such as a death, lose current membership and the number of new members decreases. These are all effects for which insurance does not provide.

Equipment and Service Disruption

Insurance provides funding for repairs and replacement of vehicles. However, how many reserve trucks does your organization have in service? Most organizations do not have top-notch vehicles sitting in reserve, and some organizations do not have any in reserve. When one vehicle is involved in a mishap, that unit will be down for anywhere from a few days to years. If the vehicle is involved in a serious collision, the vehicle most likely will be impounded until the investigation is complete. These investigations may take months to years, depending on the incident. Insurance funds may be tied up in the interim, affecting the ability of the organization to provide services.

CHAPTER REVIEW

Summary

Insurance is a great tool for assisting an individual or an organization in placing a monetary risk with another source; however, insurance does not cover every aspect of an occurrence. A number of factors limit the insurance policy. There are areas where insurance does not cover the loss.

It is imperative to recognize the services provided by an insurance carrier. Take the time to meet with the organization's insurance agent and discuss the policies your organization has in effect. Keep the organization's policy up to date. Be sure your insurance company is a reputable one that is familiar with EMS. Now is the time to review policies and look at insurance coverage your organization has in effect.

WHAT WOULD YOU DO? Reflection

After studying this chapter and reading this text you are now more prepared to handle unfortunate situations such as a collision involving an emergency vehicle. You know that you will need to get in contact with your auto insurance carrier, who will assist you in maneuvering through the process. An accident investigation needs to be performed immediately. The impact to the organization could be astronomical, depending on how the incident is handled right from the beginning.

The impact will be in direct relationship to the strength of your organization. Though each organization will be a little different, you will be able to help steer the ship from this point forward. It is important to assemble the management team and implement the plan you developed for such a tragic event. The community will respond based on the information heard. You need to take control of the release of information and be prepared to do damage control.

Review Questions

1. Describe at least three management processes ripe for improvement.
2. List at least three objectives management should have when establishing a loss control program.
3. Describe the implementation process for a strategic map for change and continuous improvement in a safety-and-health program. Use the step-by-step approach discussed in the chapter.
4. Explain the rationale for insurance today.
5. Complete a job hazard analysis for your agency based upon a hazard that potentially exists.
6. Compare and contrast two benefits and two drawbacks of insurance for your organization. Describe the effects they have on your organization.

References

Athearn, J. L., S. T. Pritchett, and J. T. Schmit. (1989). *Risk and Insurance*, 6th edition. St. Paul, MN: West Publishing Company.

Business Roundtable. (1982, January). "Improving Construction Safety Performance." Report A-3. Reprinted July 1990. (See the organization website.)

Gibbons, R. J., G. E. Rejda, and M. W. Elliot. (1992). "Insurance Perspectives: American Institute for Chartered Property." Malvern, PA: Casualty Underwriters.

Occupational Safety and Health Administration (OSHA). (n.d.–a). "Safety and Health Management Systems eTools: Obstacles to a Successful Safety and Health Program." Washington, DC: Author. (See the organization website.)

Occupational Safety and Health Administration (OSHA). (n.d.–b). "Safety and Health Management Systems eTools: Safety and Health Culture." Washington, DC: Author. (See the organization website.)

Occupational Safety and Health Administration (OSHA). (n.d.–c). "Fact Sheet: Management Leadership." Washington, DC: Author. (See the organization website.)

Occupational Safety and Health Administration (OSHA). (2007, September 7). "Safety and

Health Program Check-up." Washington, DC: Author. (See the organization website.)

Occupational Safety and Health Administration (OSHA). (2007, December 13). "Voluntary Protection Programs." "Safety and Health Management Systems eTools: Costs of Accidents." Washington, DC: Author. (See the organization website.)

Occupational Safety and Health Administration. (2009, April 16). "OSHA's Safety Pays Program." Washington, DC: Author. (See the organization website.)

Occupational Safety and Health Administration. (2009, September 29). "VPP: Voluntary Protection Programs." Washington, DC: Author. (See the organization website.)

Steffens, J. (1997). *Emergency Vehicle Driver Training Program.* York: PA: VFIS, Glatfelter Insurance Group.

Key Terms

adverse selection Occurs when the more claims an insurer pays out, the higher the premium has the potential to go.

change process A strategy intended to help focus on process rather than on individual tasks.

commercial lines Insurance policies that help to protect businesses against losses, including errors and omissions, theft, vehicle, and liability.

direct costs Costs that are paid as a result of a loss—for example, workers' compensation claims, which cover medical costs and indemnity payments for an injured or ill member.

hazard The potential for harm. In practical terms, a hazard often is associated with a condition or activity that, if left uncontrolled, can result in an injury or illness.

indirect costs Costs related to added administrative time, lower morale, increased absenteeism, and poorer internal and external customer relations.

insurance A social device in which a group of individuals transfer the potential cost of risk in order to combine experience, which permits mathematical prediction of losses and provides for payment of losses from funds contributed by all members who transferred risk.

job hazard analysis A technique that focuses on job tasks as a way to identify hazards before they occur, and focuses on the relationship among member, task, tools, and work environment.

liability loss exposure A set of circumstances that presents the possibility that one must spend time and money for the investigation, negotiation, settlement, defense, and/or payment of a claim or suit that arises out of a real or alleged failure to fulfill an obligation or duty imposed by law.

loss consequences The financial result of a peril that has caused property to be lost, damaged, or destroyed.

loss exposure Any condition or situation that presents a possibility of financial loss, whether or not an actual loss ever occurs.

peril The cause that might lead to loss, damage, or destruction of property.

personal lines Insurance policies that help to protect an individual's home, auto, and life.

property Item subject to loss, damage, or destruction.

strategic map An overview of an organization's strategies.

Developing a Safety Program

CHAPTER 4

Objectives

After reading this chapter, the student should be able to:

4.1 Articulate the concepts of a safety program.
4.2 Recognize the importance of a safety program.
4.3 Describe a safety culture.
4.4 Explain the process of establishing a safety committee.

Overview

This title on EMS safety and risk management has been written to assist EMS providers in the reduction of line-of-duty injuries, illnesses, and fatalities. It provides a framework for developing programs that will create an appropriate margin of health and safety for providers during the performance of EMS duties.

Key Terms

administrative controls
culture of consequences
engineering controls
expert power
hazard identification
hierarchy of controls
interim measures
Occupational Safety and Health Administration (OSHA)
personal protective equipment (PPE)
position power
safety committee
safety culture
safety program
worksite analysis

WHAT WOULD YOU DO?

Your insurance carrier has just reported on its safety audit of your organization. One of the auditor's recommendations is to create a safety committee. You have had many committees in the past, but never a safety committee. Where do you begin? What should be the safety committee's responsibilities? You have more questions than answers. The recommendation also notes that once your safety committee is formed and active, you must notify your insurance carrier in order to take advantage of related financial incentives. You know that not all insurance carriers offer this incentive and want to be able to qualify. In addition, the chief of the organization has made establishing a safety committee part of your goals and objectives for the year. You need to do a good job, but you are not sure how to get started. What would you do?

Questions

1. Where do you begin?
2. What should be the safety committee's responsibilities?
3. What assistance could the insurance company provide?

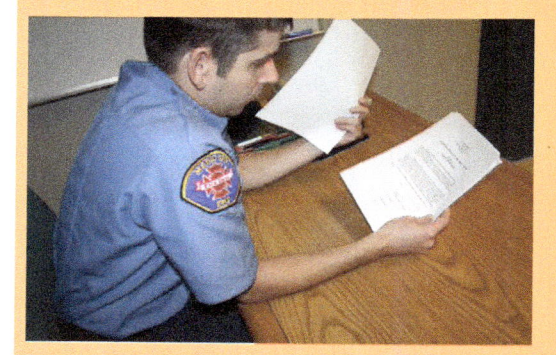

It is difficult to know where to start when you have been given a new task.
Courtesy of 24-7 EMS, a member of the HSI family of brands.

INTRODUCTION

This chapter deals with four main issues: the organization's safety program, the safety culture, the safety committee, and hazard identification. For discussion of an EMS **safety program**, this chapter in most instances focuses on the incident scene. This leads into a discussion of a **safety culture**, which can make or break a safety program. Next are the many reasons why EMS organizations should have a **safety committee**, including that it may be state mandated; some insurance companies give financial incentives for it; regardless of the financial value, a safety committee can provide a great benefit to the organization; and, most important, it can assist in the reduction of accidents. The last part of this chapter covers **hazard identification**, which will deal more with facility issues than incident scenes. Incident scenes will be discussed further in another chapter.

THE HIERARCHY OF CONTROLS

When the supervisor or safety officer identifies a hazard, it is important that one or more strategies be used to eliminate or reduce the risk of injury. Hazardous conditions include unsafe materials, machinery, vehicles, equipment, tools, and environment. Unsafe work practices include allowing untrained workers to perform hazardous tasks, taking unsafe shortcuts, horseplay, and long work schedules. To combat these hazardous conditions and unsafe work practices, a **hierarchy of controls**, comprised of your control strategies, should be developed to include engineering controls, administrative controls, personal protective equipment (PPE), and interim measures.

ENGINEERING CONTROLS

Engineering controls focus on the source of the hazard, unlike two of the other control strategies (administrative controls and personal protective equipment, which generally focus on the individual exposed to the hazard). The basic concept behind engineering controls is that, to the extent feasible, the work environment and the job itself should be designed (not necessarily by an engineer) to eliminate hazards or reduce exposure to hazards. For example, one such engineering control is using self-capping IV needles to reduce the incidence of needlesticks.

Engineering controls are considered top priority because they may effectively employ redesign, enclosure, substitution, or replacement to completely eliminate the hazard. The effective use of engineering controls eliminates the hazard, but it also eliminates the need to manage human behavior: hazard, no exposure, no accident.

If you are not able or willing to eliminate the process or procedure that creates the hazard, then the first and best strategy is to control the hazard at its source. Engineering controls do this. Engineering controls are based on the following principles:

- If feasible, design the facility, equipment, or process to remove the hazard or substitute something that is not hazardous.
- If removal is not feasible, enclose the hazard to prevent exposure in normal operations.
- Where complete enclosure is not feasible, establish barriers or local ventilation to reduce exposure to the hazard in normal operations.

Safe work practices include your organization's general workplace rules and other operation-specific rules. For example, even when a hazard is enclosed, exposure can occur when maintenance is necessary. Through established safe work practices, personnel exposure to hazards can be further reduced. Depending on the type of operations, work practices for specific **Occupational Safety and Health Administration (OSHA)** standards or to recognize hazards may be required. Some of these specific areas include the following:

- Respiratory protection (OSHA Standard 1910.134)
- Lockout/tagout (OSHA Standard 1910.147)
- Confined space entry (OSHA Standard 1910.146)
- Hazard communication (OSHA Standards 1910.1200 and 1926.59)
- Bloodborne pathogens (OSHA Standard 1910.1030)
- Hearing conservation (OSHA Standard 1910.95)

This list is not all-inclusive. Refer to the specific OSHA standards for information and guidance on the required elements for individual programs.

ADMINISTRATIVE CONTROLS

In the hierarchy of controls, the second strategy—**administrative controls**—describes control measures aimed at reducing personnel exposure to hazards, generally by designing safe work practices, scheduling, and job enrichment. Administrative controls should be used in conjunction with, and not as a substitute for, more effective or reliable engineering controls. This is because administrative controls are susceptible to human error. Controls first must be designed from a base of solid hazard analysis. Although administrative controls are a necessity and can work very well, they are only as good as the management systems that support them. Safe procedures and practices must be accompanied by good personnel training and effective consequences.

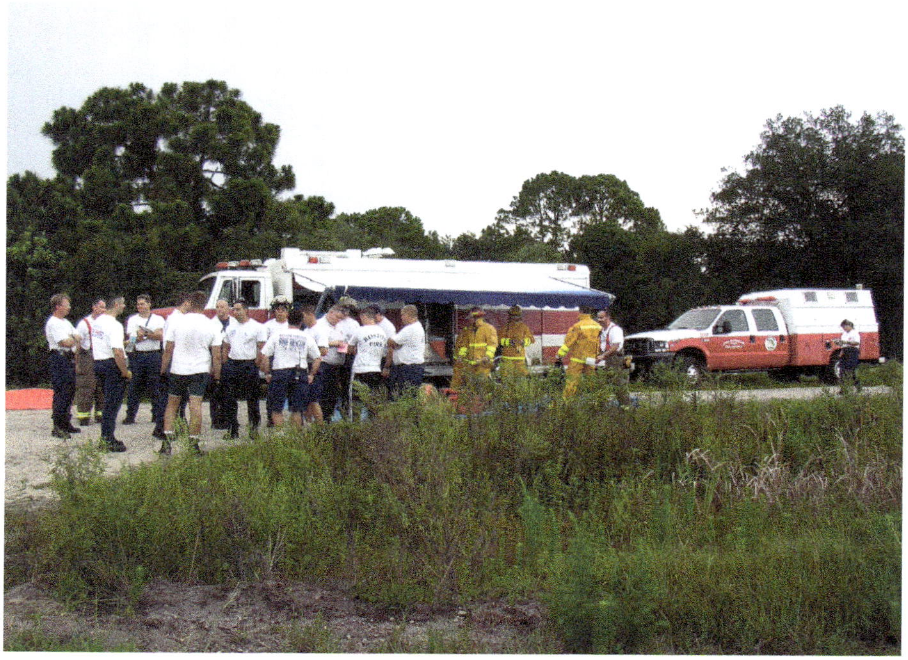

FIGURE 4.1 ■ Personnel need to take breaks and rotate during prolonged incidents. *Courtesy of Jeffrey T. Lindsey, Ph.D.*

Although safe work practices can be considered forms of administrative controls, OSHA uses the term *administrative controls* to mean other measures aimed at reducing individual exposure to hazards. These measures include additional relief personnel, breaks, and rotation of personnel (Figure 4.1). These types of controls are normally used in conjunction with other controls that more directly prevent or control exposure to the hazard.

Safe Procedures

Work procedures that are conducted in a safe manner are extremely important in preventing injuries. Job hazard analysis is an excellent tool for ensuring job tasks and procedures are free from the risk of exposure to hazards. Safe procedures include lockout/tagout procedures, chemical spill procedures, retooling procedures, confined space entry procedures, maintenance procedures, and vehicle inspection procedures.

Safe Practices

Safe practices are very general in their applicability to EMS responses and the EMS work environment. They may be a very important part of a single job procedure or applicable to many jobs in the workplace, from the administrative offices to the station maintenance shop to the incident scene. These safe practices include the following:

- Removal of tripping, blocking, and slipping hazards
- Removal of accumulated toxic dust on surfaces
- Wetting down surfaces to keep toxic dust out of the air (e.g., as in maintenance areas)
- Using personal protective equipment (PPE)

- Using safe lifting techniques
- Maintaining equipment and tools in good repair

Other safe work practices apply to specific jobs in the workplace and involve specific procedures for accomplishing a job. To develop safe practices, conduct a job hazard analysis. If during the job hazard analysis you determine that a procedure presents hazards to personnel, decide that a training program is needed. Using the job hazard analysis is recommended as a tool for training workers in new procedures. A training program may be essential if personnel are working with highly toxic substances or in dangerous situations.

Scheduling and Job Enrichment

The scheduling and job enrichment strategies use control measures that reduce member exposure to hazards by manipulating work schedules. Examples include lengthened rest breaks, exercise breaks to vary body motions, job rotation, and limited work shifts.

PERSONAL PROTECTIVE EQUIPMENT

Personal protective equipment (PPE) is used in conjunction with administrative controls to limit exposure to hazards in the workplace (Figure 4.2). Because PPE does not actually reduce or eliminate the hazard, its use may actually be considered as another administrative control.

When exposure to hazards cannot be engineered completely out of normal operations or maintenance work, and when safe work practices and other forms of administrative controls cannot provide sufficient additional protection, a supplementary method of control is protective clothing or equipment. This is collectively referred to as PPE and may also be appropriate for controlling hazards while engineering and work practice controls are being installed. For specific OSHA requirements on personal protective equipment, see OSHA's Standard 1910, Subpart I.

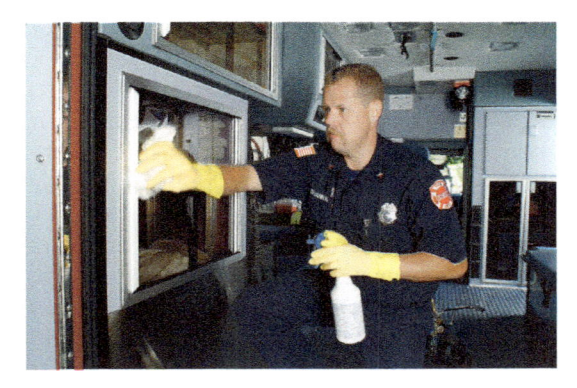

FIGURE 4.2 ■ Personal protective equipment is an important component used in conjunction with administrative controls to limit exposure to a hazard in the workplace.

The basic element of any administrative program for PPE should be an in-depth evaluation of the equipment needed to protect against hazards in the workplace. The evaluation should be used to set a standard operating procedure for personnel, and then to train personnel on the protective limitations of the PPE and its proper use and maintenance.

EMS personnel must understand that PPE does not eliminate hazards. If the equipment fails, exposure will occur. To reduce the possibility of failure, equipment must be properly fitted and maintained in a clean and serviceable condition.

INTERIM MEASURES

Interim measures or interim controls are merely temporary uses of engineering or administrative controls. In most instances, temporary measures can be taken to reduce or eliminate a hazard or exposure to a hazard until a permanent solution can be applied.

Create systems and procedures to prevent and control hazards identified through a **worksite analysis**. OSHA standards can be helpful because they address controls in order of effectiveness and preference. Whenever feasible, engineering and administrative or work practice controls should be instituted even if they do not eliminate the hazard or reduce exposure. Use of such controls in conjunction with PPE will help reduce the hazard or exposure to the lowest practical level. Where no standard exists, creative problem solving and consultant resources may help you create effective controls.

The basic formula for controlling workplace hazards, in order of preference, includes eliminating the hazard from the method, material, procedure, or facility; abating the hazard by limiting exposure or controlling it at its source; training personnel to be aware of the hazard and to follow safe work procedures to avoid it; and prescribing PPE for employees against the hazard, ensuring that they use it, and verifying that they know how to use it correctly.

Establish and provide ongoing training for personnel, supervisors, and managers to ensure that everyone at your worksite can recognize hazards and how to control them. These points are crucial to a safe and healthful workplace for you and all personnel, making it more difficult for accidents to occur and for work-related health problems to develop.

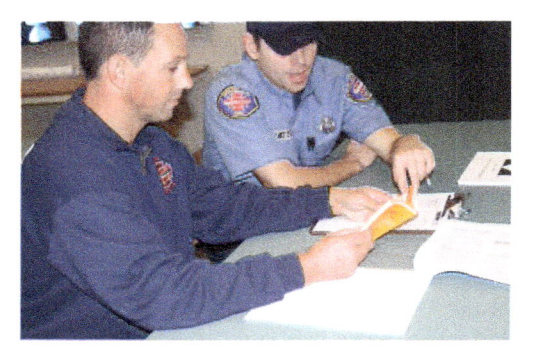

FIGURE 4.3 ■ The key aspect to a successful safety program is to create a plan. *Courtesy of 24-7 EMS®, a member of the HSI family of brands.*

SAFETY PROGRAM

A safety program is an important aspect of your organization. It is critical that it has management's commitment. Without management support, the safety program will not succeed. Safety must be first in any organization! Once you get management's support, the first step of your safety program is to create the plan (Figure 4.3).

The time to start your safety-and-health management system is now. Address the practical concerns of putting the necessary elements together and developing a program to match your work environment. Note that every organization faces different issues or has different resources available. Your plan should consider your organization's immediate needs and provide for ongoing, long-lasting protection of your personnel. Once your plan is designed, follow through and use it in the workplace so that you can anticipate, identify, and eliminate conditions or practices that could result in injuries and illnesses.

Whether you choose to work with a consultant or develop a program yourself, many publications are available. In addition to this text, a resource is your local OSHA office. OSHA will help create in great detail an effective safety-and-health program for your workplace. The rewards for your efforts will be an efficient and productive workplace with a low level of loss and injury.

DESIGNATING RESPONSIBILITY

It is essential that your organization designate an employee who is the most appropriate person to manage the safety-and-health system. This may be an individual who is dedicated to safety issues or a supervisor who assumes the safety role as part of his or her duties. The EMS safety-and-health officer is typically the person who ensures that the safety program will become an integral part of the organization. But

CHAPTER 4 Developing a Safety Program

whoever is selected to create the plan, that person should be committed to workplace safety and health, have the time to develop and manage the program, and be willing to take on the responsibility and accountability that go with operating an effective program.

The individual will need the full cooperation and support of the leadership of the organization, as ultimately the responsibility for safety and health in the workplace rests on the organization's leader.

ASK FOR HELP

Federal occupational safety and health law allows a state to develop and operate its own occupational safety-and-health program in place of the federal OSHA program. It is possible that the regulatory aspect of the law (setting of mandatory minimum standards and conducting inspections of workplaces) is being operated by your state government as opposed to federal OSHA. So, one of the first things to learn is which branch of government, federal or state, has current jurisdiction over your organization. If you are not sure what agency is responsible for administering workplace safety and health in your state, contact the nearest OSHA office to find out.

You will need to be certain that federal OSHA publications (or comparable state publications) are used in your safety-and-health activities, such as the OSHA Workplace Poster (Figure 4.4). This poster, available in English and Spanish, presents OSHA standards that apply to your organization. You need to have available for reference a copy of all OSHA standards that apply to EMS as required in your state. Standards to have on hand include the regulations that OSHA uses to inspect for compliance and should be the baseline for your inspections in determining what to do when hazards are identified; recordkeeping requirements and the necessary forms; and a copy of the Occupational Safety and Health Act of 1970.

FACTS ABOUT YOUR SITUATION

Before making changes in your safety-and-health operations, you should gather information about the current conditions and practices that comprise your safety-and-health program. This information can help you identify problems and determine what is needed to solve them. Your workplace assessment should be conducted by the person responsible for your safety-and-health management system and/or a professional safety-and-health consultant and consists of three major activities.

1. *A comprehensive safety-and-health survey of each of your facilities* will identify any existing or potential safety-and-health hazards. This initial survey should focus on evaluating workplace conditions with respect to safety-and-health regulations and generally recognized safe and healthful work practices. It should include checking on the use of any hazardous materials, observing personnel' work habits and practices, and discussing safety-and-health problems with personnel.
2. The second major activity is to complete an *assessment and evaluation of your safety-and-health program* as it relates to incident response and working at the scene of incidents. Gather as much information as you can as it relates to safety-and-health management for incident response and working at the scene of incidents.
3. The third major activity is to complete an *assessment of your existing safety-and-health program and identification of areas that work well and those that need improvement.* Gather as much information as you can that relates to safety-and-health management in the station environment and at incident scenes. You should include the following in this review:
    - *Safety-and-health activities.* Examine ongoing activities as well as those tried previously, organization policy statements, rules (both work and safety), guidelines for proper work practices and procedures, and records of training programs.

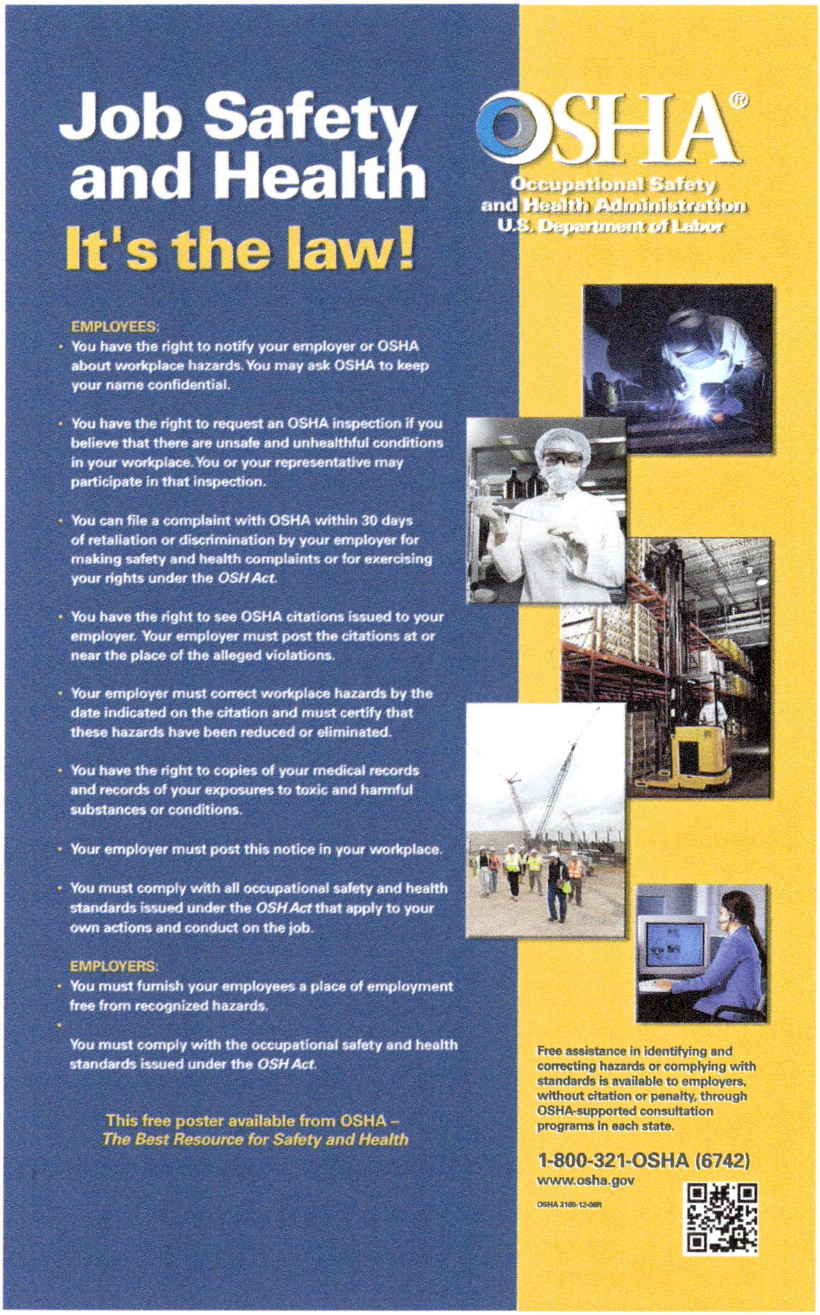

FIGURE 4.4 ■ The Job Safety and Health poster (OSHA 3165-12-06R) needs to be displayed in a prominent place in your stations and buildings. *Source: OSHA, accessed August 6, 2012, at www.osha.gov/Publications/osha3165low-res.pdf*

- *Equipment.* List your major equipment, what it is used for, and where it is located. Give special attention to inspection schedules, maintenance activities, and vehicle layouts.
- *Member capabilities.* Make an alphabetical list of all personnel, showing the date hired, job descriptions, experience, and training.
- *Accident and injury/illness history.* Review injury and illness cases and workers' compensation insurance payments and awards, and review losses. Compare your insurance rate with others; your insurance agent can be of assistance to you in gaining this information. Give special attention to recurring accidents and types of injuries.

After gathering facts, see if any major problem areas emerge, such as interruptions in your normal operations, too many individuals taking too much time off due to illness or injury, or too many damaged vehicles or equipment. General help with this kind of problem identification often can be obtained from compensation carriers, EMS associations, state agencies, major suppliers, or other EMS agencies.

If you discover a major problem, see what can be done to solve it. Once a problem is identified, work on the corrective action or a plan to control the problem. Take immediate action and make a record of what you have done. Even if you find no major problems, do not stop there; instead, develop a comprehensive safety-and-health program to avoid any major problems in the future.

SAFETY-AND-HEALTH PROGRAM

The success of any workplace safety-and-health program depends on careful planning. This means that you must take the time to analyze what you want to accomplish and develop an action plan to attain your goals. From this standpoint, you can design a step-by-step process to take you from the idea stage to an effective safety-and-health management system.

Establish your management commitment and involve personnel of the organization. No safety-and-health program will work without this commitment and involvement. The first step is to designate a person to be responsible for your safety-and-health program.

Involve your personnel as widely as possible from the beginning. They are the individuals who are the most in contact with the potential and actual safety-and-health hazards of your organization and will have constructive input on the development of your program. The ultimate success of your safety-and-health program will depend on their support.

Make sure your program assigns responsibility and accountability to all personnel in your organization. A good safety-and-health program makes it clear that each and every member, from you through to the supervisory levels to the front-line field personnel, carries responsibility for his or her part of the program. Make safety-and-health duties clear, and hold every individual accountable for his or her own safety-and-health duties.

Refer to the recommended actions to take in the worksite analysis. These will help start your program off on the right track and will help build the foundation for a successful program.

Establish and regularly conduct a worksite analysis. A successful safety-and-health program depends on an accurate identification of all the hazards and potential hazards (Figure 4.5). This is an ongoing process that includes routine self-inspections.

Worksite Analysis

A worksite analysis involves a variety of worksite examinations to identify not only existing hazards, but also conditions and operations in which changes might create hazards (Figure 4.6). Effective management actively analyzes the work and the worksite to anticipate and prevent harmful occurrences.

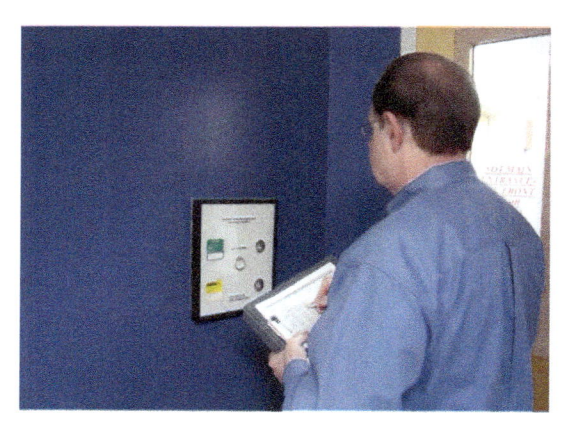

FIGURE 4.5 ■ It is important to conduct a worksite analysis in order to identify hazards and potential hazards that exist. *Courtesy of Jeffrey T. Lindsey, Ph.D.*

To identify all worksite hazards:

- Conduct a comprehensive, baseline survey for safety and health and periodic, comprehensive update surveys.
- Conduct a change analysis of planned and new facilities, processes, materials, and equipment.
- Perform routine job hazard analyses.
- Conduct periodic and daily safety-and-health inspections of the workplace.

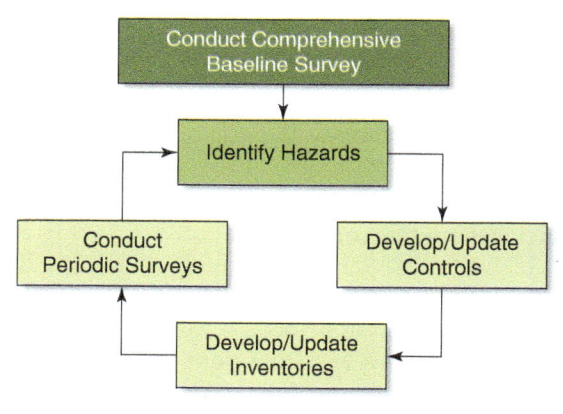

FIGURE 4.6 ■ Worksite analysis flowchart. *Source: OSHA Safety and Health Management Systems eTools, accessed August 56, 2012, at www.osha.gov/SLTC/etools/safetyhealth/comp2.html*

These major actions form the basis from which good hazard prevention and control can develop.

Comprehensive Surveys. Many workers' compensation carriers and other insurance companies offer expert services to help their clients evaluate safety-and-health hazards. Numerous private consultants provide a variety of safety-and-health expert services.

Change Analysis. Anytime something new is brought into the workplace—whether it be a piece of equipment, different materials, a new process, or an entirely new building—new hazards may unintentionally be introduced. Before considering a change for a worksite, it should be analyzed thoroughly. Change analysis helps in heading off a problem before it develops. You may find change analysis useful in various situations, such as building or leasing a new facility, purchasing new equipment, purchasing or leasing a new vehicle, starting up new processes, and when staffing changes occur.

Trend Analysis. Another action recommended under worksite analysis is analysis of injury and illness trends over time, so that patterns with common causes can be identified and prevented. Review of the OSHA injury and illness forms is the most common form of pattern analysis, but other records of hazards can be analyzed for patterns. Examples are inspection records and member hazard reporting records, including the following:

> *Injury and illness records analysis.* Since there must be enough information for patterns to emerge, small organizations may require a review of 3 to 5 years of records. Larger organizations may find trends useful yearly, quarterly, or monthly. When analyzing injury and illness records, look for similar injuries and illnesses.

These generally indicate a lack of hazard controls. Look for where the injury or illness occurred, what type of work was being done, time of day, type of incident, or type of equipment.

Analysis of other records. Repeat hazards, just like repeat injuries or illnesses, mean that controls are not working. The use of inspection reports, maintenance reports, injury and illness reports, and so on can be used to more quickly track patterns that could identify the potential occurrence of an accident or incident before it happens. Upgrading a control may involve something as basic as improving communication or accountability.

Develop and Implement Your Action Plan

Developing an action plan to build a safety-and-health program can serve as a step-by-step guide to take your program to where you want it to be. An action plan tells you what has to be done, the logical order in which to do it, who is responsible, and where you want to be when you finish. It describes problems and solutions, but is not ironclad. An action plan can and should be changed to correspond with changes in the work environment.

A good action plan has two parts:

- A list of major changes or improvements to make your safety-and-health program effective. Each item should be prioritized, have a target date for completion, and identify who is responsible for implementation.
- A specific plan to implement each major change or improvement, including what you want to accomplish, the steps required, who will be assigned to do what, and a schedule for completion.

Once a plan is established, put it into action, beginning with the highest-priority item. Ensure that it is realistic, manageable, and addresses the steps you have planned for that item. A detailed description of the steps required will help you keep track of your

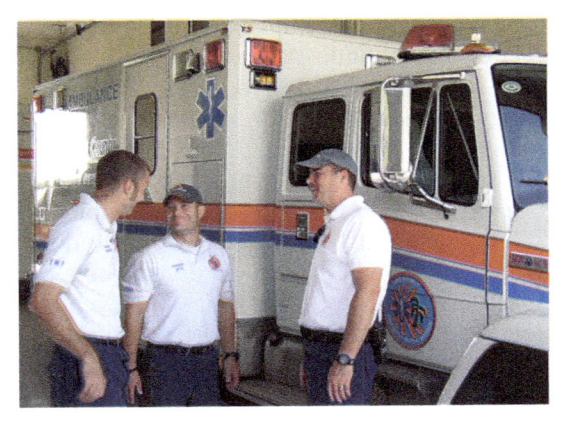

FIGURE 4.7 ■ As an EMS safety officer, it is important to have an open relationship with the personnel of the organization. *Courtesy of Jeffrey T. Lindsey, Ph.D.*

progress. Keep in mind that you can work on more than one item at a time and that priorities may change as other needs are identified or as your organization's resources change.

Open communication with personnel is crucial to the success of your efforts (Figure 4.7). Their cooperation depends on them understanding what the safety-and-health program is all about, why it is important to them, and how it affects their work. The more you do to involve them in the changes you are making, the smoother the transition will be. Putting the action plan into operation at your workplace will be a major step toward implementing an effective safety-and-health program. Remember, a safety-and-health program is a plan put into practice. Keep your program on track by periodically checking its progress.

Any good management system requires periodic review. Take a careful look at each component of the safety-and-health program to determine what is working well and what changes are needed. Any necessary improvements can be turned into new safety-and-health objectives for the coming year. Developing new action plans to implement these improvements will continue progress toward an effective safety-and-health program, reduce your safety-and-health risks, and increase efficiency and profit.

Remember to document your activities. The best way to evaluate the success of your safety-and-health program is to refer to documentation of what you have done, which can illustrate how you can make it work even better. Technical assistance may be available to you through your insurance carrier, your fellow EMS colleagues, suppliers of your equipment and vehicles, and many local, state, and federal agencies.

Establishing a quality safety-and-health management system will take time and involve some resources, but you should be pleased with the results. Personnel will feel reassured because of your commitment to their safety and health on the job. You may save money through lower absenteeism and reduced workers' compensation insurance costs. You may gain increased respect in your community. The tangible and intangible rewards for a solid safety-and-health program far outweigh the cost of an accident, injury, or workplace fatality.

Self-Inspection

The most widely accepted way to identify hazards is to conduct safety-and-health inspections because the only way to be certain of an actual situation is to look at it directly from time to time. Begin a program of self-inspection in your own workplace. Self-inspection is essential if you are to know where probable hazards exist and whether they are under control.

Figure 4.8 contains lists designed to assist you in self-inspection fact finding. These lists can give you some indication of where to begin taking action to make your organization safer and more healthful for all of your personnel. These lists are by no means all inclusive, and not all of the lists will apply to your organization. You might want to start by selecting the areas that are most critical to your organization, and then expand your self-inspection lists over time to fully cover all areas that pertain to your organization. Remember that a checklist is a helpful tool, not a definitive statement of what is mandatory. Use checklists only for guidance.

Do not spend time with items that have no application to your organization. Make sure that each item is seen by you or your designee, and leave nothing to memory or chance. Write down what you do or do not see and what you think you should do about it.

Add information from your completed checklists to injury information, employee information, and process and equipment information to build a foundation to help you determine what problems exist. It will be easier for you to determine the actions needed to solve these problems.

Self-Inspection Scope

Your self-inspections should cover safety-and-health issues in the following areas:

Receiving and storage—equipment, job planning, layout, heights, floor loads, material handling and storage methods, training for material handling equipment

Building and grounds conditions—floors, walls, ceilings, exits, stairs, walkways, ramps, platforms, driveways, aisles

Housekeeping program—waste disposal, tools, objects, materials, leakage and spillage, cleaning methods, schedules, work areas, remote areas, storage areas

Electricity—equipment, switches, breakers, fuses, switchboxes, junctions, special fixtures, circuits, insulation, extensions, tools, motors, grounding, National Electrical Code compliance

Lighting—type, intensity, controls, conditions, diffusion, location, glare and shadow control

CHAPTER 4 Developing a Safety Program 59

VFIS
1-800-461-8347

SELF-INSPECTION FORM
FOR EMERGENCY SERVICE ORGANIZATION BUILDING & GROUNDS

IMPORTANT: Periodic inspection of your organization's buildings and grounds can alert you and your maintenance staff to hazards which may cause damage and accidents to your buildings and those who use it. This form is provided for periodic self-inspection and is recommended for use on a quarterly basis to assist you in discovering hazards before an accident can occur. Correct all negative conditions immediately.

This self-inspection form does not intend to point out all hazards and exposures which may be found at your building. It is intended to be used as a guide to highlight major areas of exposure which are common to most emergency service organization buildings. The use of this form does not warrant that all hazards will be found and corrected.

INSTRUCTIONS: Please check Yes, No or NA (not applicable) answers to all questions below. All "No" answers indicate an area of **unsatisfactory conditions** and comment regarding same should be made in the space provided on the back of this form. Use a separate sheet for each building.

NAME OF ORGANIZATION: _____
BUILDING LOCATION: _____
(Street Number) (City)
(County) (State) (Zip Code)

NAME OF INSPECTOR: _____ **DATE OF INSPECTION** _____

★ ★ ★

SECTION I - GROUNDS
1. Are parking areas, walkways, stairs, driveways, etc. free from conditions that may cause slipping or falling?
   ☐ YES ☐ NO ☐ NA
2. Is exterior lighting adequate in all areas?
   ☐ YES ☐ NO ☐ NA
3. Are all exterior stairs provided with handrails which are in good condition?
   ☐ YES ☐ NO ☐ NA
4. Are exterior fire escapes in good condition?
   ☐ YES ☐ NO ☐ NA
5. Is exterior storage of trash and rubbish at least 25 feet away from the building?
   ☐ YES ☐ NO ☐ NA
6. Are daily inventory records kept for your underground fuel storage tank to insure that there is no leakage?
   ☐ YES ☐ NO ☐ NA

SECTION II - INTERIOR DOORS AND STAIRWAYS
1. Are all exit doors properly marked?
   ☐ YES ☐ NO ☐ NA
2. Are all exit doors easily accessible?
   ☐ YES ☐ NO ☐ NA
3. Do all exit doors open outward?
   ☐ YES ☐ NO ☐ NA
4. Are all exit doors equipped with panic hardware?
   ☐ YES ☐ NO ☐ NA
5. Are all doors easily opened and closed?
   ☐ YES ☐ NO ☐ NA
6. Are all doorways and areas adjacent to them free of obstructions?
   ☐ YES ☐ NO ☐ NA
7. Are full length, clear glass doors and windows properly identified?
   ☐ YES ☐ NO
8. Do all interior stairs have anti-slip treads?
   ☐ YES ☐ NO ☐ NA
9. Are stairway and exit doors kept closed at all times?
   ☐ YES ☐ NO ☐ NA
10. Do all interior stairways have properly secured hand rails?
    ☐ YES ☐ NO ☐ NA
11. Are interior stairways kept free of storage and obstructions at all times?
    ☐ YES ☐ NO ☐ NA
12. Are interior stairways properly lighted?
    ☐ YES ☐ NO ☐ NA
(reference-NFPA #101 Life Safety Code)

13. Is the emergency lighting system tested on a monthly basis?
    ☐ YES ☐ NO ☐ NA
14. Is the emergency power generator tested on a weekly basis?
    ☐ YES ☐ NO ☐ NA

SECTION III - HEATING AND AIR CONDITIONING EQUIPMENT
1. Has heating equipment been thoroughly inspected by a qualified service man within the past year?
   ☐ YES ☐ NO ☐ NA Service Date_____
2. Is heating equipment (including flues and pipes) properly insulated from combustible materials?
   ☐ YES ☐ NO ☐ NA
3. Are heating and air conditioning equipment rooms free of storage?
   ☐ YES ☐ NO ☐ NA
4. Are heating and air conditioning rooms restricted areas
   ☐ YES ☐ NO ☐ NA
5. Is air conditioning equipment cleaned and serviced annually?
   ☐ YES ☐ NO ☐ NA

SECTION IV - ELECTRICAL EQUIPMENT & CONTROL PANELS
1. Has the electrical system been inspected within the past five years by a certified electrician or electrical inspector?
   ☐ YES ☐ NO ☐ NA
2. Are electrical panels always kept closed?
   ☐ YES ☐ NO ☐ NA
3. Are electrical panels always kept clear of storage and obstructions?
   ☐ YES ☐ NO ☐ NA
4. Is circuitry adequate to handle load demand (not requiring frequent fuse replacement or circuit breaker resetting)?
   ☐ YES ☐ NO ☐ NA
5. Was electrical system installed by a competent electrician?
   ☐ YES ☐ NO ☐ NA
6. Is electrical system regularly maintained by a competent electrician?
   ☐ YES ☐ NO ☐ NA
7. Are all electrical appliances properly grounded and cleaned?
   ☐ YES ☐ NO ☐ NA
8. Are electric motors adequately ventilated to prevent overheating and are they cleaned regularly?
   ☐ YES ☐ NO ☐ NA
9. Are proper size electrical cords used and are they in good condition?
   ☐ YES ☐ NO ☐ NA
(reference-NFPA #70 National Electric Code)

FIGURE 4.8 ■ The use of checklists can be helpful. *Reprinted with permission of VFIS.*

SECTION V-KITCHEN EQUIPMENT-COMMERCIAL TYPE

1. Is all commercial cooking equipment protected as recommended by NFPA #96?
   ☐ YES   ☐ NO   ☐ NA
2. **Is hood and duct exhaust system installed according to** NFPA #96 guidelines?
   ☐ YES   ☐ NO   ☐ NA
3. Are grease filters U.L. listed for grease extraction and installed according to NFPA #96?
   ☐ YES   ☐ NO   ☐ NA
4. Are the hood and duct system cleaned at least on a semi-annual basis?
   ☐ YES   ☐ NO   ☐ NA
5. Are the kitchen appliance protected with an automatic fire extinguishing system?
   ☐ YES   ☐ NO   ☐ NA
6. Is the fire extinguishing system serviced and inspected at least on a semi-annual basis?
   ☐ YES   ☐ NO   ☐ NA

SECTION VI-HOUSEKEEPING

1. Are storage and supply rooms kept clean and orderly?
   ☐ YES   ☐ NO   ☐ NA
2. Are trash and rubbish stored in metal containers?
   ☐ YES   ☐ NO   ☐ NA
3. Are all flammable items (paint, lacquer, paint thinner, etc.) kept in safety containers and stored in approved metal cabinets?
   ☐ YES   ☐ NO   ☐ NA
4. Are adequate ash trays and metal waste receptacles provided in each room?
   ☐ YES   ☐ NO   ☐ NA
5. Are only non-flammable cleaning agents used throughout the entire building?
   ☐ YES   ☐ NO   ☐ NA
6. Is ready disposal of combustible wastes provided?
   ☐ YES   ☐ NO   ☐ NA
7. Are areas used for public meetings or other functions always thoroughly checked before securing?
   ☐ YES   ☐ NO   ☐ NA
8. Are rags, cloths, etc. used in cleaning stored in an approved, self- closing metal container?
   ☐ YES   ☐ NO   ☐ NA

SECTION VII-FIRE PROTECTION

1. Are all the fire extinguishers tagged, serviced and inspected annually?
   ☐ YES   ☐ NO   ☐ NA
2. Are all fire extinguishers tagged with latest service record and inspection date?
   ☐ YES   ☐ NO   ☐ NA
3. Are fire extinguishers located within 75 feet from any point on each floor?
   ☐ YES   ☐ NO   ☐ NA
4. Are extinguishers properly protected from damage and freezing?
   ☐ YES   ☐ NO   ☐ NA
   (reference NFPA #10)
5. Is building protected with smoke/heat detection system?
   ☐ YES   ☐ NO   ☐ NA
6. Is smoke/heat detection system tested and inspected on a monthly basis?
   ☐ YES   ☐ NO   ☐ NA
   (reference NFPA #72E)
7. Is there a two inch drain test performed on the sprinkler system on a quarterly basis?
   ☐ YES   ☐ NO   ☐ NA

COMMENTS: (If an explanation is needed for the above questions, please comment below. If any "NO" block is checked, indicate action taken and date to be corrected.)

_____
_____
_____
_____

SECTION NUMBER:	ITEM NUMBER:	ACTION TAKEN:	CORRECTION BY:	DATE CORRECTED:

FIGURE 4.8 ■ (*Continued*)

Heating and ventilation—type, effectiveness, temperature, humidity, controls, natural and artificial ventilation and exhausting

Machinery—points of operation, flywheels, gears, shafts, pulleys, key ways, belts, couplings, sprockets, chains, frames, controls, lighting for tools and equipment, brakes, exhausting, feeding, oiling, adjusting, maintenance, lockout/tagout, grounding, work space, location, purchasing standards

Personnel—training, including hazard identification training; experience; methods of checking machines before use; type of clothing; PPE; use of guards; tool storage; work practices; methods for cleaning, oiling, or adjusting machinery

Hand and power tools—purchasing standards, inspection, storage, repair, types, maintenance, grounding, use, and handling

Chemicals—storage, handling, transportation, spills, disposals, amounts used, labeling, toxicity or other harmful effects, warning signs, supervision, training, protective clothing and equipment, hazard communication requirements

Fire prevention—extinguishers, alarms, sprinklers, smoking rules, exits, personnel assigned, separation of flammable materials and dangerous operations, explosion-proof fixtures in hazardous locations, waste disposal, and training of personnel

Maintenance—regular and preventive maintenance on all equipment used at the worksite, recording all work performed on the machinery, and training personnel on the proper care and servicing of the equipment

PPE—type, size, maintenance, repair, age, storage, assignment of responsibility, purchasing methods, standards observed, training in care and use, rules of use, method of assignment

Transportation—motor vehicle safety, seat belts, vehicle maintenance, safe driver programs

Illness/injury program/supplies—medical care facilities locations, posted emergency phone numbers, accessible first aid kits

Evacuation plan—establish and practice procedures for an emergency evacuation such as fire, chemical/biological incidents, bomb threat; include escape procedures and routes, critical plant operations, employee accounting following an evacuation, rescue and medical duties, and ways to report emergencies

■ THE SAFETY CULTURE

Culture is a combination of an organization's attitudes, behaviors, beliefs, values, ways of doing things, and other shared characteristics of a particular group of people. Culture can socialize newcomers, define influence, and determine values. A strong safety-and-health culture is the result of the following:

- Positive workplace attitudes—from the chief to the newest hire
- Involvement and buy-in of all personnel of the organization
- Mutual, meaningful, and measurable safety-and-health improvement goals
- Policies and procedures that serve as reference tools, rather than obscure rules
- Personnel training at all levels within the organization
- Responsibility and accountability throughout the organization

When those criteria are consistently and effectively aimed at accident reduction, a positive safety-and-health culture is created. The basic elements of a safety-and-health culture include the following:

- All individuals within the organization believe they have a right to a safe and healthy workplace.
- Each person accepts personal responsibility for ensuring his or her own safety and health.

- Everyone believes he or she has a duty to protect the safety and health of others.

Safety cultures consist of shared beliefs, practices, and attitudes that exist at an establishment. Culture is the atmosphere created by those beliefs, attitudes, and so on, which shape behavior. An organization's safety culture is the result of a number of factors, such as management and member norms, assumptions, and beliefs; management and member attitudes; values, myths, stories; policies and procedures; supervisor priorities, responsibilities, and accountability; actions or lack of action to correct unsafe behaviors; member training and motivation; and member involvement or buy-in.

In a strong safety culture, everyone feels responsible for safety and pursues it on a daily basis. Personnel go beyond the call of duty to identify unsafe conditions and behaviors, and intervene to correct them. For instance, in a strong safety culture any member would feel comfortable walking up to the chief and reminding him or her to wear safety glasses. This type of behavior would not be viewed as forward or overzealous but would be valued by the organization and rewarded. Likewise other personnel routinely look out for one another and point out unsafe behaviors to each other.

An organization with a strong safety culture typically experiences few at-risk behaviors; consequently it has low accident rates, low turnover, and low absenteeism. Such organizations usually are extremely successful because they excel in all aspects of EMS business and practices.

Creating a safety culture takes time. It is frequently a multiyear process. A series of continuous process improvement steps can be followed to create a safety culture. EMS agencies and member commitment are hallmarks of a true safety culture where safety is an integral part of daily operations.

An EMS organization at the beginning of developing a safety culture may exhibit a level of safety awareness consisting merely of safety posters and warning signs. As more time and commitment are devoted to safety, an organization will begin to address physical hazards and may develop safety recognition programs, create safety committees, and start incentive programs.

Top management support of a safety culture often results in designating a safety-and-health officer, providing resources for accident investigations, and safety training. Further progress toward a true safety culture also requires accountability systems. Such systems establish safety goals, measure safety activities, and charge costs back to the units that incur them. Ultimately, safety becomes everyone's responsibility, not just the safety-and-health officer's. Safety becomes a value of the organization and an integral part of operations. Management and personnel are committed and involved in preventing losses. Over time the norms and beliefs of the organization shift focus from eliminating hazards to eliminating unsafe behaviors and building systems that proactively improve safety-and-health conditions.

BUILDING A SAFETY CULTURE

Any process that brings together all levels within the organization to work on a common goal that everyone holds in high value will strengthen the organizational culture. Worker safety and health comprise an area in which this may be accomplished. Such an effort is one of the few initiatives that offer significant benefits for front-line field personnel. As a result, buy-in can be achieved, enabling the organization to effectively implement change. (Note that obtaining front-line buy-in for improving member safety and health is much easier than it is getting buy-in for improving quality or decreasing costs.) When the needed process improvements are implemented, a culture develops that supports continuous improvement in all areas.

It is human nature to put one's whole focus on accomplishing a task, such as training everyone on a particular concern or implementing a new procedure. However, organizations that focus on processes, rather than tasks, generally are far more successful at meeting goals for change and improvement. Such organizations can see the forest and not just the trees, and thus can foresee as well as make midcourse adjustments as needed. They never lose sight of their intended goals; therefore, they tend not to get distracted or allow obstacles to interfere with their mission. In effect, processes themselves account for task implementation and ensure that the appropriate resources are provided and priorities are set.

IMPROVING MANAGEMENT PROCESSES

To address the management processes that are typically ripe for improvement, do the following:

Define safety responsibilities for all levels of the organization, such as safety is a line management function.

Develop upstream measures, such as the number of reports of hazards/suggestions, number of committee projects/successes, and so on.

Align management and supervisors by establishing a shared vision of safety-and-health goals and objectives.

Implement a process that holds managers and supervisors accountable for visibly being involved, setting the proper example, and leading a positive change for safety and health.

Evaluate and rebuild any incentives and disciplinary systems for safety and health as necessary.

Ensure the safety committee is functioning appropriately, including membership, responsibilities/functions, authority, meeting management skills, and so on.

Provide multiple paths for personnel to bring suggestions, concerns, or problems forward.

One mechanism should use the chain of command and ensure no repercussions. Hold supervisors and middle managers accountable for being responsive.

Develop a system that tracks and ensures timeliness in hazard correction. Many organizations have been successful in building this in an already existing work order system.

Ensure reporting of injuries, illnesses, and near misses. Educate employees on the accident pyramid and importance of reporting minor incidents. Prepare management for an initial increase in incidents and a rise in rates. This will occur if underreporting exists in the organization. It will level off, then decline as the system changes take hold.

Evaluate and rebuild the incident investigation system as necessary to ensure that it is timely, complete, and effective. It should get to the root causes and avoid blaming personnel.

SAFETY COMMITTEE

Although everyone acknowledges that a safety committee process is never perfect, imagine the benefit of having personnel and management coming together on a regular basis to identify and solve everyday safety-and-health problems.

Effective safety committees that prevent workplace injuries and illnesses are the best reason for starting one. In addition, some states require safety committees in order to keep injuries and illnesses low. Many workers' compensation carriers require insureds to have a safety committee in order to receive certain discounts, which can help keep overall costs low as well.

ROLES AND RESPONSIBILITIES

You do not have to climb a mountain and sit on a big rock for six days to envision a safety committee or your place in it. But, it is important that you develop a clear vision about how you and the safety committee can most effectively complement the mission of your organization.

The purpose of a safety committee is to bring personnel and managers together to achieve and maintain a safe, healthful workplace. It is easy to start a safety committee, but to develop an effective one—one that achieves and maintains a safe, healthful workplace—requires personnel and managers committed to achieving that goal. Once you understand the role, purpose, and function of your safety committee, you will be better able to start, develop, and maintain a successful team.

One way of looking at the role of the safety committee is to think of it as a consultant firm that would be hired by your organization to do several things, such as identify workplace hazardous conditions and work practices, determine the root causes for those conditions and practices, develop solutions and submit recommendations to correct problems and improve systems, and monitor the progress of recommendations and the quality of safety programs and activities.

Note that none of these responsibilities requires the safety committee to actually control safety programs or people. When the safety committee assumes the role of a consultant group within an organization, it is not expected to control a budget, safety training, or purchasing equipment (Figure 4.9). These responsibilities are more properly carried out by the appropriate individuals, such as the assistant chief or supervisor.

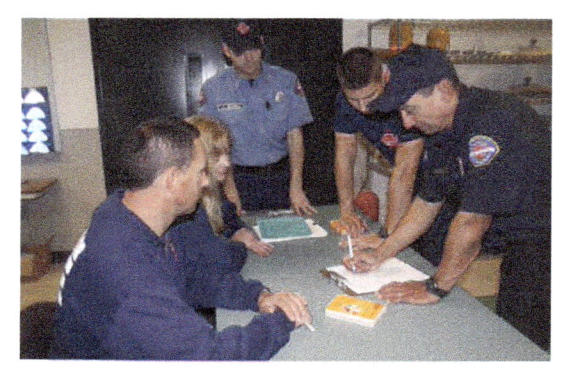

FIGURE 4.9 ■ The role of the safety committee should be to control safety programs or people. *Courtesy of 24-7 EMS®, a member of the HSI family of brands.*

THE COMMITTEE'S PURPOSE

The purpose of the safety committee also might be viewed as its mission. The purpose of a safety committee is to bring personnel and management together in a nonadversarial, cooperative effort to promote safety and health. A safety committee assists the EMS organization and makes recommendations for change.

One of the committee's most important responsibilities is to promote a nonadversarial relationship and increase trust between labor and management. Read W. Edwards Deming's book, *Out of the Crisis* (1986). In it, he details 14 elements of Total Quality Management (TQM). He states that for any sound management system to work, you must first eliminate fear in the workplace before embarking on the other elements. Safety people need to be sure that their actions are reducing fear (adversarial relationship) in the workplace.

As consultant, one of the most important jobs of the safety committee representative is to act as a liaison: to receive and report employee safety concerns and provide regular feedback to the EMS provider regarding the status or response to those concerns. Not providing adequate feedback to providers may render a safety committee ineffective, in the view of providers, in its ability to communicate and effectively carry out its purpose.

The safety committee also performs consultative duties upstream to management. This is done primarily through the written recommendation process. Just because the organization is required by law or by its insurance carrier to form a safety committee does not necessarily mean the organization is going to invest much time and money in the committee. To get top management's respect and commitment, the safety committee must earn it. The safety committee must provide management with useful information, and the committee must make informed decisions. Effective recommendations educate management and result in greater respect and commitment to the safety committee.

Among the safety committee's most important purposes are these:

> Help protect EMS providers by receiving, reporting, responding to safety concerns in a timely manner and by being a safety leader through example.

> Help protect the organization by writing effective recommendations that propose solutions to surface and root causes, and state a strong arguments for taking corrective action by emphasizing the costs versus benefits, which is the bottom line.

> Help the organization maintain a safety-conscious workplace by evaluating and assisting in developing an effective and comprehensive safety management system.

> Help the organization create a **culture of consequences** by evaluating and assisting in developing effective accountability and recognition/reward processes.

> Bring labor or its personnel and management together in a cooperative effort and on a regular basis to discuss and solve safety problems.

All of these purpose statements emphasize the safety committee's responsibility to assist, not actually do, all the work for the organization. The safety committee need not control programs, activities, budgets, and so on. The committee's primary purpose is to assist the organization by problem solving and communicating.

If the safety committee does not effectively carry out its intended purpose, it may actually (and unintentionally) function to hurt the organization's safety-and-health effort. For instance, the safety committee may intend to communicate effectively with management, but if its personnel do not have the knowledge, skills, or abilities to accomplish its purpose, the unintended or actual result may be a dismal failure to communicate with management.

The safety committee may have the best intentions, but if it cannot follow through effectively with its plans, it may actually function to harm a safety program or activity rather than help it. Without education and training, safety committee personnel may not have the basic knowledge, skills, and abilities to perform their responsibilities. Given proper education and training, the safety committee is more likely to function to carry out its intended purpose.

The safety committee may be feeling very positive about the design of a program or process. It may have wonderful goals and objectives that support those programs or processes. Yet if the safety committee does not have the knowledge, skills, and ability, for whatever reason, to meet those goals, it will have great difficulty in carrying out its stated purpose. The safety committee may unintentionally function to fail, or fall short of meeting its purpose.

STARTING THE SAFETY COMMITTEE

If your organization does not currently have a safety committee, start one. But how do you sell the idea to management? In many instances you will need to talk about the bottom-line benefits to get management's attention.

Some organizations think of safety as merely one of the costs of doing business. They believe the safety committee is a cost center activity that drains the organization of money it needs for other purposes. If this is the case, think about selling management on the safety committee by first making a commitment to ensuring that the safety committee is a savings center activity and that you only will conduct activities and make recommendations that can be shown to save money for the organization. Promise not to do things that waste time and money or otherwise duplicate what EMS providers, supervisors, and managers should be doing as part of their jobs. For private-sector EMS agencies, this helps improve the overall profit margin. For public-sector organizations, this helps conduct services within budget.

Benefits

The safety committee performs the role of consultant to the organization. If your organization hired an external consultant, it would cost thousands of dollars long term for the same service the safety committee can provide in-house. Every hazard the safety committee identifies and is directly involved in eliminating results in significant savings in potential accident costs. In addition to saving costs, the safety committee acts as a forum for management and labor to communicate safety-related concerns. The benefits from improved communication may be hard to quantify, but they may be substantial.

The safety committee can serve as a valuable problem-solving group that addresses workplace conditions, morale, and quality. By developing solutions, the safety committee improves the organization's stability. It also provides an excellent opportunity for providers to improve their professional skills in communications, human relations, problem solving, meeting management, and analysis. Since supervisors and managers should be informed about occupational safety and health, the safety committee is a natural starting place for preparation of future supervisors and chiefs.

Costs versus Benefits

Side Bar

The National Safety Council publishes the average economic costs of injuries and deaths in the United States. The following data illustrate the costs for death, injuries, or crashes for 2007.

Average Economic Cost per Death, Injury, or Crash, 2007

Death	$1,130,000
Nonfatal Disabling Injury	$61,600
Property Damage Crash (including nondisabling injuries)	$7,500

Average Economic Cost by Injury Severity, 2007

Incapacitating injury (A)	$65,000
Nonincapacitating evident injury (B)	$21,000
Possible injury (C)	$11,900

Average Comprehensive Cost by Injury Severity, 2007

Death	$4,100,000
Incapacitating injury	$208,500
Nonincapacitating evident injury	$53,200
Possible injury	$25,300
No injury	$2,300

Average Economic Cost of Fatal and Nonfatal Injuries by Class of Injury, 2007

Home injuries (fatal and nonfatal) per death	$3,380,000
Public nonmotor-vehicle injuries (fatal and nonfatal) per death	$3,240,000
Work injuries (fatal and nonfatal) per death:	
without employers' uninsured costs	$30,350,000
with employers' uninsured costs	$33,350,000

Average Economic Cost by Class and Severity, 2007

	Death	Disabling Injury
Home injuries	$1,000,000	$9,900
Public injuries	$1,000,000	$6,700
Work injuries:		
without employer costs	$1,260,000	$39,000
with employer costs	$1,270,000	$43,000

Source: National Safety Council. (2007). Estimating the Costs of Unintentional Injuries. (See the organization website.)

Statistics such as those from the National Safety Council (2007) can be used by the safety committee to write strong recommendations that emphasize the bottom line by contrasting the costs versus the benefits. Your insurance company can also provide you with valuable data for this purpose. Including cost versus benefit analysis with each recommendation can show how much money your safety committee helps save the organization every time it uncovers and improves a hazardous condition, unsafe work practice, or inadequate procedure.

Every dollar spent by your organization on proactive safety, including safety committee activities, may return hundreds. You have got to convince management that an effective safety committee not only saves lives, but also saves money.

Make sure the safety committee has a written plan that includes all of the following sections:

* Role or purpose(s) of the safety committee
* Reasons for establishing the safety committee
* Need for management and member participation
* Need for support by all areas of the organization
* Responsibilities of the committee
* Duties of committee personnel

An example of a written plan that you can use as a template for your safety committee is offered in Figure 4.10. Be sure you modify it to meet the unique needs of your safety committee.

Makeup of the Safety Committee

If one of the purposes of the safety committee is to bring management and personnel together in a cooperative effort to improve the safety and health of workers, it just makes business sense to include representatives from management ranks as well as the personnel.

The safety committee becomes a forum for arriving at mutual solutions to problems that help to ensure both management and member acceptance. It is important for the safety committee not to be dominated by management in general or by any one individual, be it the safety officer, chairperson, or safety committee member. To make sure this does not happen, establish ground rules and techniques for decision making that promote group consensus.

Management representatives and the chairperson will be the primary conduits of communication between the safety committee and the organization. Committee members are the primary communicators with providers. It is very important that communication occurs in both directions.

How to Increase Involvement. To ensure a high level of motivation in the safety committee, it is important for it to be composed of both managers and personnel who understand their roles and responsibilities and are interested in its success. It is equally, if not more, important for the organization's culture to support committee activities. But for one reason or another, EMS organizations experience difficulty generating enthusiasm for the safety committee.

XYZ Emergency Medical Services
SAFETY COMMITTEE PLAN

Introduction. XYZ EMS is committed to accident prevention in order to protect the safety and health of our 50 employees. Injury and illness losses due to hazards are needless, costly, and preventable. To prevent these losses, a joint management/member safety committee will be established. Personnel involvement in accident prevention and support of safety committee members and activities are necessary to ensure a safe and healthful workplace.

Purpose. The purpose of our safety committee is to bring workers and members together in a nonadversarial, cooperative effort to help our organization promote and maintain a safe and healthful workplace.

Organization. There will be at least two management representatives to XYZ's EMS safety committee. One member representative from each shift and one member representative from administration also will be elected or encouraged to volunteer as a safety committee member. Managers and personnel are encouraged to volunteer as members of the committee.

Membership. The safety committee chairperson will be elected from the committee membership and will serve at the pleasure of the committee. Safety committee members will serve a continuous term of at least one year. Length of membership will be staggered so that at least one experienced member is always serving on the committee.

Membership in the committee will be considered professional development and annotated in each member's performance appraisal. XYZ EMS considers membership in the committee as a prerequisite for advancement to management positions.

Responsibility. The safety committee has the following responsibilities:

- Meet regularly to discuss safety and health.
- Communicate with committee members and the organization.
- Identify hazardous conditions and unsafe work practices.
- Recommend strategies to eliminate hazards.

Recommendations. Safety committee recommendations will be put in writing and submitted to management. Management will respond to recommendations according to the following schedule:

- Fatality: *immediate*
- Serious physical harm: *immediate*
- Minor injury: *14 days*
- Administrative, not applicable: *30 days*

Procedures. The committee's plan of action requires procedures by which the committee may successfully fulfill its role. Procedures developed should include meeting date, time, and location; election of chairperson and recorder; order of business; and records.

Duties of each member should include:

- Report unsafe conditions and practices.
- Attend all safety and health meetings.

FIGURE 4.10 ■ EMS Safety Committee Plan Sample.

- Review all accidents and near misses.
- Recommend ideas for improving safety and health.
- Set an example by working in a safe and healthful manner.
- Observe how safety and health are enforced in the workplace.
- Complete chairperson/committee assignments.
- Represent member safety interests.

Getting Organized. The safety committee is to be composed of a number of people from management and personnel. What kind of structure should the safety committee take? That really depends on the mandate the committee has received from the organization, the management system, size of the organization, and the organization's culture. But, generally safety committees are composed of the following positions: member representative, management representative, chairperson, recorder, and treasurer.

The elected chairperson has some very important duties to fulfill. They are as follows:

- Prepare an agenda for meetings.
- Arrange for a meeting room.
- Notify members of meeting dates/times.
- Distribute the agenda.
- Delegate responsibilities.
- Make assignments.
- Preside and conduct the meeting.
- Enforce committee ground rules.
- Communicate with the organization.
- Report the status of recommendations.

Duties of the safety committee recorder include the following:

- Assist the chairperson with the agenda.
- Record minutes of the meeting.
- Distribute and post the minutes.
- Assume the chairperson's duties if necessary.

Duties of safety committee members include the following:

- Receive suggestions, concerns, reports from personnel.
- Report personnel suggestions, concerns, reports to committee.
- Report back to personnel on their suggestions, concerns, reports.
- Attend all safety committee meetings.
- Receive training on safety and health subjects.
- Review injury and illness reports.
- Monitor safety and health programs and system.
- Set example by working safely.
- Conduct safety inspections.
- Make recommendations for corrective action.
- Assist in communicating committee activities to all members.

Figure 4.10 ■ (*Continued*)

Lack of Interest. There are many reasons that might explain why managers and personnel may have no interest in a safety committee. Among them are the following:

Why join the safety committee? Who cares?

Apathy toward the safety committee is common in many EMS organizations. There may be many reasons, but usually it is due to some form of nonsupport or a lack of interest by top management, which is a common complaint. As discussed earlier in this chapter, the safety committee members may want to reflect first on their own ability to carry out their purposes before they blame management; for example, who is going to be interested in attending and actively participating in safety committee activities when those activities may actually somehow threaten a person's job security or continuance to volunteer with the organization?

I was "volunteered."

It goes without saying that safety committee members should be volunteers. They always will be more effective as a group of interested volunteers who participate because they want to and not because they have to. But when personnel do not volunteer, management feels obligated to do something, so it selects and "volunteers" the personnel needed.

We don't have any money.

This is a common misconception made by safety committee members. As we learned earlier, safety committees are consultant groups that help develop and implement, but do not need to control safety programs.

Meetings are boring.

Personnel may feel that meetings seem like uninspired and unproductive gripe sessions.

I'm not properly trained.

Personnel are expected to help in safety, but they see that management does not make a commitment to training. They may acknowledge that they perform quarterly inspections, but without understanding the specific hazards or how to correct them, which leads them to believe that it is all just a waste of time.

I'm too busy.

Some may say that all their time is spent on what they are paid to do. Or in the case of volunteers, they may say that their volunteer work does not leave them any extra time for additional duties.

The chairperson hasn't got a clue.

When the chairperson does not have or take the time to plan a meeting, the consequence usually is a lack of structure. Frustration and other negative feelings about the committee are allowed to proliferate.

One person dominates meetings.

When the safety manager or another person is consistently overbearing, "always gets his way," or discounts the ideas of others, participants lose their will to contribute.

We never get anything done.

Committee members believe that they contribute good ideas in the meetings, but follow-through is absent or it takes months to finally get it addressed.

We're just a pack of watchdogs.

People do not like to be called a snitch or to be distrusted by their peers.

Even if you already have a great safety committee, it is likely that at least one of the signs listed above is present to some degree in your organization. So, what's the secret to eliminating those objections? Consequences. We do what we do in the workplace because of consequences, not just because someone tells us to do it.

The key is to design positive consequences into the safety management system and, more specifically, into safety committee participation. That means developing a culture that recognizes and rewards discretionary behaviors. Job security is enhanced, not threatened, when people participate in safety activities. If you do this effectively, personnel will be knocking down the door to join the safety committee.

Management Commitment

Commitment is serious time, money, and concern (TMC). Real commitment requires that management invest time and money into safety activities. Real concern for safety is expressed formally through the mission statement, policies, job descriptions, and performance appraisals. Commitment is expressed informally through word of mouth: Supervisors and managers set the highest examples, they insist that everyone else does also, and they apply appropriate consequences when personnel fail or excel. When management expresses a concern for safety, but hesitates or fails to invest time and money, it is a demonstration of nothing more than moral support for safety—which is nice but ineffective.

How is commitment to the safety committee demonstrated? Here are some possibilities:

- Allow members of the safety committee more than an hour each month to work on their safety responsibilities.
- Promote those who serve on safety committees, because they have increased knowledge and skills in safety and health.
- Respond to the recommendations made to correct hazards.
- From time to time attend (as observers) safety committee meetings.

When a safety committee member complains that he or she lacks "top management commitment," hold up a mirror and say, "Here's the answer to your problem." The cause of the problem may be that the safety committee, through lack of ability or action, lacks credibility. To be believable, committee members must have a clear understanding of their role, purpose, duties, and responsibilities. They need to understand where their responsibility ends, and where management's responsibility takes over (helping versus doing).

How can management encourage personnel to volunteer? The answer to that question is simple. It is done by providing the WIIFM (what's in it for me)—that is, by rewarding members of the safety committee with both tangible and intangible incentives.

Tangible rewards are external. They might consist of monthly merit pay increases or bonuses for taking on additional professional responsibilities. Membership on the safety committee might be recognized informally, with a thank-you and a pat on the back, or more formally on performance appraisals under "Professional Development." If you are serving in a volunteer organization, you may consider a special parking space or gift certificates to certain restaurants. However, it is essential that you do not set up your committee for failure; that is, you do not want individuals joining for money or prizes. Developing a culture of safety and health may be in itself enough of a benefit for individuals to want to participate on the safety committee.

The safety committee is a tool to be used to improve the safety of the organization. However, nothing is foolproof. There are situations that even the best safety committee may not be able to prevent. The bottom line is to consider offering an incentive, but do so wisely.

Intangible rewards are internal. They might include increased self-esteem, pride, a feeling of satisfaction of a job well done. Management also might let it be known formally and informally that it is to a member's advantage for career or promotional advancement to have had experience on the safety committee. After all, a member of the safety committee gains additional professional skills in communication, meeting with management, problem solving, occupational safety-and-health programs, hazard identification, accident investigation, recommendation writing, and so on. Consequently, safety committee membership should make a member more qualified for advancement.

Power

People and groups exercise various types of "power" to get what they want. A well-liked leader is able to take advantage of charismatic power to get his or her followers to perform. The nonleader in a position of responsibility may threaten people in order to influence their behaviors. However, to increase credibility, it is important for the safety committee to use two other forms of power—expert power and position power.

Expert power stems from the realization that members of the safety committee play the role of internal consultant to the organization. They know that their credibility depends on the expertise they bring to the role. How do you gain expertise? By increasing knowledge, skills, and abilities through experience. Proposing effective recommendations to management is crucial if credibility is to be gained. The most effective recommendations will include costs and benefits, talk the bottom line to management, and offer reasonable options for correcting workplace hazards, unsafe work practices, and ineffective administrative controls.

Another power that is used often is **position power**. If you find out who has the ear of the chief, then you know who has position power. The safety committee has the greatest position power when the chairperson regularly meets with the person at the top who is making the decisions for the organization.

Communication is the key here. Personnel see the safety committee as a communications conduit to management. When a member informs or makes a suggestion to the safety committee representative, he or she expects to get some sort of feedback soon after and wants to see action. To the EMS provider, it is an immediate need. If the safety committee representative takes the information to the safety committee, but neglects to give the member feedback, what is the member to think, but that the safety committee is a bunch of do-nothings and a waste of time? Therefore, to gain credibility with providers, communicate regularly and often with them. If a hazard cannot be fixed for a while, let the personnel know why. Even if it is not the answer personnel want to hear, they will appreciate the fact that the safety committee is doing its job.

Another good idea is to brag about safety committee accomplishments formally and informally. That does not mean that members of the committee should go out and literally boast about how great they are. Instead it means to let the workforce know about safety committee bottom-line accomplishments, and to do so with some excitement and pride.

SAFETY COMMITTEE TRAINING

Once volunteers do become members of the committee, they must be properly trained to be effective and motivated (Figure 4.11). Safety committee members who lack effective training will "spin their wheels" a lot, but rarely get much done. Lacking adequate knowledge and skills, they will not be able to fulfill their most important role as a consultant group that assists the organization in making improvements to the safety management system: the root causes for all safety problems.

Training will help each member to:

- Understand the role and purpose of the safety committee.
- Understand and carry out individual responsibilities.
- Understand and carry out organization safety plans, policies, and processes.
- Understand important safety-and-health concepts, principles, and methods.
- Improve personal safety leadership and communication skills.
- Improve meeting management skills.

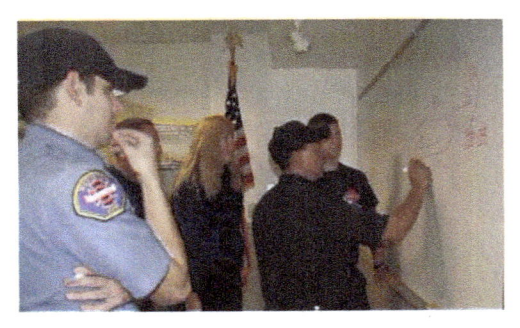

FIGURE 4.11 Training is an essential process for an effective safety committee. *Courtesy of 24-7 EMS®, a member of the HSI family of brands.*

- Improve analysis, evaluation, and problem-solving skills.
- Improve writing skills.
- Improve the ability to successfully submit proposals.
- Increase their value to the organization.
- Increase the opportunity for career advancement.

Training will help the safety committee to:

- Fulfill its mission to assist the organization.
- Improve its status within the organization.
- Work together as a problem-solving team.
- Submit high-quality recommendations to correct hazards.
- Have a positive impact on lowering claims costs.

A well-trained safety committee will help the organization to:

- Demonstrate effective safety leadership and management.
- Lower injury and illness rates.
- Improve morale.
- Correct hazards in a timely manner.
- Gain a better understanding of the positive impact of safety.
- Maintain a fair system of accountability.
- Develop a successful recognition program.

The field of occupational safety and health has many specialized and highly technical subject areas. Your safety committee will benefit if its members are familiar, at least to some degree, with safety subjects such as hazard communication, lockout-tagout, confined space entry, construction safety, and ergonomics (manual material handling), and with health subjects such as bloodborne pathogens, hazardous waste and emergency response, hazardous atmospheres, hearing conservation, ventilation, and ergonomics (repetitive motion).

Minimum Requirements

For a safety committee to operate successfully, its members must be properly trained in at least three very important areas: (1) safety committee operations and how to conduct meetings; (2) hazard identification and control concepts and methods; and (3) accident investigation procedures.

Operations

Safety committee members should be trained in how the safety committee operates and what is expected of them as members. Any training method might work for new safety committee members, but one-on-one, hands-on training is most effective. The chairperson can best convey clear expectations and answer any questions the new member might have if the training is done during a brief one-on-one session. It would be important to cover the general requirements contained in any standard operating policies and applicable laws with the new member.

SAFETY MEETINGS

Safety meetings need to be conducted on a regular basis. Meetings should be 1 hour or less, unless the majority of the committee agrees to extend it. You should cover the following:

- Review safety-and-health inspection reports to help correct safety hazards.
- Evaluate the accident investigations conducted since the last meeting to determine if the

cause(s) of the unsafe situation was identified and corrected.
- Evaluate your workplace accident-and-illness prevention program and discuss recommendations for improvement, if needed.
- Document attendance.
- Write down subjects discussed.

The meetings also should be recorded. Prepare minutes from each safety committee meeting, preserve them for 1 year, and make them available for review.

HAZARD IDENTIFICATION AND CONTROL

A hazard is an unsafe workplace condition or practice that could cause an injury or illness to an employee. If you look around your work environment, whether it is the station (Figure 4.12) or at the scene of an incident (Figure 4.13), you will be able to locate a few hazardous conditions or work practices without too much trouble.

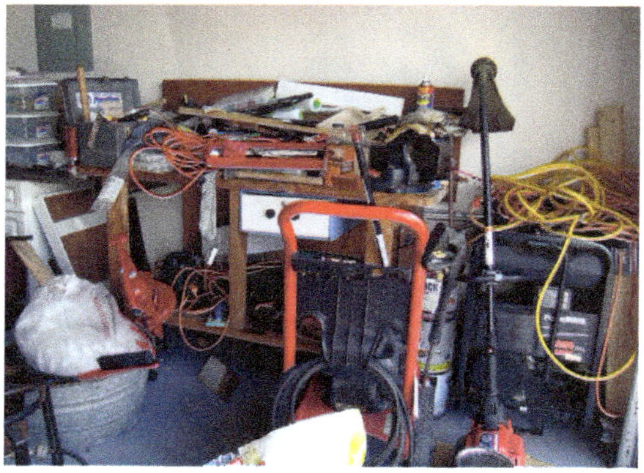

FIGURE 4.12 ■ The station may have a number of hazards. *Courtesy of Jeffrey T. Lindsey, Ph.D.*

HAZARD ANALYSIS

Hazard analysis techniques can be quite complex. Although they are necessary in some cases, frequently a basic, step-by-step review of the operation is sufficient. One of the most commonly used techniques is the job hazard analysis

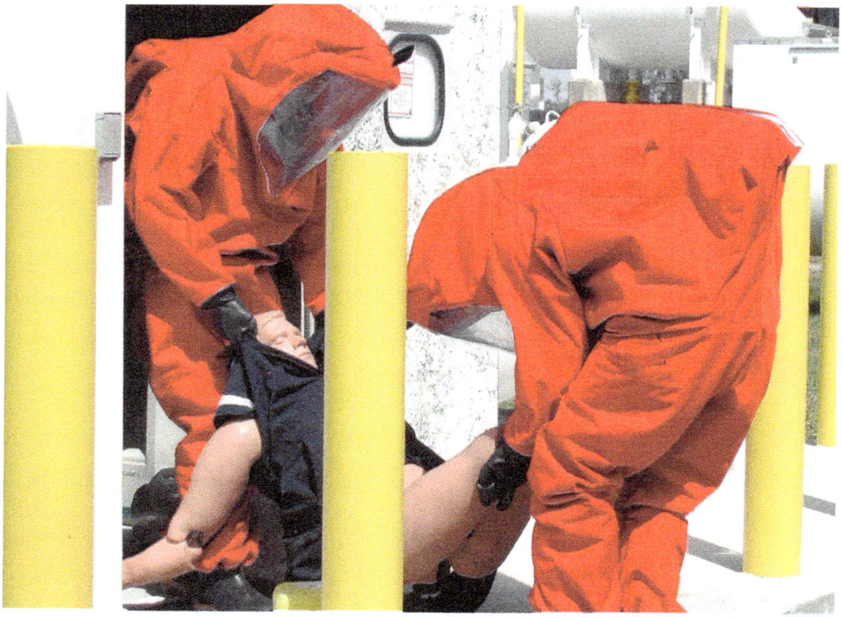

FIGURE 4.13 ■ The incident typically has multiple hazards. *Courtesy of Estero Fire Rescue.*

CHAPTER 4 *Developing a Safety Program* **75**

Best Practices

The National Highway Traffic Safety Administration (NHTSA) supports programs to ensure the safety of first responders working on the nation's roads. Traffic incidents involving fire, emergency medical services (EMS), and law enforcement personnel are routine occurrences on U.S. roads. NHTSA endeavors to improve the safety of first responder personnel on the roadside.

The Safe, Accountable, Flexible, and Efficient Transportation Equity Act: A Legacy for Users (SAFETEA-LU), Sec. 2014, First Responder Roadside Vehicle Safety requires that NHTSA develop and implement a comprehensive program to address the safety of first responders. The statute directs the agency to:

- Promote compliance with state and local laws intended to increase the safe and efficient operation of first responder vehicles;
- Compile a list of best practices by State and local governments to promote compliance with the laws;
- Analyze state and local laws intended to increase the safe and efficient operation of first responder vehicles; and
- Develop model legislation to increase the safe and efficient operation of first responder vehicles

In November 2006, NHTSA hosted a meeting of law enforcement, prosecutors, emergency responders, and other interested parties to assist in the development of a comprehensive model program for use by states to address first responder safety. This effort included development of a model law on first responder safety. Additionally, NHTSA has developed training materials for all first responders that focus on first responder roadside safety.

With its law enforcement, EMS, and fire service partners, NHTSA was involved with the Emergency Vehicle Safety Initiative, an effort spearheaded by the U.S. Fire Administration (USFA) with support from the Department of Transportation. As a separate part of this cooperative effort, the International Association of Chiefs of Police (IACP) researched and evaluated state best practices in first responder roadside safety.

NHTSA also worked closely with the National Conference of State Legislatures (NCSL) and the National Committee on Uniform Traffic Laws and Ordinances (NCUTLO) to develop a "move over" model law. As of 2008, 40 states have instituted "move-over" laws. The goal of such legislation is to ensure the safety of emergency personnel while working in or around the roadway. Although laws vary in terms of specific provisions and penalties, they specify that traffic must slow down and, if possible, move over to an adjacent traffic lane. Both the IACP and the National Sheriffs' Association (NSA) have adopted resolutions in support of uniformity in "move-over" laws.

Source: National Highway Traffic Safety Administration. "First Responder Roadside Vehicle Safety." (May 21, 2008). Washington, DC: NHTSA. (See the organization website.)

(JHA). Jobs that were initially designed with safety in mind may now include hazards or improper operations. When done for every job, this analysis periodically puts processes back on the safety track. Other, more sophisticated techniques are called for when complex risks are involved. These techniques include the following:

What-if checklist.

This is a broadly based hazard assessment technique that combines the creative thinking of a selected team of specialists with the methodical focus of a prepared checklist. The result is a comprehensive process hazards analysis that is extremely useful in training operating personnel on the hazards of the particular operation.

Hazard and operability study (HAZOP).

This is a formally structured method of systematically investigating each element of a system for all of the ways in which important parameters can deviate from the intended design conditions to create hazards and operability problems. The hazard and operability problems are typically determined by a study of the diagrams by a team of personnel who critically analyze the effects of potential problems arising in the operation.

Failure mode and effect analysis.

This analysis is a methodical study of component failures. It starts with a diagram of the process that includes all components that could fail and conceivably affect the safety of the process.

Fault tree analysis.

This is a quantitative assessment of all of the undesirable outcomes that could result from a specific initiating event. It begins with a graphic representation (using logic symbols) of all possible sequences of events that could result in an incident. The resulting diagram looks like a tree with many branches, each branch listing the sequential events (failures) for different independent paths to the top event. Probabilities (using failure rate data) are assigned to each event and then used to calculate the probability of occurrence of the undesired event.

HAZARD CLASSIFICATIONS

All workplace hazards exist in four general areas: materials; equipment, machinery, and tools; environment; and people. When you conduct a walk-around inspection, you are usually looking for hazardous materials, equipment, and environmental factors. These represent hazardous physical conditions in the workplace. The people category refers to personnel of the workforce at any level who may be using unsafe work behaviors or practices. Actually, personnel who are distracted in any way from the work they are doing should be considered a "walking" hazardous condition that increases the likelihood of an unsafe behavior.

Typically, most accidents are caused by the combination of work processes and management dysfunction that allows the unsafe or unhealthy behavior to exist or continue. The reason that a workforce member has an accident is that the behavior and decision making are condoned or never characterized as wrong. Ultimately, management is responsible, not the employee's behavior.

PRINCIPLES OF HAZARD IDENTIFICATION AND CONTROL

To be effective, safety committee members must know basic hazard identification and control concepts and methods. One of the duties a member of the safety committee might have is to conduct quarterly (or more frequent) walk-through safety inspections. Safety inspections can be effective in spotting workplace hazards, but only if those doing the inspecting know what they are looking for and what they are doing.

Once hazards have been found, safety committee members should be able to help take corrective action to eliminate or reduce the hazard. The most common strategy for eliminating hazards is to apply the hierarchy of controls, which were explained earlier in the chapter.

PROCESSES TO IDENTIFY HAZARDS

Your ability to identify hazardous conditions and unsafe work practices can be very effective if you are given the correct tools.

Formal Observation Process

One of the most effective methods to collect useful data about hazards and unsafe behaviors in the workplace is the formal observation process. In this process EMS providers are assigned the task of completing a minimum number of observations of safe and unsafe behaviors during a given period of time. These data are gathered and analyzed to produce graphs and charts reflecting the current status of and trends in provider behaviors. Just posting the results of these observations tends to increase awareness and lower injury rates. But, more important, the data give important clues about the safety-management system weaknesses that exist.

Observation processes like this are important because they can effectively identify behaviors that account for 95% of all workplace injuries. One caution: An important requirement for a successful process is that disciplinary action is never linked to observations.

The Safety Inspection

Three important points should be remembered when conducting the safety inspection audit:

- Use a checklist.
- Know what you are doing. Only competent individuals should conduct safety inspections. They should be aware of the different types of hazards in the workplace. Unsafe materials, tools, equipment, station design, noise, atmospheres, temperature extremes, and work practices should be evaluated. The inspector should know what to look for and how to look for it. Training is essential.
- Allow enough time to conduct a thorough inspection. The more time you give to complete the safety inspection, the more likely it is that you will uncover the hazard waiting to injure someone. A short inspection conducted once a quarter by an untrained employee may not be worth the time spent to conduct it.

There are advantages and disadvantages of using the safety inspection checklist. An important advantage is a properly constructed checklist that helps you inspect for hazardous conditions and unsafe work procedures in a structured, systematic manner. If a well-conceived checklist is not used, it is more likely that quality will suffer over time. Without any checklist, the conduct of the inspection will vary widely from person to person, depending on expertise.

Simply put, an important disadvantage is that same checklist. It takes time to construct, time you may not have, although the long-term advantages far outweigh the short-term effort. A second disadvantage is that using a checklist might cause the dreaded "tunnel vision" syndrome, which occurs when an inspector overlooks a hazard in the workplace because it was not addressed in the checklist. The cure for this common disease is to merely place a "catch-all" question into the checklist that asks the inspector to decide whether or not there are any other hazards that need to be corrected.

Boilerplate safety checklists are available. Check with your insurance company to see if they offer them.

Routine safety-and-health site inspections are designed to catch hazards missed at other stages. This type of inspection should be done at regular intervals, generally on a weekly basis. In addition, procedures should be established that provide a daily inspection of the work area. You can use a checklist already developed or make your own, based on past problems, standards that apply to EMS, input from everyone involved, and your organization's safety practices or rules.

It is important to remember that inspections should cover every part of the worksite. They should be done at regular intervals, and safety officers and organization supervisors should be trained to recognize and control hazards and to track those identified hazards to correction. Information from inspections should be used to improve the hazard prevention and control program.

An Organized Workplace

Poor housekeeping can contribute to low morale and sloppy work. Most safety action programs start with an intensive cleanup campaign in all areas of the workplace. The EMS station can be a hazard all unto itself. Get rid of unnecessary items, provide proper waste containers, store flammables properly, make sure exits are not blocked, mark aisles and passageways, provide adequate lighting, and so on. Get everyone involved and impress upon employees that you want to make the workplace safer, more healthful, and more efficient.

CATCHING HAZARDS

After hazards are recognized and controls are put in place, additional analysis tools can help ensure that the controls stay in place and other hazards do not appear. These other tools include provider reports of hazards, accident and incident investigations, and injury and illness trend analysis.

Member Reports of Hazards

EMS personnel play a key role in discovering and controlling hazards that may develop or already exist in the workplace. A reliable system for member reporting is an important element of an effective safety-and-health system. The workplace must not only encourage reporting, but must also value it.

It is often helpful to establish multiple ways to report hazards so that, depending on comfort level and the nature of the issue, several avenues are available to get concerns addressed. Examples include supervisor chain of command, safety-and-health committee member, voice mail, and a suggestion box. An effective reporting system should have a policy that encourages personnel to report safety-and-health concerns, and timely and appropriate responses should be given to the reporting personnel. Also, timely and appropriate action should be taken where valid concerns exist and required hazard corrections should be tracked. The effective system should also protect reporting personnel from any type of reprisal or harassment.

Accident/Incident Investigations

Accident/incident investigations are another tool for uncovering hazards that were missed earlier or that slipped by the planned controls. But they are only useful when the process is positive and focuses on finding the root cause, not someone to blame. All accidents and incidents should be investigated. Near misses are considered an incident, because given a slight change in time or position, injury or damage could have occurred.

Six key questions should be answered in the accident investigation and report: Who? What? Where? When? How? Why? Thorough interviews with everyone involved are necessary.

In many companies, safety committees will review and evaluate accident reports. It is important that safety committee members understand what an effective accident report looks like. The primary purpose of the accident/incident investigation is to prevent future occurrences. Therefore, the results of the investigation should be used to initiate corrective action.

Injury and Illness Trend Analysis

Hazards found during worksite analysis should be reviewed to determine what failure in the safety-and-health system permitted the hazard to occur. The system failure should then be corrected to ensure that similar hazards do not reoccur. The OSHA 300 log is probably the best statistical tool available for analyzing hazardous conditions and unsafe work practices trends. More than 25 important injury and illness trends have been identified using the OSHA 300 log.

Take a look at each column of your company's OSHA 300 log and ask the following questions to determine trends:

Who is getting hurt? Is someone getting hurt over and over, and is it the same kind of injury?

What actually caused the injuries? This question looks for the basic cause of the physical trauma to the body.

Where are personnel getting hurt? Are they doing their regular jobs, or are they doing other jobs when they get hurt? Are personnel getting injured more in certain incidents or areas of the workplace, or in particular locations?

When are workers getting hurt? Look for trends:

- A particular time of the day?
- Early or late in the work shift?
- A particular day of the week? Mondays? Fridays?
- A particular week of the month? Just before payday?
- A particular month of the year? December?
- A particular quarter of the year? Last quarter of the budget?
- A particular season of the year? Just before hunting season?

How was the member injured? This question is directed toward hazardous conditions and unsafe work practices. Were hazardous materials, tools, or equipment being used? What was the member not using (PPE)?

Why was the member injured? Are work shifts too long? Were personnel using unsafe practices? Are personnel getting hurt as a result of factors at or outside of work, and were they factors the organization can or cannot control?

Take the information you gain from this analysis to draw conclusions about where your greatest effort needs to be directed. Most lost-workday claims are due to strains and sprains. Your log may reflect this trend. At any rate, analyzing the OSHA 300 log allows you to act on facts, not hunches.

HAZARDOUS MATERIALS

For the purposes of this chapter, the term *hazardous materials* refers only to those found in the station or EMS facilities and include the following:

> Liquid and solid chemicals such as acids, bases, solvents, explosives, and so on. The hazard communication program is designed to communicate the hazards of chemicals to all EMS personnel and to make sure safe work practices are always used.

> Solids such as metal, wood, plastics. Raw materials used to manufacture products are usually bought in large quantities, and can cause injuries or fatalities in many ways.

> Gases such as hydrogen sulfide and methane. Gas may be extremely hazardous if leaked into the atmosphere.

> Personnel should know the signs and symptoms related to exposure to hazardous gases in the workplace.

HAZARDOUS EQUIPMENT

Hazardous equipment includes machinery and tools. Hazardous equipment should be properly guarded so that it is virtually impossible for a member of the workforce to be placed in a danger zone around moving parts that could cause injury or death. A preventive maintenance program should be in place to make sure equipment operates properly. A corrective maintenance program is needed to make sure equipment that is broken and causing a safety hazard is fixed immediately. Tools also need to be in good working order, properly repaired, and used for intended purposes only. Any maintenance person will tell you that accidents can occur easily if tools are not used correctly. Tools that are used while broken also are very dangerous.

Hazardous work practices include taking unsafe shortcuts or using established procedures that are accidents waiting to happen. As mentioned earlier, hazardous work practices represent about 95% of the causes of all accidents in the workplace. Management may unintentionally promote unsafe work practices by establishing policies, procedures, and rules (written and unwritten) that ignore or actually direct unsafe work practices. These safety policies, plans, programs, processes, procedures, and practices are called system controls and ultimately represent the causes of about 95% of all workplace accidents.

SYSTEMS TO TRACK HAZARD CORRECTIONS

An essential part of any safety-and-health system is the correction of hazards that occur despite the overall prevention and control program. For larger organizations, documentation is important so that management and personnel have a record of the correction. Many EMS organizations use the form that documents the original discovery of a hazard to track its correction. Hazard correction information can be noted on an inspection report next to the hazard description. Member reports of hazards and reports of accident investigation should provide space for notations about hazard correction.

Frequently, EMS organizations will computerize the hazard tracking system, which can be as simple as adding a few items to an existing commercial database.

PREVENTIVE MAINTENANCE SYSTEMS

Good preventive maintenance plays a major role in ensuring that hazard controls continue to function effectively. It also keeps new hazards from arising due to equipment malfunction. Reliable scheduling and documentation of maintenance activity are necessary (Figure 4.14). The scheduling depends on knowledge of what needs maintenance and how often. The point of preventive maintenance is to get the work done before repairs or replacements are needed. Documentation is a good idea, but it is also a necessity in larger companies.

Medical Programs

A company's medical program is an important part of the safety-and-health system. It can deliver services that prevent hazards that can cause illness and injury, recognize and treat illness and injury, and limit the severity of work-related injury and illness. Medical programs consist of everything from a basic first aid and CPR response to sophisticated approaches for the diagnosis and resolution of ergonomic problems.

EMS has not been particularly proactive about putting together a comprehensive medical program for personnel. Though NFPA 1582 is a standard for firefighters for physical exams, there is no set standard for EMS personnel. Nonetheless, it is important to develop a comprehensive physical exam program and a return-to-work program.

Whatever the type of medical program, it is important to use medical specialists who have occupational health training. (See OSHA standard 1910.151[b] for first aid requirements. Also, the Bloodborne Pathogens Standard has requirements to protect employees who provide emergency response [1910.1030].)

Safety-and-Health Training

Does everyone in the workplace know what the workplace plan is in case of a fire or other emergency? When and where PPE is required? What are the types of chemicals used in the workplace and the precautions to use when handling them? Training can help to develop

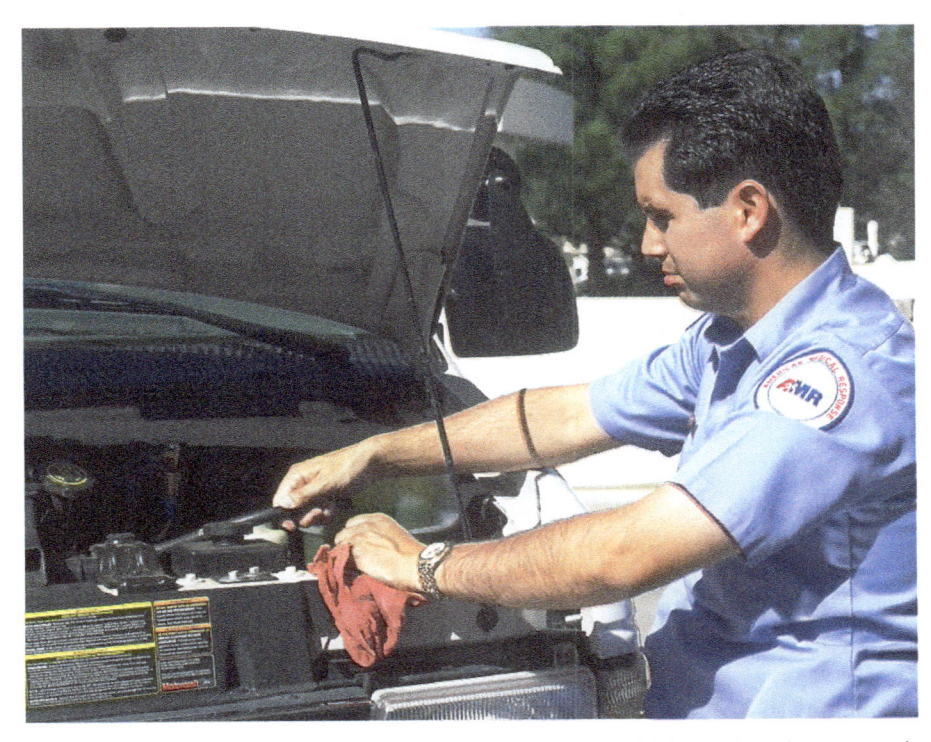

FIGURE 4.14 ■ Preventive maintenance is essential to ensure that vehicles and equipment are in working order.

the knowledge and skills needed to understand workplace hazards and safe procedures. Training is most effective when integrated into an organization's overall training in performance requirements and job practices (Figure 4.15).

The content of an organization's training program and the methods of presentation should reflect the needs and characteristics of the particular workforce. Therefore, identification of needs is an important early step in training design. Involving everyone in this process and in the subsequent teaching can be highly effective.

The following five principles of teaching and learning should be followed to maximize program effectiveness:

- Trainees should understand the purpose of the training.
- Information should be organized to maximize effectiveness.
- People learn best when they can immediately practice and apply newly acquired knowledge and skills.
- As trainees practice, they should get feedback.
- People learn in different ways, so an effective program will incorporate a variety of training methods.

The types of safety-and-health training needed include orientation training for personnel; Job Safety Analysis, Standard Operating Procedures, and other hazard recognition training; required training; accident investigation training; and drills. Training should target everyone in the organization, including managers and supervisors. Training for managers should

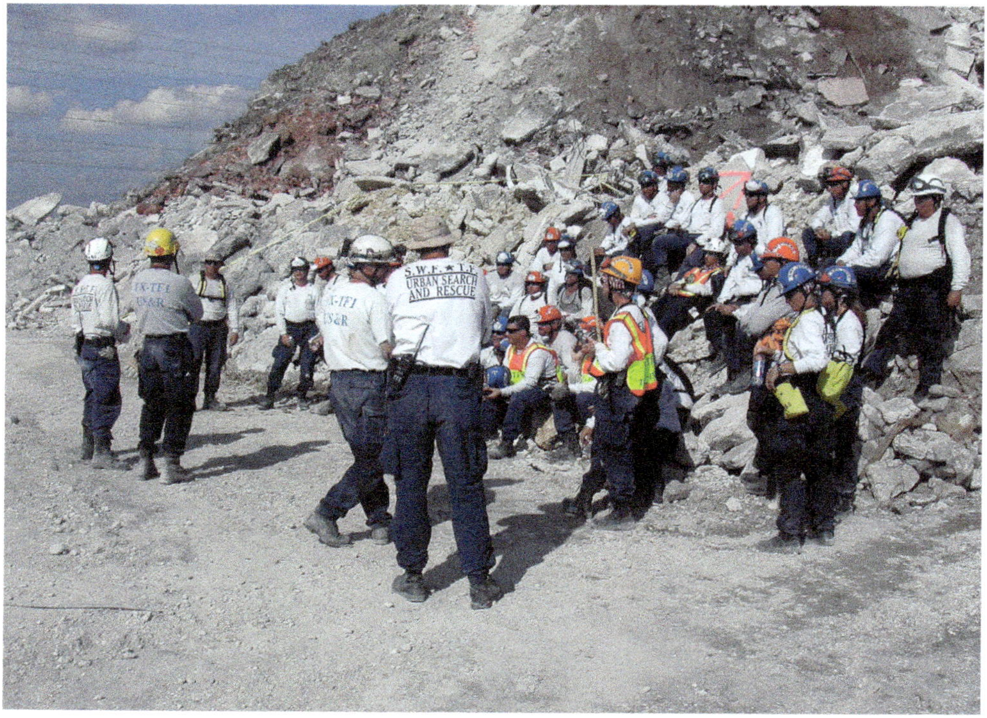

FIGURE 4.15 ■ Training is critical for demonstrating hazards and safety procedures to members of the organization. *Courtesy of Estero Fire Rescue.*

emphasize the importance of their role in visibly supporting the safety-and-health program and setting a good example. Supervisors should receive training in the organization's policies and procedures, as well as hazard detection and control, accident investigation, handling of emergencies, and how to train and reinforce training.

A plan to evaluate the training program should be constructed when a training is initially designed. If the evaluation is done correctly, it can identify the program's strengths and weaknesses and provide a basis for future program changes.

Keeping training records will help ensure that everyone who should get training does. A simple form can document the training record for each employee.

CHAPTER REVIEW

Summary

This chapter should have prepared you to handle the case study that was discussed at the beginning of the chapter. You should be able to establish a safety committee, which is an integral part of a safety program. The safety committee is not a discipline committee, but rather a committee to review accidents to determine if there are ways to do things better. The committee also looks at administrative controls, including policies and training.

In addition, this chapter has given an overview of the goals of a safety program. It detailed the various components of a safety program. This gives you the basic foundation of how to develop your own safety program. The safety culture of the organization is very important not only to the organization but also to the viability of the safety program. There are various ways to create a safety culture, and this chapter has given you some ways to create a positive safety culture in your organization.

EMS is not exempt from required postings. The chapter discussed the various posters that are required for your organization. Your specific state may have additional posting requirements.

The safety program is the foundation for the safety officer. Creating and maintaining such a program takes work and diligence. It is well worth the effort. The goal should be to provide the safest work environment for EMS personnel.

WHAT WOULD YOU DO? Reflection

The first step in starting your safety committee is to put together a plan. Figure 4.10 can serve as a template. In addition, your supervisor must buy into the plan. In most instances when an outside force such as your insurance carrier recommends that you do something, your organization's management tends to be more cooperative and willing to start new programs. In this situation, the chief has made it one of your goals. Your insurance carrier also is a resource to assist you in the startup of your safety committee. Once your plan is in place, the next step is to get personnel to serve on the committee. From there, you call your first meeting, and begin the work of the committee.

Review Questions

1. Describe the hierarchy of controls and the four general strategies.
2. Describe the three major activities of a workplace assessment.
3. Explain the composition of a safety culture.
4. What is the role and responsibility of the safety committee?
5. What are the purposes of the safety committee?
6. What are the definitions of the terms *expert power* and *position power*?
7. What is a hazard?
8. Describe the questions to ask when using the OSHA 300 log to trend losses.
9. What are the five principles of teaching and learning to maximize your safety program effectiveness?

References

Agency for Healthcare Research and Quality. (2001, July). "Making Health Care Safer: A Critical Analysis of Patient Safety Practices." Evidence Report/Technology Assessment, No. 43. AHRQ Publication No. 01-E058. Rockville, MD: Author. (See the organization website.)

Demings, W. (1986). *Out of the Crisis: Quality, Productivity, and Competitive Position.* Cambridge, UK: Cambridge University Press.

National Highway Traffic Safety Administration. (2008, May 21). "First Responder Roadside Vehicle Safety." Washington, DC: Author. (See the organization website.)

National Safety Council. (2007). Estimating the Costs of Unintentional Injuries. (See the organization website.)

Occupational Safety and Health Administration. (n.d.). "Bloodborne Pathogens—1910.1030." From Part Number 1910, "Occupational Safety and Health Standards: Toxic and Hazardous Substances." (See the organization website.)

Occupational Safety and Health Administration. (n.d.). "Hazard Communication—1910.1200." From Part Number 1910, "Occupational Safety and Health Standards: Toxic and Hazardous Substances." (See the organization website.)

Occupational Safety and Health Administration. (n.d.). "Hazard Communication—1926.59." From Part Number 1926, "Safety and Health Regulations for Construction: Occupational Health and Environmental Controls." (See the organization website.)

Occupational Safety and Health Administration. (n.d.). "Medical Services and First Aid—1910.151." From Part Number 1910, "Occupational Safety and Health Standards: Medical and First Aid." (See the organization website.)

Occupational Safety and Health Administration. (n.d.). "Occupational Noise Exposure—1910.95." From Part Number 1910, "Occupational Safety and Health Standards: Occupational Health and Environment Control." (See the organization website.)

Occupational Safety and Health Administration. (n.d.). "Permit-Required Confined Spaces—1910.146." From Part Number 1910, "Occupational Safety and Health Standards: General Environmental Controls." (See the organization website.)

Occupational Safety and Health Administration. (n.d.). "Respiratory Protection—1910.134." From Part Number 1910, "Occupational Safety and Health Standards: Personal Protective Equipment." (See the organization website.)

Occupational Safety and Health Administration. (n.d.). "The Control of Hazardous Energy (Lockout/Tagout)—1910.147." From Part Number 1910, "Occupational Safety and Health Standards: General Environmental Controls." (See the organization website.)

Occupational Safety and Health Administration. (n/d). "Safety and Health Management Systems eTools." Washington, DC: Author. (See the organization website.)

Oregon OSHA. (n.d.). "Oregon OSHA Online Course 101: Safety Committee Basic Training." (See the organization website.)

Safe, Accountable, Flexible, Efficient Transportation Equity Act: A Legacy for Users. Public Law No. 109–59. 119 STAT. 1857. (2005, August 10). (See the organization website.)

National Ag Safety Database. (n.d.). "Safety Committee." (See the organization website.)

Washington State Department of Labor and Industries. (n.d.). "Core Rules: Safety Committees and Safety Meetings—WAC 296-800-130." (See the organization website.)

Key Terms

administrative controls Control measures aimed at reducing exposures to hazards, generally by designing safe work practices, scheduling, and job enrichment; should be used in conjunction with, and not as a substitute for, more effective or reliable engineering controls.

culture of consequences An environment in which individuals are rewarded or recognized and held accountable for their actions.

engineering controls To the extent feasible, the work environment and the job itself should be designed (not necessarily by an engineer) to eliminate hazards or reduce exposure to hazards.

expert power A concept that stems from the realization that individuals who are considered experts in their fields play the role of an internal consultant to the organization.

hazard identification The process of identifying hazards or unsafe processes or conditions.

hierarchy of controls Four general strategies for managing hazards: engineering controls, administrative controls, personal protective equipment (PPE), and interim measures.

interim measures Temporary uses of engineering or administrative controls.

Occupational Safety and Health Administration (OSHA) The federal agency that oversees the safety of all occupations in the United States.

personal protective equipment (PPE) Equipment such as eye and hearing protection, gloves, and respiratory filters used in conjunction with administrative controls to limit exposure to a hazard in the workplace.

position power A concept that stems from the realization that a person can be in a position to have influence on a decision maker.

safety committee Personnel and management coming together on a regular basis to identify and solve everyday safety-and-health problems.

safety culture A combination of an organization's attitudes, behaviors, beliefs, values, ways of doing things, and other shared characteristics about safety.

safety program A program made up of the practical concerns of putting together the elements necessary to create a safe environment for personnel and patients.

worksite analysis A variety of worksite examinations that identify not only existing hazards, but also conditions and operations with a potential for hazards.

CHAPTER 5 Risk Management Process

Objectives

After reading this chapter, the student should be able to:

5.1 Identify risk management components.
5.2 Explain the need for effective risk management concepts in an EMS agency.
5.3 Examine the history and development of risk management.
5.4 Evaluate methods of risk management.
5.5 Identify roles and responsibilities of leaders in risk management.
5.6 Identify the role of EMS personnel in risk management.
5.7 Describe the benefits of risk management.

Overview

This title on EMS safety and risk management has been written to assist EMS providers in the reduction of line-of-duty injuries, illnesses, and fatalities. It provides a framework for developing programs that will create an appropriate margin of health and safety for providers during the performance of EMS duties.

Key Terms

exposure	**relative risk**	**risk retention**
goals	**risk**	**risk transfer**
objectives	**risk avoidance**	**severity**
probability	**risk management**	**speculative risk**
pure risk	**risk manager**	

CHAPTER 5 *Risk Management Process* **87**

WHAT WOULD YOU DO?

The equipment committee is looking at new equipment and procedures for your EMS service. Committee members want to begin providing transports for high-risk neonatal patients. A variety of special equipment must be purchased in order to provide the service. You are asked to do a risk assessment to determine the level of risk this new service will impose on your organization. You are more than willing to help out, but have no idea where to begin. Your report is due in 2 weeks.

Questions

1. Where would you begin?
2. What would the prioritization formula look like for this issue?
3. What would be your final recommendation?

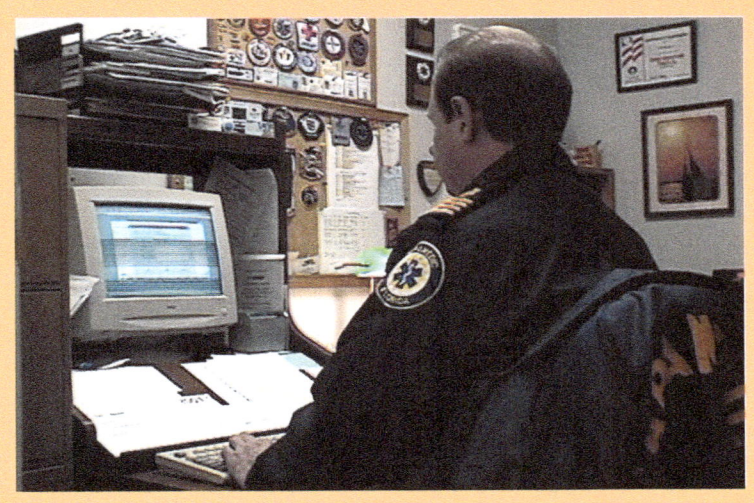

Prior to committing to new services, you should look at the risk that may be created by providing the service. *Courtesy of Jeffrey T. Lindsey, Ph.D.*

INTRODUCTION

There are various levels of risk in any type of organization. Therefore, risk management must be an integral part of any organization. Every individual in the organization also should be part of the risk management team. Every risk has to be managed to a certain level. The acceptable level of risk you tolerate for the organization will depend on your position in the organization. This chapter establishes a process that can manage the risk based on the *EMS Risk Management Resource Guide* developed by the Pennsylvania Emergency Health Services Council (2004) and funded under a contract with the Pennsylvania Department of Health.

RISK

The term **risk** is literally defined as the possibility of meeting danger or suffering harm or loss, or **exposure** to harm or loss. With this in mind, the concept of applying the term to the EMS profession brings about certain challenges, given that the nature of the work is sometimes inherently dangerous.

Three interrelated concepts are used in determining risk: the **probability** that an event may occur, a detrimental or undesirable consequence related to the event, and the **severity** of the potential harm of the event.

RISK ASSESSMENT

Relative risk is judged by specific undesirable events along a broad scale of undesirability. For example, an on-the-job injury could range from a minor occurrence to a fatal injury. Regardless, both of these outcomes are undesirable. It is without deliberation that the minor occurrence would be a much better alternative than a fatal injury. In this situation, the person who was injured or who had a close call will consider the probable and potential consequences. He most likely then will adjust his behavior to minimize or alleviate the risk of such an event occurring in the future.

The way to assess risk is by determining the probability of an occurrence and the effect that the occurrence has on the organization or components of the organization. To understand the data that are compiled, a risk assessment is expressed in various terms. The best way to describe the probability of an occurrence is to use subjective terms (Table 5.1).

Probability and consequence can be combined and expressed mathematically as the product of loss probability. An example of this is an insurance company that considers an asset worth $2 million but decides there is a low risk of ever having to pay that amount.

TABLE 5.1 ■ Risk-Related Terminology

Topic	Examples of Related Terms
Describing the probability of an occurrence	• Rare vs. high • 1 in 10 • A percentage
Describing undesirable consequences	• Death • Injury • Disaster
Talking about a financial loss	• Combined costs of payments
Writing a workers' compensation claim	• Loss of productivity

When discussing the probability of risk, it is important to understand that risk probability is bidirectional. That is, it illustrates the chance that something undesirable may occur, and it illustrates the probable outcome rated on a scale of negative consequences. (This concept will be reviewed later in the chapter.) As an example: Statistically you can predict the number of ambulance crashes that occur annually. You also can predict the number of injuries and fatalities that arise from those crashes. However, the statistics are neither able to predict where or when a crash will occur, nor can they provide an assessment of the seriousness of the crash.

Every situation an EMS professional enters carries with it a certain amount of risk. The integration of probability and consequence will assist in guiding the EMS profession into a proactive approach to risk management.

RISK MANAGEMENT

Risk management refers to activities that involve the comparison and/or evaluation of risks and development of methods that will effect change in the probability or consequence of an act. Identification and evaluation of risks as well as the identification, selection, and implementation of control measures make up the complete process of risk management.

Community Risk Management

In contrast to fire protection and law enforcement, EMS is not often viewed as contributing to controlling risk in a community. However, the simple fact of having specialized equipment and trained personnel on hand shows that EMS is a valued asset to a community's response to risk.

Although most EMS organizations focus on treatment and transport of the sick or injured during or after an emergency, the medical role of EMS is still based on the need to protect the community's population. With this in mind, any EMS organization can be viewed as part of a community's risk management program; that is, it exists to assist in limiting the loss from illness and injury when an emergency occurs.

As a whole, EMS organizations often are reactive in terms of risk management in the community. This means that EMS will change behaviors or conditions only after an unfortunate incident has occurred. Also, effort is needed in the areas of prevention and public education, which can help to reduce both the severity and frequency of emergencies. For example, EMS can make citizens aware of the risks in the community and promote prevention. It also can increase understanding of potential hazardous situations, medical emergencies, and more effective responses to emergencies. Educational and outreach programs are well received by the public and include such programs as community CPR classes, helmet awareness, falls in the elderly, and specific hazard recognition and avoidance (Figure 5.1).

EMS Organizational Risk Management

Multiple publications and other resources provide a wide range of methods for risk management. The means by which risk management

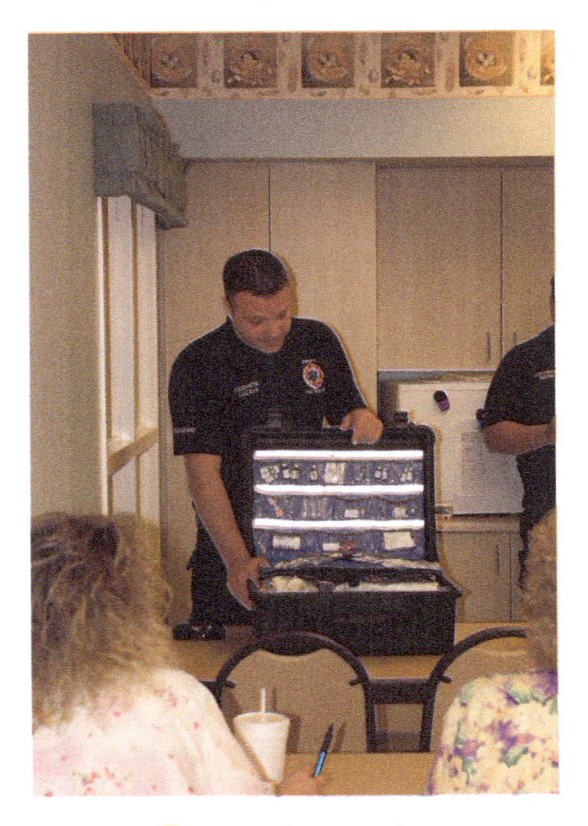

FIGURE 5.1 ■ Community outreach programs are a key component for EMS organizations. *Courtesy of Estero Fire Rescue.*

is undertaken is determined by the individual organization. However, the risk management process must be properly managed, evaluated continuously, and upgraded as needed.

Risk Manager

An organization's **risk manager** typically has responsibility for handling relations with outside agencies, such as insurance companies. Depending on an organization's size and revenue, the risk manager may have to wear many hats. He may be a supervisor with risk management responsibilities along with responsibility for several other equally important tasks. In this case, a risk management team may be an option that an organization can use. The risk management team should not be confused with a safety team. Although some responsibilities may overlap, their missions are different. It also should be understood that although an organization utilizes a risk management team, one member of that team should have overall responsibility for decision making.

Risk Management System

Risk management is a dynamic process. As in any effective system, goals and objectives must be clearly stated, understood by all relevant persons, attainable, and measurable. Risk managers or other individuals who are responsible for the goals being met should be an integral part of the process.

Goals and Objectives

When developing goals and objectives, it is important to keep in mind the differences between them. **Goals** are benchmarks that are established to affect a certain outcome (e.g., reduce the number of back injuries). **Objectives** are the means by which a goal is obtained (e.g., conduct body mechanics training annually and make additional personnel available as needed for lifting assistance).

■ THE RISK MANAGEMENT PROCESS

The risk management process involves five steps: identifying and analyzing loss exposures, examining the feasibility of alternative risk management techniques, selecting the best risk management techniques, implementing the techniques, and monitoring the program (Figure 5.2).

IDENTIFYING AND ANALYZING LOSS EXPOSURES

Identifying and analyzing essentially comprise the process of detecting potential loss

Five Steps of Risk Management

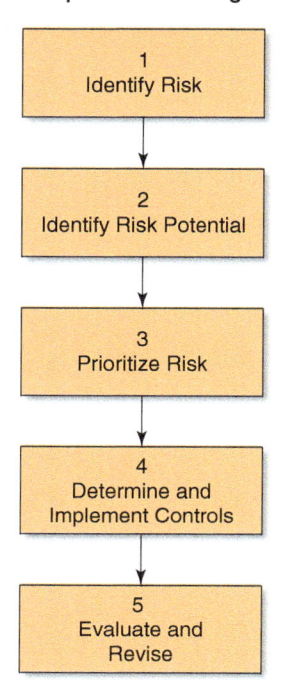

1. Identify Risk
2. Identify Risk Potential
3. Prioritize Risk
4. Determine and Implement Controls
5. Evaluate and Revise

FIGURE 5.2 ■ Risk management flowchart.

exposure. The daily vehicle checklist is a great example. When the vehicle check is conducted, a checklist is used to help identify potential problems. Once a potential problem has been identified, the crew must determine the level of corrective action needed.

There is some potential for risk involved in all aspects of EMS (Table 5.2). The purpose of identifying it is to determine what types of things create risk so that they and the associated costs can be avoided or dealt with successfully in the future.

When identifying risk in the workplace, you should use documentation that already exists, such as current injury reports, accident reports, and disciplinary or other action-type reports. Neighboring organizations as well as a multitude of industry and trade journals are available to assist with the identification of risk.

TABLE 5.2 ■ Broad Areas of Potential Risk in EMS

Area	Risks
Personnel	• On the job illness, injury, exposure, fatality • Workplace violence • Diversity awareness
Vehicles	• Operator error • Vehicle collisions • Mechanical problems
Equipment	• Damage and routine wear • Loss of equipment • Misuse of equipment
Facilities	• Fires • Natural disasters • Housekeeping • Lighting

Note: An EMS organization should consider any and all risks, especially those that may be specific to the organization.

FEASIBILITY OF ALTERNATIVE RISK MANAGEMENT TECHNIQUES

A number of areas must be considered when examining the feasibility of alternative risk management techniques. They include exposure avoidance, loss prevention, separation of loss exposures, duplication, insurance, and retention.

Exposure Avoidance

An EMS organization could provide a number of services but may not want to because of costs and potential costs of providing such services. For example, some organizations only provide BLS-level services and allow other organizations to provide ALS care. Another example is extrication. Some agencies have elected to perform auto extrication, although others have opted out until the patient has been extricated and turned over to them for emergency medical care. Others fall somewhere in between.

Loss Prevention

An organization may elect to provide ALS services; one example is airway management via endotracheal intubation (Figure 5.3). To reduce the loss potential, the EMS service may implement procedures for endotracheal intubation and provide the tools to assist in recognizing the difference between successful and unsuccessful intubations. In addition, the agencies may provide responders with alternative airway devices, such as a laryngeal mask airway or King Tube.

Separation of Loss Exposures

Many agencies provide BLS transport services only. ALS then is provided by a separate unit or through the fire service. Another separation would be to place stations strategically throughout a district or to utilize the system status management. Either method of unit distribution may be viewed as a means to separate loss exposures of the organization.

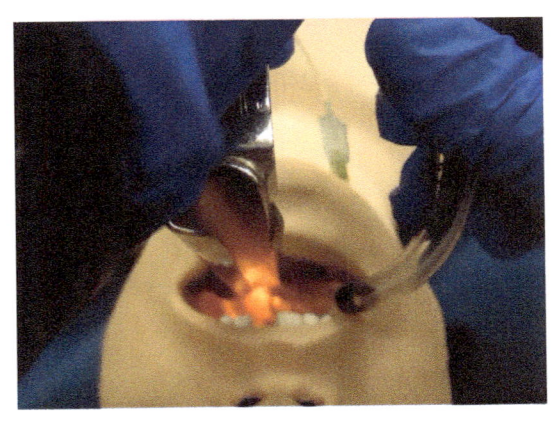

FIGURE 5.3 ■ Endotracheal intubation is one way among many to provide airway management. *Courtesy of Jeffrey T. Lindsey, Ph.D.*

Duplication

Many organizations have duplicate resources, such as one or two units in reserve for use when primary vehicles need maintenance. However, for many organizations the cost of duplicating resources is virtually prohibitive. So there are other options, some quite creative. One example is called a mutual-aid agreement, which requires an agency's command officer to make a specific request for assistance from a neighboring jurisdiction. Another example is an automatic-aid agreement, which also arranges for a neighboring jurisdiction to assist, but without a specific request from a command officer. Instead it allows the dispatch center to send or request resources based on the information provided in the initial emergency call.

Insurance

An alternative risk management technique is to purchase an insurance policy, which will fund a loss as specified in the contract. Essentially, the risk is being transferred financially to another company to provide for instances related to the policy coverage. In other words, you are not transferring the risk to the insurance company; the risk is still there. However, if an incident occurs, the damages incurred can be financially covered by the insurance coverage.

Retention

Retention may take many forms, intentionally or unintentionally. One form is self-funding, where the organization has set aside funds to cover losses or the deduction part of the insurance policy. Consider what a potential loss may be and determine how much in reserves must be maintained for such an occurrence. If the method your organization selects is self-funding, then your organization will need to set aside enough money in a reserve account to cover any claims that may occur.

Self-funding requires you to allocate or retain earnings in order to pay for a certain level of loss. When an organization is financially able to establish a bond to cover all losses, then it would be considered 100% self-insured. This is rare, however, in EMS. The amount you put in reserve is typically not the whole amount of the potential loss. Instead, EMS agencies should purchase a supplemental insurance policy that would cover the difference between the level of self-funding and the total potential loss.

To properly evaluate risk, one must determine the probability or likelihood that a harmful event may occur. When evaluating probability, look at the number of times a specific incident has occurred over a given period. With this information, decide into which one of the four categories in Figure 5.4 the incident belongs. However, it is important to remember that usually the most severe incidents are the least common.

During the risk evaluation, the following questions should be answered: What is the risk? Has the risk occurred locally? What is known regarding the national occurrence, and how does this organization compare? What is the probability of different outcomes? What are the consequences if these outcomes occur?

Retention of risk is a difficult process. A variety of considerations should be taken into account when determining the amount

High Frequency Low Severity	High Frequency High Severity
Low Frequency Low Severity	Low Frequency High Severity

FIGURE 5.4 Risk management evaluation chart.

Best Practices

Charleston County, South Carolina, takes risk management very seriously. In 2007, the county won three awards in safety and risk management from the South Carolina Association of Counties: 2007 Safety Achievement Award, 2007 Sustained Excellence in Risk Management Award, and 2007 Service Award. The following is an excerpt from the press release.

2007 Safety Achievement Award

The 2007 Outstanding Safety Achievement Award was awarded to Charleston County for the combined effort between the Safety and Risk Management Department and Emergency Medical Services (EMS). The award was given because the number of back injuries to EMS paramedics and emergency medical technicians was reduced by over 70 percent after the County implemented 23 new hydraulic ambulance stretchers.

"The new stretchers can mechanically and safely lift patients weighing up to 650 pounds, which has greatly reduced the repetitive and heavy daily lifting done by our emergency responders," said Larry Hodge, Director of Charleston County's Safety and Risk Management Department.

The County purchased the new stretchers after its successful use of stair chairs, which can safely transport patients down flights of stairs. "Since the County began using stair chairs two years ago, not one EMS employee has received a back injury while using the equipment," Hodge said. "Prior to the implementation of the stair chairs, EMS employees were challenged daily to lift patients down flights of stairs, which in historic buildings and homes, are often narrow and sometimes uneven."

2007 Sustained Excellence in Risk Management Award

The 2007 Sustained Excellence in Risk Management Award was given to Charleston County for its continued strain injury reduction campaign initiative, which was introduced by the Safety and Risk Management Department. Charleston County also received this award for achieving the lowest number of on-the-job injuries since joining the South Carolina Counties Workers Compensation Trust in 1991.

The year 2007, marked the third consecutive year that the County experienced a reduced number of on-the-job injuries, which has been a major factor in reducing its workers compensation insurance costs. "This accomplishment is projected to save $400,000 in workers compensation insurance costs for next year's County budget," Hodge said.

2007 Service Award

The 2007 Service Award was given to Charleston County's Safety and Risk Management Department for assisting other South Carolina counties with their safety and risk management concerns. The award was also given for the department's oversight during Habitat for Humanity's Women Build Week. The department helped keep the County's female employees safe as they volunteered to build homes for citizens in need.

"During the past two years of participating in the Habitat for Humanity homebuilding projects, not one Charleston County employee has been injured while working on these home building projects," Hodge said. "We were present at the build site, but we also trained our employees in advance so they can safely work electrical equipment and other tools needed for the job."

The Safety and Risk Management Department also assisted during the Palmetto Police Motorcycle Skills Competition, which was sponsored by the Charleston County Sheriff's Office. "This was the second consecutive motorcycle skills competition hosted in Charleston, and again we saw no injuries, thanks to the excellent pre-planning and on-site management of this event by the Sheriff's Office and Safety and Risk Management staff," Hodge said. Safety is one of Charleston County's core values: "Shared accountability for the safety

(Continued)

of risk an organization retains. Among the considerations is the amount of cash needed to keep in reserve for self-funding the risk. Sometimes not providing a certain level of service is better option. Regardless, a well-thought-out decision is an important part of the process.

SELECTING THE BEST RISK MANAGEMENT TECHNIQUES

When selecting a risk management technique, you need to take into account a number of considerations. The first is the cost-benefit analysis, during which three points should be considered:

- The frequency and severity projections of expected losses for your organization
- For each feasible combination of risk management measures, a forecast of the expected effect on the frequency, severity, and punctuality of the projected losses
- A projection of costs involved in applying the various measures; for example, the cost of insurance premiums or loss prevention devices

Nonfinancial considerations must be taken into account as well, such as what the ethical implication of the decision might be.

The minimum expected cost method also must be considered. In other words, what is the impact to the service if a loss occurs? It may still be possible to provide services if the station burns to the ground, but a unit being totaled in a collision may have a dramatic impact on the services provided. This is especially true if the service has only one unit.

The next step is to prioritize or rank the areas that need to be addressed. As a rule, the risks with the highest frequency and highest severity will be addressed first with the outcomes less likely to occur following. Prioritizing risk is accomplished by determining the potential outcome based on three factors: *severity* (the expected severity of an incident that could occur), *probability* (the chances that given an exposure to a hazard an accident will result), and *exposure* (the exposure to the hazard). When determining the risk for a given hazard, the following formula may be utilized:

$$\text{Total Risk} = (S)\text{everity} \times (P)\text{robability} \times (E)\text{xposure}$$

When prioritizing risk, the first step is to identify the hazard. When identifying the hazard, it is important to state what the hazard is and what the result could be. Tables 5.3 through 5.6 will provide a value and a recommended action for that value.

TABLE 5.3 ■ Risk Analysis Value: Severity (S)

Incident Severity (S)

0 No potential for damage or injury
1 Slight < 5%, no lost time
2 Minimal 5% to 24%, lost time, no hospitalization
3 Significant 25% to 50%, requires care
4 Major 50% to 74%, permanent injury
5 Catastrophic >74%, fatalities

TABLE 5.4 ■ Risk Analysis Value: Probability (P)

Incident Probability (P)

0 Impossible incident
1 Remote or unlikely under any conditions
2 Unlikely under normal conditions
3 P = 50 (probability 50%) under normal conditions
4 P > 50 (probability greater than 50%) for occurrence
5 Very likely to happen

TABLE 5.5 ■ Risk Analysis Value: Exposure (E)

Incident Exposure (E)

0 No exposure
1 Below average amount of exposure
2 Average exposure
3 Above average exposure
4 Great exposure

TABLE 5.6 ■ Recommended Actions

$Risk = S \times P \times E$

Values	Risk Level	Action
80–100	Very high	Stop
60–79	High immediate	Correct
40–59	Substantial	Correction required
20–39	Significant	Possible attention needed
1–19	Slight	Possibly acceptable
0	None	None

IMPLEMENTING THE TECHNIQUES

After you consider all possibilities, the next step is to implement the decision. As with most plans, you must monitor the decision and alter the program to meet the needs of the organization. Organizations change on a regular basis, and so must risk management plans and techniques.

Insurance as a Risk Management Technique

As discussed previously, risk can be transferred in many ways. By paying a rate otherwise referred to as the premium, insurance is one way to transfer the cost of the risk to another party, but not all loss exposures are insurable. The ideal characteristics of an insurable exposure include the following:

- The exposure involves **pure risk** rather than **speculative risk**.
- Uncertainty exists as to the time or probability of loss.
- The occurrence, time of the occurrence, and amount of an insured's loss can typically be determined.
- A large number of exposures are insured.
- A loss will not simultaneously affect many insureds.
- Insurance is economically feasible.

Insurance applies to only pure risks. The difference between pure risks and speculative risks can be defined as follows: *Pure risk* presents only two possible outcomes: financial loss or no financial loss. The result is either undesirable (loss) or neutral (no loss), but it is not beneficial in any case. In contrast, a *speculative risk* may have three potential outcomes: a financial loss, no financial loss, or financial gain. An example of speculative risk is the stock market. A purchase is made in hopes that the stock will go up; however, there may be no financial gain or, in some instances, a financial loss.

Financial management historically has not been considered by EMS organizations.

It is common in commercial business management and can provide a positive influence on EMS organizations. In today's economic environment, it is even more critical to take financial management into consideration. This is accomplished by comparing the cost to the benefit. In other words, is it fiscally prudent to continue to provide the level of service based on the benefit of the service to the patient?

Many EMS organizations may see a financial loss due to lack of business (Figure 5.5). That is because there is no way an EMS agency can predict how many individuals will become ill or get injured. The service must be available 24/7 with no certainty about the number of requests. This is a speculative risk. However, whether or not the vehicle responding reaches the patient and returns without an incident is a pure risk. There is no gain should the vehicle be in a mishap, but it is a necessary tool of the business.

Essentially, insurance is a means to cover unexpected events that cannot be predicted based on the probability of an occurrence or the time the event may occur. If the probability of the loss or the time of the loss can be predicted, then insurance is not necessary. So, probability or time of loss are two areas that need to be determined.

Determining control measures is based on the results found in risk potential and the prioritizing of the steps in the risk management flowchart (Figure 5.2). Control measures must be determined prior to implementation, so the cost and associated benefits may be considered. You should consider a number of factors when determining control measures.

> *Predicted effect.* What effect will occur when considered in conjunction with the cost to implement the control?
>
> *Time.* This is the time it would take to implement the control measure. Could the resources used to control the risk be used more efficiently

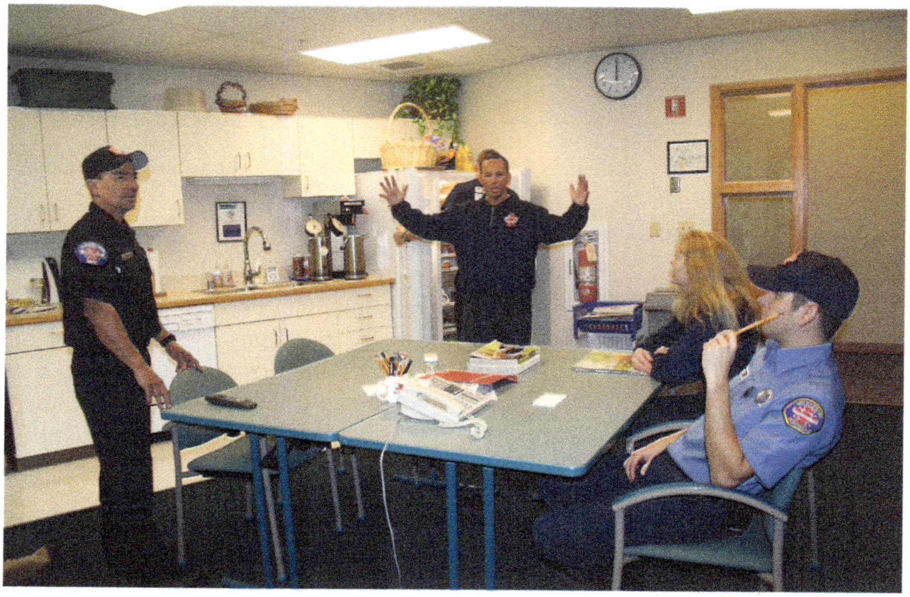

FIGURE 5.5 ■ EMS organizations can see a financial loss due to lack of business. *Courtesy of 24-7 EMS®, a member of the HSI family of brands.*

and effectively during the implementation time period? Will any other efforts be compromised?

Time to results. What is the time period between the implementation of a control and the actual results from implementation? If the control measure is a long-term goal, then this should be clearly expressed in the proposal for the control.

Effort. What is the ease or difficulty with which a control measure is implemented? Can the effort be better applied to other programs? Are there multiple solutions? Will less effort be required for one solution than another? The personnel that a risk affects the most should be involved in decision making when more efficient ways to control a risk are addressed.

Implementation cost. What is the actual cost of implementation? What is the cost should the implementation not occur? Cost is often the deciding factor regarding whether a measure is implemented or rejected. The cost for implementing a control measure always will affect the priority of the implementation.

Insurance cost. Does implementing the control measure reduce or increase the insurance cost? Estimating potential losses are how insurance costs are established. The costs are generally derived from reviewing losses in a generic sense from a common industry as well as from reviewing customer-specific losses.

Funding. Funding for risk management can be expressed in two categories: **risk retention** and **risk transfer**. Risk retention is dependent on internal funding, such as budgeted operating expenses, reserve funds for losses, and borrowing funds to pay for unanticipated losses. Risk transfer includes commercial insurance purchase and indemnity clauses.

Cost-benefit analysis. This is the process by which risks are prioritized through some type of ranking system. A cost-benefit analysis almost always deals with the safety and health of personnel. However, if the implementation costs use real dollars, then a balance sheet will have to be prepared that outlines the cost of the implementation and prospective savings from the implementation.

Risk control can be placed in three categories: administrative, engineering, and personnel protection. See Table 5.7, which assists in defining the risk control categories.

Essentially, the methods of risk control include risk avoidance, risk reduction, and risk transfer. Risk control should be completed only after all risks of an operation have been identified. Note that risks during emergencies cannot be completely controlled; however, the severity of those risks can be addressed and minimized.

TABLE 5.7 ■ Risk Control Categories

Controls	Comprised of	Intentions
Administrative	Guidelines, policies, and procedures to limit, reduce, or eliminate losses.	Make the task safe for the worker.
	Examples: SOP, training requirements, safe work practices, and regulations and standards.	
Engineering	Engineered systems that remove or limit hazards.	Make the task safe for the worker.
	Examples: apparatus design and mechanical ventilation.	
Personnel Protection	Equipment, clothing, and devices designed to protect the worker.	Make the worker safe form the hazards.
	Examples: helmets, gloves, SCBA, and tools.	

Risk avoidance is the complete elimination of a particular risk in order to prevent an undesirable event from occurring. An example of this is avoiding an area with unstable roadways, which would eliminate any potential risk. It is a good practice to avoid risk whenever possible. EMS personnel can do so in many situations, even though EMS is a high-risk job. For example, instead of EMS crews blindly bolting into the scene of an unknown emergency to search for ill or injured patients, they can stop, size-up the scene for potential dangers, and, call for the assistance of, if available, law enforcement to secure the scene before they enter. This is an example of risk avoidance.

You can accomplish risk reduction by testing, planning, training, and enforcement of safety and risk-management-related issues. The reevaluation of risk management programs and a proactive approach are essential to reducing risk.

Risk transfer is the final means of mitigating risk potential. The concept of risk transfer is the complete removal of a risk by transferring it to a separate party. Risk transfer can be used for any real hazards or for financial risk. An example of risk transfer for a real hazard would be if an EMS organization decided that a procedure was too dangerous to complete and an outside contractor was hired to complete the task, thereby transferring and eliminating the potential risk. An example of risk transfer for a financial risk would be the purchase of insurance for equipment, thereby alleviating the financial risk. It should be understood that financial risk transfer does not eliminate or reduce the risk; it simply offers compensation should a loss occur.

MONITORING THE PROGRAM

For a risk management program to be truly effective, evaluation and revision are necessities. The intention of a risk management program is improvement of problem areas. Evaluation should mirror the points that were identified previously in risk identification, with some type of follow-up to determine if the desired outcome was achieved.

LOSS CONTROL

Loss control for EMS is a rather new idea. For years, loss control was a concept that was fairly exclusive to the insurance and commercial industries. With an openly litigious society and the increasing need to operate EMS services as a business, loss control has become an invaluable tool to be used by all services.

An effective and proactive loss control program is essential for maintaining and improving a company's financial success, customer service, management, personnel morale, and equipment serviceability. Loss control encompasses all management activities directed at the prevention, reduction, or elimination of the pure risks of business. It can be described as the concept by which an organization deters loss from occurring. It can be accomplished by means of evaluation of the workplace environment, job performance, practices, and coordinated efforts to reduce lost work hours, property, and inventory.

Loss control is a program whereby the organization initiates measures that control the loss. Once the loss occurs, the organization must ensure the losses do not go out of control. An example of loss control involves a responder who hurts his back. The organization sends the responder to the designated panel physician, who is familiar with the organization and able to return the injured person back to work in 2 days on modified duty (Figure 5.6). Compare that example to one in which the organization does not identify a panel physician. That individual is allowed to choose his own doctor, who takes him off work for 6 weeks. The control of the

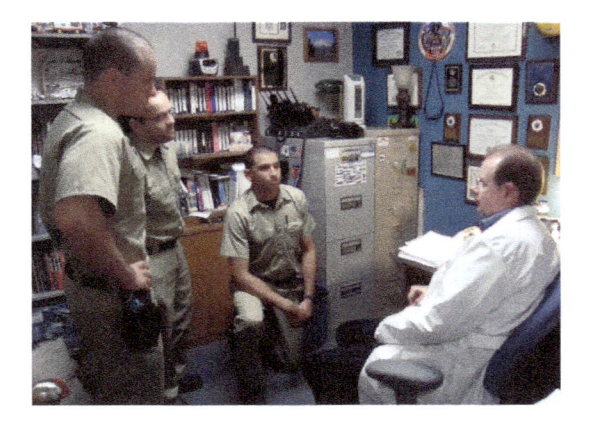

FIGURE 5.6 ■ Find a physician who understands the job of an EMS professional in order to provide the most appropriate care and to get him back to active duty as soon as possible. *Courtesy of Jeffrey T. Lindsey, Ph.D.*

TABLE 5.8 ■ Examples of Hidden Costs

- Time lost from work by injured
- Lost time by other workers
- Lost time by supervisor
- Hiring costs
- Overtime costs
- Overhead cost while work is disrupted
- Loss of earning power
- Loss of efficiency
- Loss of public confidence
- Training costs
- Clerical time
- Damage to tools and equipment

financial loss is gone. Loss control is about managing the loss that has occurred. The overall strategy comes down to four elements:

- Risk management—identification and prevention
- Risk control—decision making and elimination
- Loss control—control of loss that has occurred
- Loss management—getting the organization back to the original state

FINANCE

Although insurance carriers cover the costs of incidents and injuries, a multitude of hidden costs are incurred by the EMS organization. Hidden costs are those costs that are not covered by the insurance carrier. A conservative means by which to determine hidden costs to the EMS organization is to figure that the hidden cost is at least equal to the total paid for the incident or injury by the insurance carrier. Examples of hidden costs are listed in Table 5.8.

In order for an EMS organization to recover from the financial burden created by an unintentional injury, it must increase revenue by an equal amount. The payment of hidden costs typically comes from an EMS organization's operational budget. With the funds being used to cover hidden costs, the money is no longer available for other expenses such as payroll, new equipment, and other expenses.

CUSTOMER SERVICE

Relating customer service to loss control may be a new idea to some, but taken in the context that crashes, injuries, and other losses directly impact performance, attention to customer service is an essential part of loss control.

To explain further, customer service is linked to loss control by being a tool that is used in attracting and maintaining customers. An EMS service operates essentially in a glass house and is usually under constant public scrutiny. With this being the case, the general public, contractors, and other services will not view a service as reliable or able to provide quality care if the service displays a poor image by not having vehicles that are appropriately maintained or involved in vehicle crashes. The success of an EMS organization is directly linked to the confidence the public has in the ability to deliver quality care.

LEADERSHIP AND SUPERVISION

Ineffective management can contribute to accidents, just as effective management can contribute to an accident-free workplace. To be most effective, managers must model the behaviors and attitudes they expect in personnel. If EMS personnel see management taking dangerous shortcuts or engaging in other risky behaviors, they may do so as well, creating an environment that will lead to injuries. The converse also is true. When EMS personnel see management actively participating in safety and loss control, personnel are more likely to strive to maintain the same high standards.

Proper training and education are essential for all management and supervisory personnel. To effectively administer safety and loss control, management and supervisory personnel must become resident experts in the EMS organization's safety standards, loss control programs, and safety programs. If an organization does not have such standards or programs, it must commence to implement them and demonstrate to personnel the commitment to safety and loss control.

SAFETY AND PREVENTION

Safety and prevention are utilized in conjunction with a loss control program. Although there are several similarities in the programs, each has its own characteristics and purpose. Whereas loss control deals mostly with the management aspect of controlling company losses, a safety/prevention program deals with the actual performance of work. For a safety program to be effective, safety concerns must be identified.

Key issues essential for the implementation and management of a safety/prevention program include safety inspections, legal responsibility, acceptance of risk, and consensus standards.

SAFETY INSPECTIONS

Safety inspections can be separated into two categories: informal and formal. Informal inspections should be performed daily by personnel, supervisors, and management under the principle that all personnel have some responsibility for safety. These types of informal inspections are observed through personnel's routine job functions. Should personnel observe an unsafe condition or act, it should be reported immediately to a supervisor or someone else who has safety responsibilities and administrative authority.

Formal inspections are planned events and generally are conducted by the safety/risk manager. These inspections are calculated and typically are conducted with a checklist. Formal inspections also provide the opportunity to review previously identified safety concerns and determine the effectiveness of any corrections.

Standard Operating Procedures

Standard operating procedures (SOP) provide descriptions of specific job functions. SOPs are formal written guides that identify personnel by job title and describe various job functions, the sequence of functions, and steps by which these functions are carried out. The usual format of an SOP is a standardized company tool that outlines routine and nonroutine tasks. SOPs serve not only as tools for training, but also to ensure that a specific procedure is carried out in an approved manner. SOPs should be considered for use in the following situations:

- Repetitive procedures that must be performed the same way each time
- Critically important procedures that must be performed by following detailed, step-by-step instructions
- Standardization of procedures to ensure quality control

Reporting Policy

An effective reporting policy is essential and supplies the very best means of disseminating hazard information. EMS personnel work daily with equipment and in various situations. They know and understand potential risks associated with work performance. For a reporting policy to be successful, it should be simple because people are less likely to report an issue in a complicated format. The policy should provide for direct feedback to EMS personnel and include company notifications should a policy or procedural change occur. In addition, a mechanism should be in place for personnel to provide feedback to management about policy and program performance. The way in which feedback occurs should be anonymous and accomplished in a nonthreatening manner. Management should show support for the reporting policy through its active role in the reporting policy program.

Safety Committee

Safety committees are an important part of a safety and health program. When a company decides to establish a safety committee, representatives from management as well as supervisory and field workers should be considered. The committee's goal should be a proactive approach to safety and prevention by reviewing existing company safety policy and procedures, and developing and revising new policies should deficiencies be discovered. The committee should routinely make the meetings productive by having a clear agenda and the authority to enact changes that are recommended. Additional benefits of a safety committee are that the committee will serve as a platform for personnel to see efforts come to fruition. The company will receive both cost savings through a decrease in accidents and injuries and potential cost reductions in workers' compensation insurance rates should the committee become certified through the state.

LEGAL RESPONSIBILITY

An organization is held legally responsible for any acts or omissions that result in harm to individuals, property, or the environment. Organizations also are expected to perform in a responsible manner. They never should expose the public or individuals to an unreasonable risk. This principle could apply to a wide variety of areas, including but not limited to physical injury, fatality, public or private property damage, environmental damage, revenue impact on an organization or individual, damage to a reputation, and malpractice.

Organizations are legally responsible to provide a safe and healthy workplace for all personnel. Occupational Safety and Health (OSHA, a federal agency) laws and regulations define an employer's minimum responsibility in providing a reasonably safe and healthy workplace; this includes volunteer organizations. As stated previously, some inherent risk will always be involved in the performance of emergency medical duties. The nature of the work places EMS personnel into and forces them to deal with situations that are unplanned and many times uncontrolled.

Even though the risk involved in some emergency situations may not be foreseen and certainly may be beyond a responder's control, the types of risk generally are predictable. The anticipated risks should be planned for and steps taken to mitigate or minimize those risks, and all work should be conducted as safely as reasonably possible.

It should be noted that the preceding information only applies to emergency situations. The responsibility to provide a reasonably safe and healthy workplace applies to EMS organizations, when personnel are working at a location that is routinely under the control of the organization.

Documentation is a critical step when dealing with the legalities of risk management.

Documentation of all patient contacts is essential from medical and legal standpoints. Other essential documentation includes training, such as training on local regulations, applicable standards, and protocols, as well as certification and recertification.

ACCEPTANCE OF RISK

EMS practitioners knowingly accept an increased risk of accidents, injuries, and sometimes fatalities. EMS practitioners as well as other emergency services providers knowingly work in an environment with elevated risk (Figure 5.7). There may be some concern regarding an EMS practitioner bringing suit against either an EMS organization or an individual for injury or death resulting from an emergency.

Legal precedent protects organizations from negligence suits brought by emergency service workers. The reasoning behind these precedents is that the emergency worker was aware of the risk and knowingly accepted those risks. However, those precedents do not relieve the EMS organization of reasonable protective measures regarding risk and safe performance of duties.

CONSENSUS STANDARDS

Standards governing EMS are issued from multiple organizations. These organizations include OSHA and the National Fire Protection Association (NFPA). The differences between those organizations are that in many states OSHA has legal authority to fine and in some instances to close an organization for

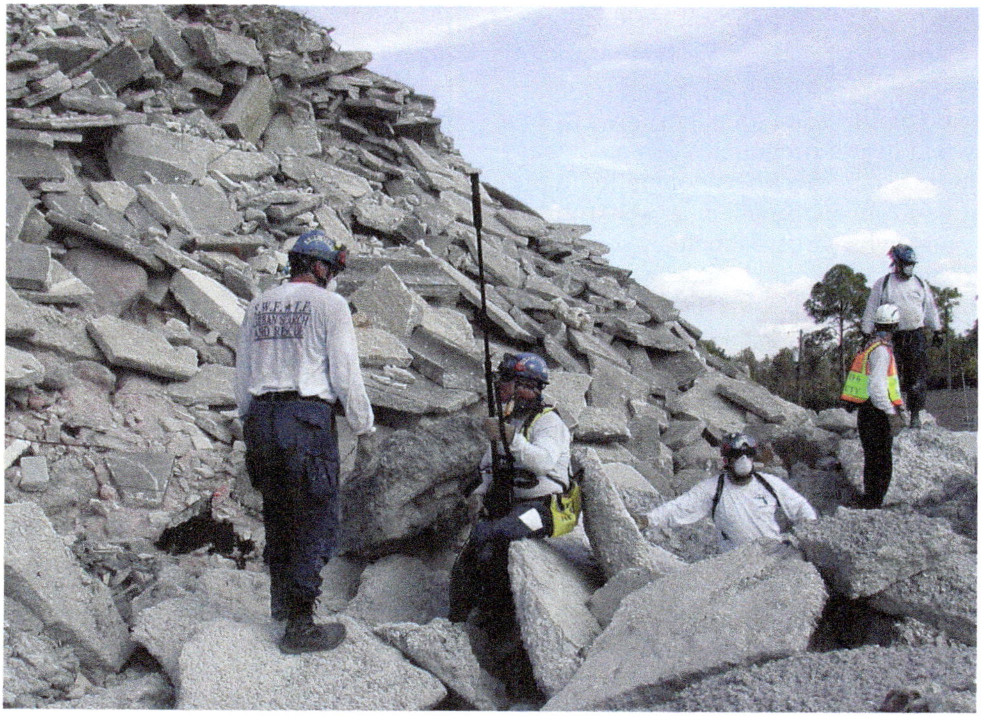

FIGURE 5.7 ■ EMS personnel work in high-risk areas. *Courtesy of Estero Fire Rescue.*

safety violations, whereas NFPA develops best practices recommendations. However, from a legal standpoint both are accepted industry standards and are viewed as such should any type of legal action be taken either for or against an organization or individual.

Having well understood and practiced policies and standard operating guidelines that coincide with accepted industry standards is a sound practice in maintaining adherence to consensus standards. Maintaining close adherence to accepted standards will assist in ensuring that the organization will be protected from fines and other legal action for failure to exercise appropriate risk management practices.

CHAPTER REVIEW

Summary

Risk management is not new, but it has not been embraced by EMS organizations to a level that would lead to a benefit. This chapter has provided a look at risk management and how to implement a risk management program in your EMS organization. EMS personnel work in an inherently dangerous environment. This does not mean there are not ways to reduce the potential liability related to working in this environment. EMS will never avoid or eliminate the entire risk, but managers can take a proactive approach to help reduce the risk.

WHAT WOULD YOU DO? Reflection

You have used the prioritization formula to do your calculations. You are now ready to report to the equipment committee. The report to equipment committee on high-risk neonate transports looks like this:

Severity: What is the expected severity of an incident that could occur? *Probability:* What are the chances that given an exposure to a hazard an accident will result?

Exposure: What is the exposure to the hazard?

Total Risk = (S)everity × (P)robability × (E)xposure

Risk Analysis Values

Incident Severity (S)
5, catastrophic > 74% fatalities. High-risk neonate transports have a high potential for deaths.

Incident Probability (P)
3, P = 50 (probability 50%) under normal conditions. Research shows a 50/50 likelihood of an incident happening.

Incident Exposure (E)
3, above average exposure. After speaking to our insurance risk manager, it is determined we have an above-average exposure. Training, equipment, and protocols are critical.

Risk = S × P × E
Risk = 5 × 3 × 3
Risk = 45

Values Risk Level Action
40–59, Substantial. We are subjecting ourselves to substantial risk and need to consider the value of providing this service.

Review Questions

1. What are three interrelated concepts that are used in determining risk?
2. Describe the typical responsibilities of a risk manager in an EMS organization.
3. Diagram the risk management process.
4. What are some of the areas of consideration when examining the feasibility of alternative risk management techniques?
5. Select a topic to do a risk evaluation for your organization. Put together a risk evaluation in the format of a report. Be sure to answer the appropriate questions.
6. Complete the following table:

Controls	Comprised of	Intentions
Administrative		
		Make the task safe for the worker.
	Equipment, clothing, and devices designed to protect the worker, such as helmets, gloves, SCBA, and tools.	

7. What are some of the ideal characteristics of an insurable exposure?
8. Cite several examples of hidden costs.

References

Pennsylvania Emergency Health Services Council. (2004, April). *Emergency Medical Services Risk Management Resource Guide: An Adjunct to an EMS Safety Program.* Harrisburg, PA: Pennsylvania Department of Health. (See the organization website.)

FEMA, U.S. Fire Administration. (1994). "Incident Safety Officer (Revised) (F729). Washington, DC: Author. (See the organization website.)

International Association of Fire Fighters. (n.d.). *EMS Safety: Techniques and Applications.* FA-144. Emmitsburg, MD: U.S. Fire Administration. (See the organization website.)

Mitterer, D., and R. Patrick., (n.d.). "Risk Management for EMS and the Ambulance Transport Industry." York, PA: VFIS.

U.S. Fire Administration. (1996, December). "Risk Management Practices in the Fire Service. FA-166." (See the organization website.)

Key Terms

exposure An act of subjecting or an instance of being subjected to an action or an influence on a hazard.

goals Benchmarks that are established to affect a certain outcome.

objectives The means by which a goal is obtained, by establishing plans that support the completion of the goal.

probability The chances that, given an exposure to a hazard, an accident will result.

pure risk Refers to only two possible outcomes: financial loss or no financial loss.

relative risk Risks that are judged by specific undesirable events along a broad scale of undesirability.

risk The possibility of meeting danger or suffering harm or loss; exposure to harm or loss.

risk avoidance The complete elimination of a particular risk in order to prevent an undesirable event from occurring.

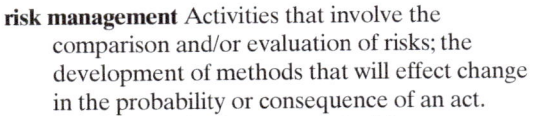

risk management Activities that involve the comparison and/or evaluation of risks; the development of methods that will effect change in the probability or consequence of an act.

risk manager Typically, personnel with responsibility for handling relations with outside agencies such as insurance companies.

risk retention Accomplished by testing, planning, training, and enforcement of safety and risk management-related issues.

risk transfer A means of mitigating risk potential.

severity The degree of harshness or seriousness of an incident.

speculative risk A type of risk in which there may be a financial loss, no financial loss, or financial gain.

CHAPTER 6: Vehicle Driving and Fleet Maintenance

Objectives

After reading this chapter, the student should be able to:

6.1 Identify and assess safety needs for both emergency and nonemergency situations.
6.2 Identify and analyze the major causes involved in line-of-duty deaths related to vehicle operations.
6.3 Discuss the process of selecting and training an emergency vehicle driver.
6.4 Describe the proper format to conduct a vehicle inspection check.
6.5 Discuss the importance of vehicle maintenance as it pertains to safety.

Overview

This title on EMS safety and risk management has been written to assist EMS providers in the reduction of line-of-duty injuries, illnesses, and fatalities. It provides a framework for developing programs that will create an appropriate margin of health and safety for providers during the performance of EMS duties.

Key Terms

acquired abilities
crisis maintenance
driver proficiency
driver selection
driver training
emergency vehicle technicians (EVTs)
full check inspection
human aspects
personnel records
preventive maintenance
quick check inspection
routine maintenance
scheduled maintenance
vehicle characteristics

WHAT WOULD YOU DO?

The training officer is preparing to post a notice for new drivers. She approaches you to find out what safety factors you think should be taken into consideration. The organization has never had a formal process to qualify drivers to drive the ambulances. In the past all that was needed to qualify as an ambulance driver was a valid driver's license and the training captain riding around town with the person to ensure good driving habits. There have been an increase in accidents in your organization, and now the chief wants a formal program. The training officer asks you to tell her.

Questions

1. What qualifications the driver should possess?
2. What type of training should the driver go through that demonstrates a safe approach to driving?
3. Should the safety officer serve on the selection committee?
4. What other issues should she consider?

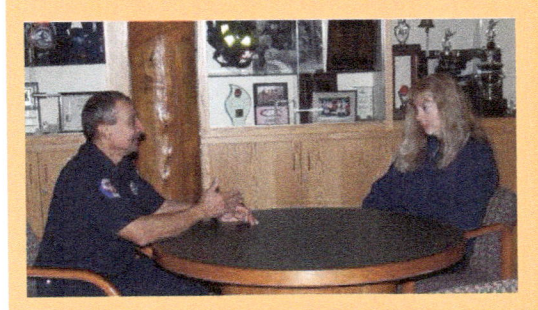

Safety officers should be an integral part of the driver selection process. *Courtesy of 24-7 EMS®, a member of the HSI family of brands.*

INTRODUCTION

Department commitment to driver competency and accountability can have a profound effect on reducing crashes, injuries, and fatalities. Through attitude and behavior, EMS safety officers must reflect the importance of safety in all aspects of dealing with emergency vehicles, the agency's vehicle fleet, and all organizational policies and training. This chapter will cover the selection of emergency vehicle drivers, including the training essential to prepare them and to maintain their driving proficiency, and it will conclude with a look at the importance of vehicle maintenance.

CRASH INJURY AND FATALITIES

Ambulance crashes have received some attention in EMS and other trade media, but few peer-reviewed analytical accounts exist.

THE RESEARCH

The peer-reviewed studies pertinent to this topic include the following studies.

A study by Auerbach, Morris, Phillips, Redlinger, and Vaughn (1987) analyzed a very small sample of ambulance crashes in Tennessee. Notably, despite their known effectiveness in reducing injury and death, only about half of the vehicle drivers and front-seat occupants were wearing occupant restraints; over half of the patients lying prone on a stretcher were restrained, whereas only 15% of bench-seat occupants were wearing restraints. Almost all rear-compartment occupants sitting in the jump seat were wearing restraints.

A study conducted by Pirrallo and Swor (1994) examined ambulance crashes in four years of Fatality Analysis Reporting System (FARS) data, and provided an overview of the earlier literature, including a series of sporadic government reports. Few characteristics differentiate fatal ambulance crashes during emergency responses and nonemergency responses.

Biggers, Zachariah, and Pepe (1996) conducted a retrospective study of one year of ambulance crash data from the fire department of Houston, Texas. An important finding from this study was that a driver history of prior EMS vehicle crashes is a key risk factor for future crashes.

A study by Kahn, Pirrallo, and Kuhn (2001) analyzed 1987 to 1997 FARS data, finding that unrestrained rear occupants were most at risk for fatal and/or incapacitating injuries.

In two other studies (Cook Jr., Meador, Buckingham, and Groff, 1991; and Larmon, LeGassick, and Schriger, 1993), field data monitoring restraint use suggests that there is frequent suboptimal use of the standard restraint systems fitted in ambulances for both crew and patients.

A review by Gershon, Vlahov, Kelen, Conrad, and Murphy (1995) conducted on EMS worker injuries focused mostly on injury type rather than injury cause, although motor-vehicle collisions were noted as a source of the most serious EMS worker injuries.

5. Citizenship and respect for law and order (obeying traffic ordinances)
6. Spirituality (subtle connectedness among traffic users)
7. Morality and rationality (people's rights in public places)
8. Empathy and sympathy (showing solidarity with other traffic users)
9. National unity and integration (identifying with positive symbols)
10. Creative driving practices (multitasking, recreation, artistic expression)

The studies noted above have shown that there is an underlying problem with ambulance crashes. However, additional research is needed to determine the full extent of the causes of ambulance crashes. The results of the research should drive changes in the ambulance industry. Though EMS continues to see the results of poor ambulance design and lack of safety, few in the industry have made significant strides to change the design of the ambulance.

HUMAN FACTORS

Four categories of human factors contribute to vehicle crashes:

Knowledge. Drivers may lack knowledge of traffic laws, which are the physical laws that govern the vehicle operation, or they may lack awareness of potential dangers.

Skills. Inadequate skills in handling vehicles may be the result of insufficient training, lack of hands-on training, or inexperience.

Ability. The driver may have poor judgment or slow or improper reactions.

Attitude. Failure to obey laws or take proper precautions, improper use of the roads, allowing excitement to lead to impulsive actions, dangerous shortcuts, and irresponsible or reckless behavior all contribute to emergency vehicle crashes and fatalities.

Side Bar

Traffic Psychology

Developed by Dr. Leon James at the University of Hawaii, traffic psychology refers to how a driver learns to modify his own style of conduct in traffic situations and to monitor the impact of the individual's driving behavior on other road users. The benefits of this idea include perfecting character by teaching interpersonal skills that encourage the following:

1. Chivalry (being polite to strangers)
2. Charity (caring for the feelings of other road users)
3. Freedom (self-responsibility)
4. Family values (being nice to your passengers)

Other factors include inattentiveness, failure to concentrate on driving tasks, and the emotional sense of power and urgency that accompanies running the emergency vehicle lights and siren. The latter factor especially can block out reason and prudence and lead to the reckless operation of the emergency vehicle.

A review of the U.S. Fire Administration's "Firefighter Fatalities in the United States" (Fahy, LeBlanc, and Molis, 2008) report suggests that age appears to be a factor not only in fire apparatus crashes but also in ambulance crashes. For example, many of the younger firefighters who enter the emergency services have only 2 to 3 years of normal driving experience. Though the older driver has more experience, he also may have slowed responses. The suggested minimum age of 21 has been established for emergency vehicle drivers. In some cases, the organization's insurance company may suggest this age limit.

Another factor that contributes to emergency vehicle crashes is improper or no background checks of the potential drivers. According to Kahn, Pirallo, and Kuhn (2001), 41% of ambulance drivers involved in fatal accidents had prior citations on their driving records (Figure 6.1).

■ THE SAFE DRIVER

The three most important aspects of emergency driving are personnel, personnel, personnel (Figure 6.2). Without the right personnel, the organization is subject to a variety of issues surrounding the operation of the organization. Selecting and keeping a qualified driver behind the wheel are essential to the safe and efficient operation of the emergency vehicle.

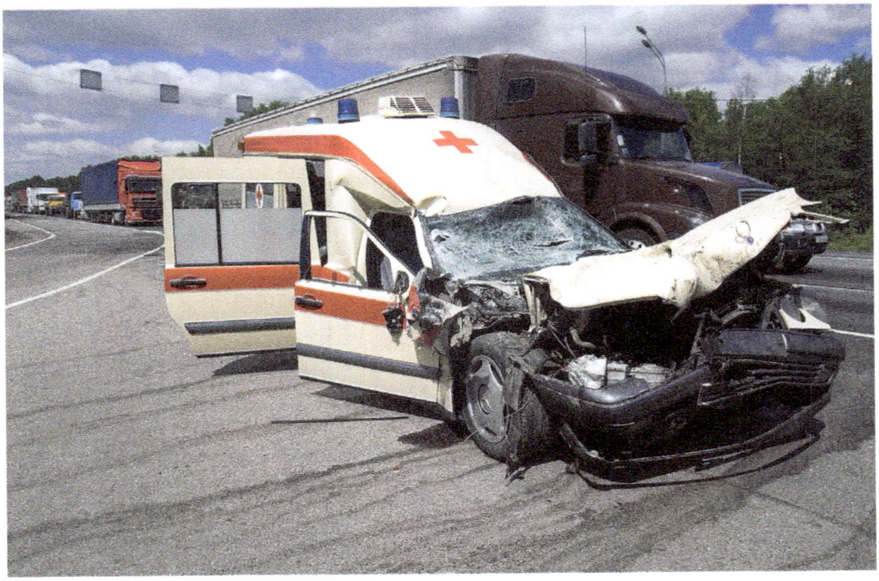

FIGURE 6.1 ■ In 41% of vehicle accidents involving ambulances, ambulance drivers had prior citations.
Source: Fotolia/© Alexander Sayganov.

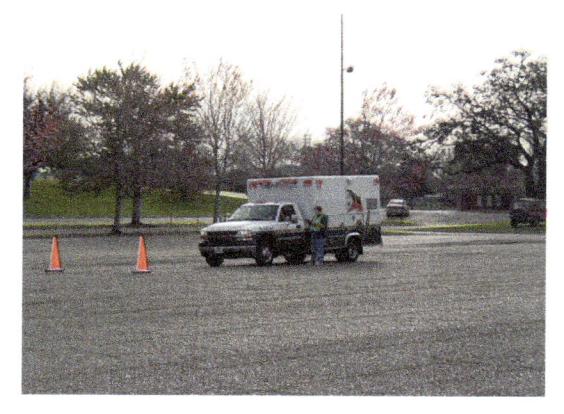

FIGURE 6.2 ■ The EMS safety officer plays an important role in the selection of personnel to drive and operate emergency vehicles. *Courtesy of Jeffrey T. Lindsey, Ph. D.*

In emergency vehicle driving, there are three principles of safe operation: **driver selection**, **driver training**, and **driver proficiency**.

DRIVER SELECTION

A comprehensive approach to the selection of emergency vehicle drivers is the key element to developing and maintaining safe emergency vehicle operations. The four major considerations of such a program are **human aspects**, **acquired abilities**, **vehicle characteristics**, and **personnel records**.

Human Aspects

With appropriate training, human attitudes and activity can be altered. However, human nature is impossible to change. So, to select the best possible candidates for drivers of emergency vehicles, include among your considerations the candidate's driving records, physical fitness, judgment, knowledge, attitude, personal appearance, and hygiene.

It is important to note that an overall evaluation of the human aspects should be done on a continuing basis after a candidate is hired. Close scrutiny of an organization's emergency vehicle drivers is a necessity. Major changes in one or more of the human aspects can occur at any time. Negative changes are usually triggered by a significant emotional event. The degree of impact and the length of time that a negative influence can persist are unique to each individual.

Driving Records. Prior to employment or volunteering, the department should verify driving records by having the applicant sign a consent form to allow the department to check records with the state. The applicant's driving record should be reviewed for the number of moving violations over the past 36 months, any driving under the influence (DUI) convictions, reckless driving citations, and license suspensions. Evaluation of driver education certificates, specialized driving license (such as commercial driver's license [CDL]), and physical qualifications (such as vision and hearing) can help reduce the number of vehicular incidents that occur each year.

Physical Fitness. Consistently good health is vital for all emergency vehicle drivers. Sufficient rest and nutrition, physical fitness, and freedom from controlled substances are essential requirements for emergency vehicle drivers. Therefore, a medical examination performed by a licensed physician should be conducted to determine if someone is physically able to perform the job of driver under all conditions. The medical exam should reveal no medical or physical condition that would prove detrimental to operating an emergency vehicle. The presence of a medical condition alone may not indicate an impaired operator. However, it can identify an area to consider when determining a person's medical fitness to operate an emergency vehicle.

The examination should identify cardiovascular disease' neurological and neurovascular disorders; insulin-dependent diabetes; and rheumatic, arthritic, orthopedic, muscular, neuromuscular, or vascular diseases, which if left untreated or if severe enough could interfere with the ability to control and operate an emergency vehicle. The examination also should identify disqualifying conditions such as those associated with sudden loss of consciousness, as well as mental illness and substance abuse/dependency.

Being physically fit is an important aspect of driving an emergency vehicle. A driver's physical condition will substantially impact his ability to drive competently. Some questions that can be asked when determining physical fitness include these: Do you have trouble looking over your shoulder to change lanes or looking left and right to check traffic at intersections? Do you have trouble moving your foot from the gas to the brake pedal? Do you have trouble turning the steering wheel? Have you fallen down once or more in the previous year—not counting a trip or stumble? Do you walk less than one block per day? Do you have trouble raising your arms above your shoulders? Do you feel pain in your knees, legs, or ankles when going up or down a flight of stairs consisting of ten steps?

Because a variety of motor skills are necessary to accomplish an intended action, the potential candidate's coordination should also be assessed. Drivers must make split-second decisions in reaction to a traffic situation and execute those decisions smoothly. For instance, if a child runs into the road, the driver will have to simultaneously steer and brake (and perhaps clutch and shift gears), while watching for other potential hazards on the road, such as oncoming traffic, bystanders, or parked cars.

Age also must be combined with physical fitness when evaluating an individual as a potential driver of an emergency vehicle. For example, at age 18 an individual usually has only a maximum of 2 years of driving experience. At age 65 or older an individual may have begun to lose certain aspects of his vision or hearing and may have increasing physical limitations.

It should be recognized that age, maturity, and experience, as well as other human aspects, are all different and not necessarily related.

Judgment. Judgment involves the ability to make good decisions. Some qualities that should be considered when evaluating a potential driver's judgment might include these:

Excitability. Does this person get overly excited or agitated in a critical situation?

Maturity. Does the candidate have the ability to keep emotions in check while driving?

Also consider the candidate's ability to make a decision. Is the individual decisive? If yes, does the individual typically assume an offensive or a defensive posture? Many times this is reflected in a personnel file. Excessive aggressiveness may be documented in the form of counseling sessions or disciplinary action.

Knowledge. Knowledge is an individual's clear perception of truth, fact, or a series of issues relating to a specific subject. A potential emergency vehicle driver must not have wrong information or misconceptions about emergency vehicle driving. An emergency vehicle driver's knowledge of the emergency vehicle he operates is vital and must include the vehicle's features and operational characteristics.

Attitude. Attitude is the individual's disposition toward driving and maintenance. Some types of unwanted attitudes that have been identified (Lindsey and Patrick, 2007) include the following:

Immature attitude. This person only cares about his own safety.

> **Side Bar**
>
> **Ambulance Safety**
>
> Dr. Nadine Levick has dedicated much of her time to the research and education of ambulance safety. Dr. Levick is known for her passion in the research of ambulance safety. She has published a number of papers and is currently the only researcher to take an active role in conducting research on ambulance crashworthiness by conducting crash tests on ambulances. Dr. Levick advocates that the research on ambulance design and safety must be in concert with the traffic and automotive engineers who understand the dynamics of vehicles.
>
> Dr. Levick maintains a website (www.objectivesafety.net) that hosts various research projects along with access to the summits on ambulance safety hosted by the Transportation Research Board. Dr. Levick chairs the EMS committee and has been active in the dissemination of ambulance safety through this committee.

Brazen/show-off. This person is more concerned about image than reality.

Laid back. This person is so laid back that reaction time may be hours or days late.

Comic attitude. This person does not panic, but he also does not take dangerous situations seriously.

When selecting drivers, consider the applicant's attitude. Expect the candidate to be mature and appropriate, modest but realistic about his skills, alert and focused on task, and serious about the safety of others as well as his own.

Personal Appearance and Hygiene. A driver's appearance, including his personal hygiene, tells a great deal about his level of professionalism. His bearing should be a credit to the organization and inspire the community's confidence in his ability to handle an emergency. A professional appearance also includes taking all appropriate precautions against the spread of infection—to patients as well as to himself and his crew. If a driver gets sick, he will not be of much use to the organization or to the patient.

Professional appearance relates not only to the person but also to the equipment. Clean, properly stowed equipment makes the task—driving the emergency vehicle and transporting patients—safer and easier, and helps to make the results more positive (Figure 6.3).

DRIVER TRAINING

Not everyone can or should be an emergency vehicle driver. The selection process for an emergency vehicle driver candidate is a critical part of the emergency vehicle driver training program.

Acquired Abilities
Manipulative skills are necessary to coordinate the steering, accelerating, and/or braking functions of maneuvering an emergency vehicle. They are based on a number of driving characteristics, which the driver has acquired from the time he began to drive. These characteristics, good or bad, will be reflected when driving an emergency vehicle. Desirable characteristics need to be reinforced, whereas a concentrated effort must be made to eliminate the bad characteristics.

New Drivers. Driving is a psychomotor skill that requires learning a certain set of skills and then practice, practice, practice until the motions become almost automatic. Although these skills are sometimes called instinctive reactions, they are not. They are learned responses. New emergency vehicle

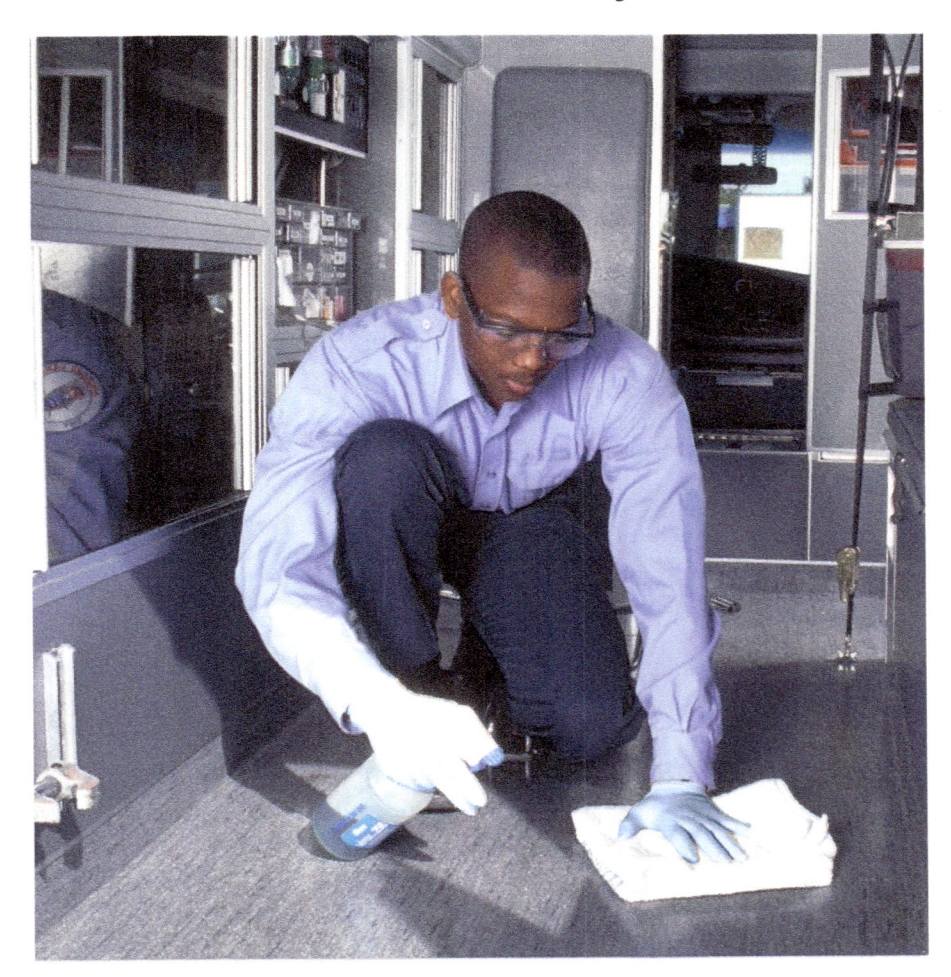

FIGURE 6.3 ■ The rear of the ambulance must be kept clean and orderly.

drivers must split their attention between basic vehicle control (such as steering, braking, and shifting gears) and the attention and concentration needed for the social and decision-making aspects of driving. Inexperienced drivers need to recognize that their ability to react effectively to traffic situations and avoid crashes will be limited until these vehicle-handling skills are mastered.

Defensive Driving. In general, adults have developed driving habits, which can influence their potential to safely and properly operate an emergency vehicle. If poor habits exist, they must be identified and corrected. These routines or mental ruts can cause them to be resistant to change, even when it makes sense to do a familiar task—such as driving—differently. Three culprits—routine, comfort, and confidence—often are at the root of this problem:

> *Routine.* "We've always done it this way" or "There was never any SOP, and the way I do it was never questioned or corrected."

Comfort. "This is the easiest way to get it done in the least amount of time."

Confidence. "I know the way I'm doing it may not be the best or the safest, but this way works. When all else fails, I use the methods that are tried and true."

Training for defensive driving is designed to illustrate that the characteristics of routine, comfort, and confidence can be used to arrive at a safer way of doing things, especially while driving emergency vehicles. An open-minded individual with the correct attitude recognizes that there is nothing wrong with developing and implementing new methods—especially when they still can retain a sense of routine but in a safer manner, a sense of comfort in knowing one is doing something as safely as possible, and a sense of confidence in new methods because they work.

What are the goals of a defensive emergency vehicle driver? One is to maintain the highest level of safety possible. Each driver is responsible for the safety of the citizens served and should be fully dedicated to the safety of fellow providers.

Another goal is to be prepared for unexpected situations and conditions that can adversely affect emergency vehicle operations. These include adverse weather, terrain, road conditions, and mechanical malfunction (Figure 6.4). The emergency vehicle driver must attempt, through learned responses, to limit the possible outcomes by controlling his reactions to these forces.

Finally, an important goal of effective training in defensive driving, and applied practice, is to avoid unnecessary legal consequences occurring as a result of emergency vehicle operations.

Defensive driving is an acquired ability and must be learned over time and constantly reinforced to ensure continued applicability. It includes successfully completing defensive driving training, which introduces and reinforces

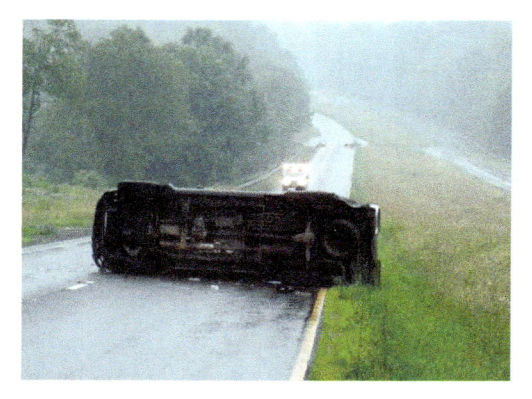

FIGURE 6.4 ■ Adverse weather is common in many areas. *Courtesy of Jeffrey T. Lindsey, Ph.D.*

concepts such as space management, following distance and rate of closure, hazard identification, correct braking techniques, and evasive maneuvers.

Driving Knowledge and Performance. The emergency vehicle driver should pass a written driving test as well as a road test. Those tests should be followed by a period of on-the-job training to evaluate the driver's performance under actual field conditions. Following successful completion of the written test, the driving test, the on-the-job evaluation, and any local requirements, the supervisor should consider the driver a qualified emergency vehicle driver.

Operator Qualifications. In addition to passing the initial driving and medical checks, the driver must maintain an up-to-date and valid driver's license, report any violation he receives when driving his personal vehicle, remain physically and mentally fit, and participate in training when available.

When a driver is first hired or begins to drive voluntarily for an organization, a review of state motor-vehicle records for the previous 3 years should be conducted. This review should check for any speeding, careless or reckless driving, driving under the influence of alcohol or other mind-altering substances, and moving violations.

In addition, many organizations do an annual motor-vehicle record check on all their personnel. The driving record should be checked for any collisions or other driving-related incidents the driver has had in the previous 5 years. The driver's license should be checked to make sure that the individual is licensed and qualified to operate the class of vehicle he must operate in EMS.

Licensing. An emergency vehicle driver with an expired state driver's license is no use to the organization. The driver must remember to renew his license before the expiration date and keep abreast of changes in licensing requirements.

Participation in Training. After the driver has been selected to be an emergency vehicle driver, his most important task is to improve his job performance at every opportunity. Training programs are a part of that experience. Often this is the beginning of several years of training.

Vehicle Characteristics

Driving any type of an emergency vehicle may be a radical change for some people (Figure 6.5). It is even more complicated if the type of vehicle is drastically different from a familiar experience. For instance, an individual placed in an emergency vehicle who has never driven a vehicle weighing over 3,500 pounds will have more to learn than just emergency vehicle driving procedures.

The ability to safely control and maneuver an emergency vehicle is one of the most critical aspects of an operator's responsibilities. While driving, the operator should be in control of the vehicle and take into consideration the vehicle characteristics, capabilities and limita-

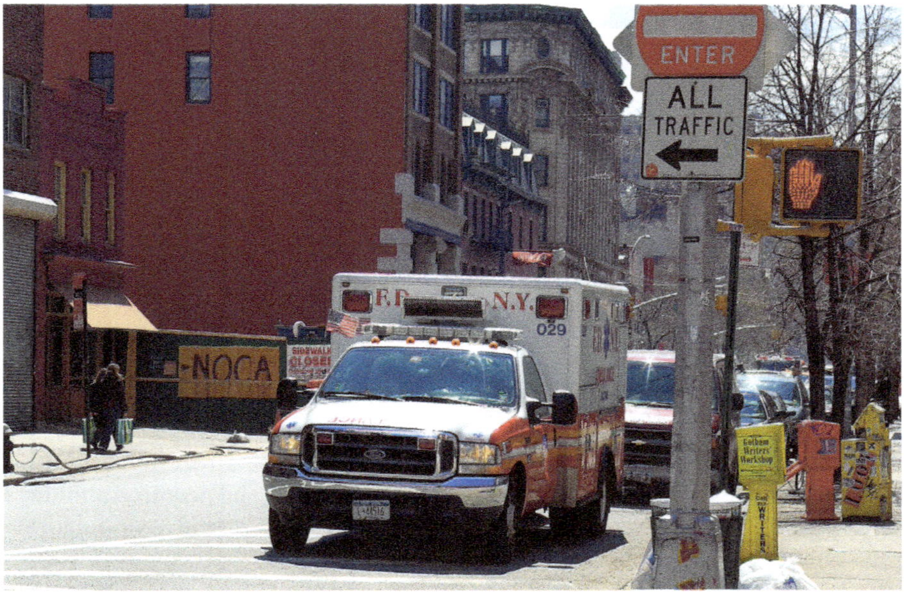

FIGURE 6.5 ■ Driving an ambulance is not like driving your personal car. *Source: Fotolia/Jean-Claude Drillon.*

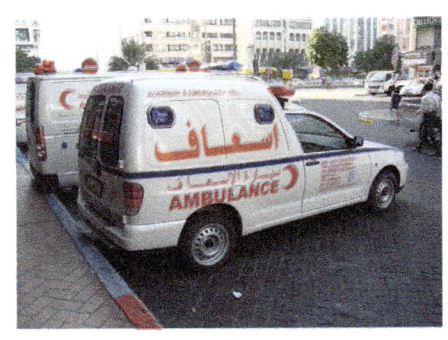

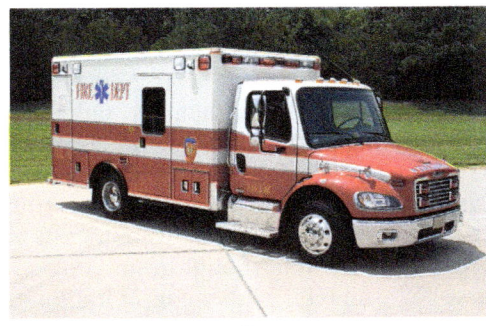

FIGURE 6.6 ■ There are various types and sizes of ambulances. *(a) Courtesy of Jeffrey T. Lindsey, Ph.D. (b) Fotolia/Rodney Earle.*

tions (such as speed, road conditions, auxiliary braking systems, and weight transfer). Operating and controlling the vehicle at a speed from which the vehicle could be safely slowed or stopped could decrease the potential for a skid and loss of control. Based on simple physics and inertia, a top-heavy vehicle is inclined to tip over if the driver turns the wheel suddenly in an effort to bring the wheels back onto the road.

Types of Emergency Vehicles. The type of emergency vehicle can have a significant influence on the amount of training necessary to instill proficiency (Figure 6.6). A new emergency vehicle driver would require more time and training than a driver moving from one type of vehicle to another. It is essential that a driver receives individual training and be proficient in driving a specific emergency vehicle.

Vehicle Components and Features. The introduction of new technologies require a special understanding of the various vehicle components and features, even for emergency vehicle drivers with years of service.

Antilock braking systems (ABS), for example, represent a major technological advance in emergency vehicle operations. Their application to emergency vehicles requires more experienced drivers to become familiar with new and revised driving procedures and habits.

Special Driver Training. Certain types of vehicles require special driver training. An example would be large bus-size vehicles. In recent years, a number of states have added one or more criteria for obtaining the privilege of driving heavy vehicles classified as commercial with laws and statutes pertinent to emergency driving. These laws establish the requirements for operating such vehicles on public highways.

Recordkeeping

Recordkeeping is an essential component of the safety program. In the event of an accident, records will be reviewed to attest to the training and abilities of the individual to ascertain whether or not he was qualified and able to perform the job.

In addition, a record of each individual's human aspects and **acquired abilities** should be compiled and stored in a central location that is convenient and secure for the organization. The personnel file should contain the qualifications of each individual. The information in the

Best Practices

Winter Park Ambulance Safety Design

In order to treat patients effectively, paramedics often are required to ride in the back of an ambulance unrestrained. Due to the location of the equipment and controls in older units, it was impossible to treat patients and remain safely belted. While Winter Park Fire Rescue has not experienced any serious accidents involving their ambulances, their leadership realized this environment was not designed for a safe operation. So when it was time to replace the ambulances in Winter Park, EMS Supervisor Lieutenant/Paramedic Andrew (A.J.) Isaacs led the team who are now being credited for this totally new design.

Lieutenant Isaacs looked at the workspace and performed hours of research to determine what environment would be the safest for our paramedics. It was concluded that to fix the problem, the patient area would need to be redesigned. The ergonomics of an ambulance's patient compartment had not been considered in this way before. That is when Medtec Ambulance Inc. of Goshen, Indiana, stepped up to the plate. Each vehicle now contains a much safer work space for our firefighters where in many cases they can remain seated and secured in a five-point harnessed attendant seat, a true ambulance industry first.

Others are seeing the benefit of Winter Park's safer ambulance design. Firefighters and paramedics from numerous other agencies, as well as the National Institute for Occupational Safety and Health (NIOSH), are extremely interested in incorporating many of these new safety features in their units and recommendations.

Fire Chief Jim White said of the new design, "I am very proud to see the creativity and innovative ideas of our staff come to fruition. We are convinced that the changes incorporated in these vehicles will make the job safer for our firefighters."

The Five-Point Safety Harness is the key to the redesigned Action Safe area. Paramedics can remain restrained and treat a vast majority of patients while en route to local hospitals.

These new ambulances incorporate high intensity reflective markings in a chevron pattern, making the rear of the vehicles more visible to motorists during highway operations. Video monitoring cameras are located to the rear and in the patient compartment to provide the driver/operator an additional field of vision while backing the unit. Keeping the patient compartment cool and comfortable in the hot Florida heat is vital to quality patient care. So these new units have two independent air conditioning systems. The "chassis" system operates independently from the patient compartment air conditioning system which is powered by an on-board hydraulic generator while on the road and by a shore line while in quarters.

During a busy 24-hour shift firefighters can lift more than 15 patients into the rescues. After several different field tests, a decision was made to equip the new units with a power lifting type patient stretcher. The stretcher has a capacity of 700 pounds and reduces the risk to firefighters from having to dead lift patients into the back of the rigs.

Source: Winter Park Fire Department (2008).

---

file can then be used as a means to select an emergency vehicle driver, identify an individual requiring additional training, and alert the organization to one who is in need of recertification.

Training Records. A key component of the personnel file is the training record for each individual. Most companies not only keep track of classes attended, but they also have some type of evaluative system in place so competency and proficiency can be monitored. Typically the training records include the following:

- Classes attended (proficiency not verifiable)
- Classes successfully completed (proficiency at time measured via testing or simulation)
- Certification (proficiency measured and certified by the organization)
- Licensing (proficiency measured and licensed by the agency)

Each individual's personnel file, including drivers and vehicle technicians, becomes a legal document. It can be used either on behalf of the emergency company or against the company. It should be emphasized that the absence of any documentation presents the potential for a high degree of liability and, in the opinion of some legal minds, a greater liability.

The information in the personnel file of an emergency worker should relate to his qualities and capabilities as an emergency vehicle driver. This information should address his physical ability to perform the function of an emergency vehicle driver. It also should address his driving record. This is important for two reasons: First, one's driving record is an indication of whether or not a person has demonstrated respect for motor vehicle operations and laws. Second, the action of researching a driving record serves as a protection for the person who is authorizing the candidate to be an emergency vehicle driver for the emergency company.

Some control measures that should be undertaken to determine the driving record for each potential and existing emergency vehicle driver include these:

- Checking motor vehicle records (MVRs) even before a person can begin training
- Checking MVRs on an ongoing basis, at least annually
- Making a photocopy of each emergency vehicle driver's operator's license and placing it in the driver's personnel file on a yearly basis

The organization must establish standard operating procedures/standard operating guidelines (SOPs/SOGs) to determine if a person's previous offenses prevent him from driving an emergency vehicle.

Suspected Drug and/or Alcohol Abuse.
These issues involve emergency companies just as they do society in general. However, they are particularly important to organizations entrusted with the care and transportation of the public. An EMS agency should have a substance abuse policy that includes the conditions under which an individual can be tested and disciplined if necessary.

One excellent routine for testing for drug and/or alcohol abuse in emergency operations occurs in the event of a vehicular accident: The driver must be tested. The reasoning is that the existence of the accident constitutes "reasonable cause" for the company to require testing. In addition, it provides both the emergency vehicle driver and the company with a defense of no such substance abuse if a plaintiff alleges the possibility of drug or intoxicant use by the emergency vehicle driver.

Drinking should be prohibited for all emergency personnel. Many organizations designate a set amount of time, such as 12 hours before driving an emergency vehicle, during which personnel should not consume any alcoholic beverages. Likewise, neither illegal drug use or abuse of prescription drugs is ever acceptable under any circumstances and should never occur on or off duty.

Driver Training Courses
Training is the foundation of all safe practices (Figure 6.7). The type of course, with or without integration of classroom and applied practice, and instructor qualifications all contribute to the effectiveness of training. For the average emergency vehicle driver, it generally

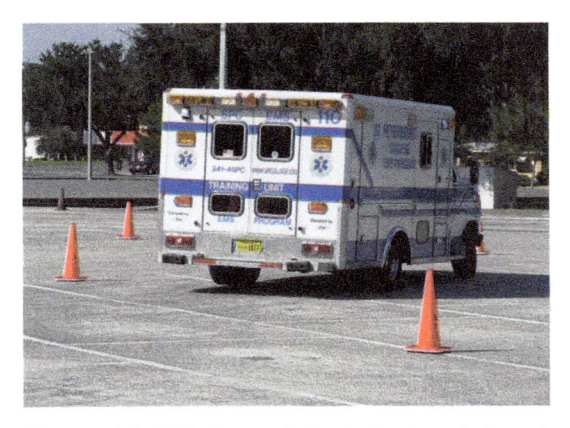

FIGURE 6.7 ■ Driver training is the foundation of reducing the liability of the agency in emergency response. *Courtesy of Fredrick H. Rogers.*

takes 8 to 24 hours of actual behind-the-wheel experience to be able to deal with the basic maneuvering of an emergency vehicle. Note that driver training is not a once-and-done process. Though EMS does not have a formal standard, NFPA standard 1451 delineates that driver training shall be provided for all personnel as often as needed, but no less than twice a year.

There is no real test to measure ability once the emergency vehicle driver is released to drive in an emergency situation, so anyone can fool themselves into believing they are a very good driver simply because they have not been involved in a crash. Emergency vehicle drivers should understand that the job requires a complex set of mental, social, emotional, and physical skills and processes. They must be able to recognize and evaluate their own driving patterns and evaluate problem driving behaviors and attitudes.

Driver training is an important element of preparing the right people to drive an emergency vehicle. A driver must be provided with driver training and education appropriate to the driver's duties.

DRIVER PROFICIENCY

An emergency vehicle driver is expected to be mentally and physically fit for every response. A driver's physical fitness may be affected by his health and the amount of rest he is getting. For example, if the driver has the flu, he may not be at his best and alert; a shoulder injury may affect his ability to maneuver the vehicle; over-the-counter medications may make him sleepy; or lack of sleep can make his response times slower. If a driver is not in good physical condition, it is best not to drive.

Driver Recertification

An individual may have excellent human attributes and acquired abilities at the time of selection. He also may demonstrate proficiency in all the varying components of driving emergency vehicles. But if these skills are not applied at regular intervals, competency decreases. Hence, the need for continual recertification is essential.

Driver recertification should be closely correlated to the characteristics of the organization. For example, if a driver is regularly driving an emergency vehicle under various conditions, recertification may be nothing more than a check ride. On the other hand, if a driver has not driven a specific emergency vehicle in over 6 months or only once in 18 months, recertification may involve a complete retesting on that vehicle.

Development of a recertification program should be based on the following:

- Actual emergency vehicle driving experience
- Observed proficiency and supervisory reports compared to performance in the field
- Length of time since last recertification
- Introduction of new emergency vehicles
- Introduction of new technology on existing emergency vehicles

Although a personalized recertification program can be developed and administered,

Best Practices

Emergency Vehicle Driver Training Programs

VFIS recommends that a formalized written statement be adopted requiring all drivers to successfully complete a driver education and training program. The program should have written objectives to specifically address the critical areas of operation for an emergency vehicle driver. Originations should reference the current applicable standards for vehicle operation (NFPA Standards, AAA Best Practices, and ASTM Standards). In addition, the program should require all emergency vehicle drivers to meet the following minimum education and training qualifications:

1. Sixteen hour driver education and training program.
   a. Eight hours of classroom education. This session should cover topics which include but are not be limited to:
      * Importance of Driver Training
      * Extent of the Problem
      * Personnel Selection
      * SOPs/SOGs
      * Map Reading
      * Vehicle positioning
      * Legal Aspects of Emergency Vehicle Driving
      * Vehicle Dynamics
      * Vehicle Inspections and Maintenance
      * Vehicle Operations/Safety
      * Written Test
   b. Successful completion of a Competency Course. Each driver should spend sufficient time on the competency course to demonstrate proficiency in the operation of a vehicle. The driver should demonstrate competency on each vehicle they operate. Specific tasks that should be measured are:
      * Use of Mirrors
      * Turning
      * Blind Right Side and Rear Positioning
      * Backing
      * Braking and Stopping
      * Depth Perception (front and rear)
      * Height Clearance
      * Proper Communication

   At a minimum, sections IA and IB should be completed by each emergency vehicle driver at least every 5 years.
2. Sufficient hands-on training (actual road driving) to effectively demonstrate handling capabilities of emergency vehicles necessary to perform duties. Additionally, organizations providing EMS transport should conduct training with an on-board patient (simulated or actual). Eight (8) hours minimum.
3. The emergency service organization driver education and training program and procedures should be based upon current recognized safety standards and departmental guidelines as well as manufacturers suggested procedures. Additionally, the utilization of maps and practical testing with maps should be used.
4. Experienced drivers should minimally receive annual (actual driving) retraining and education based upon their actual hands-on emergency vehicle driving activity. The type and length of education and training is to be determined by the chief operating officer. Factors to review include:
   a. Driving record
   b. Personnel file regarding driving related issues
   c. Number of emergency calls driven
   d. Length of service as a driver
   e. Environment driven in (rural, suburban, urban)

CHAPTER 6 *Vehicle Driving and Fleet Maintenance* 121

Best Practices (Continued)

COMPETENCY COURSE

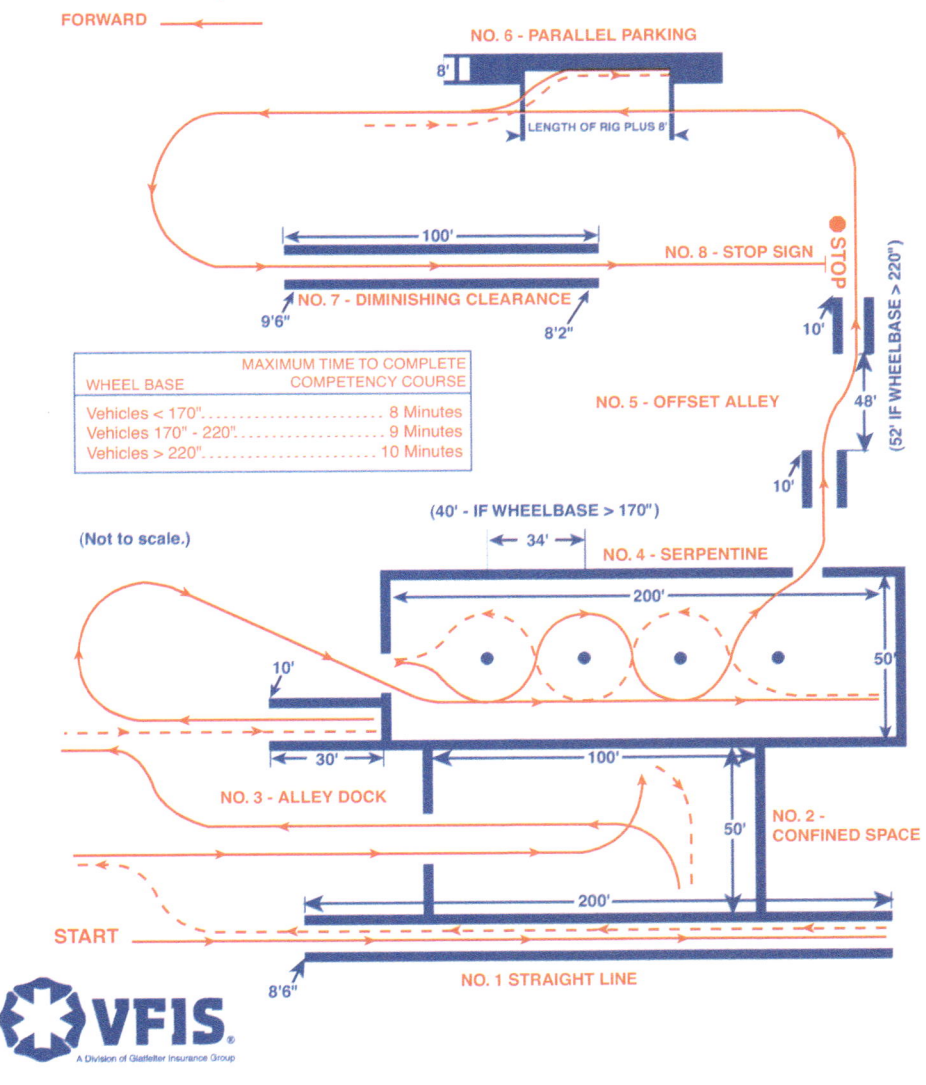

Diagram of a competency driver course. *Reprinted with permission of VFIS.*

(continued)

Best Practices (Continued)

5. Ongoing classroom education should occur at least annually and specifically address relevant safety issues (example: intersections and rollovers, private vehicle use), and review department SOPs/SOGs and new equipment/technology (minimum 4 hours).
6. There should also be a periodic review of the hands on skills of each driver. The frequency can vary dependent on a number of factors which include:
   a. Motor Vehicle Record checks
   b. Number of emergency calls driven
   c. Length of service as a driver
   d. Environment driven in (rural, suburban, urban)
   e. Age
   f. Personal Auto Liability Coverage Verification
7. Driver education and training should also be required for those individuals that are not emergency vehicle drivers (i.e. fire apparatus or ambulances drivers, etc.); but are authorized by the department or state to use red/blue lights on personal vehicles. (It is recommended that the education and training follow, at minimum, sections 1A, 3, and 5.)

Source: Content courtesy of VFIS.

---

it is both difficult and time consuming. As a result, most emergency agencies establish one or more thresholds that automatically dictate recertification. Typically, consider time, such as annually; amount of activity as a driver; observed and documented competency (or lack of); and the introduction of new technology (ABS braking) or vehicles into the organization.

Driver recertification is a vital element in maintaining a valid and professional emergency vehicle driver program. Whether a personalized program or one with established thresholds is adopted, it is important that recertification of all drivers be an integral part of the program.

Shift Work

An emergency vehicle driver's effectiveness is controlled by a number of factors, including fatigue. Both mental and physical fatigue can influence the ability of an emergency vehicle driver. Some examples include a lack of sleep or a sudden awakening from a deep sleep. Although evidence is limited or inferential, chronic predisposing factors and acute situational factors recognized as increasing the risk of drowsy driving and related crashes include the following:

- Sleep loss
- Driving patterns, including driving between midnight and 6:00 a.m.; driving a substantial number of miles each year or a substantial number of hours each day; driving in the midafternoon hours (especially for older persons); and driving for longer times without taking a break
- Use of sedating medications, especially prescribed anxiolytic hypnotics, tricyclic antidepressants, and some antihistamines
- Untreated or unrecognized sleep disorders, especially sleep apnea syndrome (SAS) and narcolepsy. (Canaan, 2000)

Those factors have cumulative effects. A combination of them substantially increases crash risk.

Driver readiness also is affected if the driver is a shift worker. Night-shift workers typically get 1.5 fewer hours of sleep per 24 hours compared with day-shifty workers. The midnight to 8:00 a.m. shift carries the greatest risk of sleep disruption because it requires workers to contradict circadian patterns in order to sleep during the day.

A study of hospital nurses reached the following conclusions. Rotating shifts (working four or more day or evening shifts and four night shifts or more within a month) caused the most severe sleep disruptions of any work schedule. Nurses on rotating schedules reported more accidents (including auto crashes, on-the-job errors, and on-the-job personal injuries due to sleepiness) and more near-miss crashes than did nurses on other schedules (Gold, Rogacz, Bock, Tosteson, Baum, et al., 1992). About 95% of night nurses working 12-hour shifts reported having had an automobile accident or near-miss accident while driving home to and from night work (Novak and Auvil-Novak, 1996).

Hospital interns and residents routinely lose sleep during on-call periods, which may last 24 hours or more. A survey of house staff at a large urban medical school found that respondents averaged 3 hours of sleep during 33-hour on-call shifts, much of which was fragmented by frequent interruptions (Marcus and Loughlin, 1996). About 25% reported that they had been involved in a motor-vehicle crash, 40% of which occurred while driving home from work after an on-call night. Others reported frequently falling asleep at the wheel without crashing, for example, while stopped at a traffic light.

Although this evidence does not demonstrate a conclusive association between shift work and crashes, it is believed that shift workers' increased risk for sleepiness is likely to translate into an increased risk for automobile crashes. Competing demands from family, second jobs, and recreation often restrict the hours available for sleep and further disrupt the sleep schedule.

Shift workers themselves can take steps to reduce the risks of drowsy driving by planning time and creating an environment for uninterrupted, restorative sleep (good sleep hygiene) (Minors and Waterhouse, 1981; Rosa, 1990). Shift workers who completed a 4-month physical training program reported sleeping longer and feeling less fatigued than did matched controls who did not participate in the program. Nurses working the night shift reported using white noise, telephone answering machines, and light-darkening shades to improve the quality and quantity of daytime sleep (Novak and Auvil-Novak 1996). However, individual response to the stresses of shift work varies (Harma, 1993), and the background factors or coping strategies that enable some workers to adapt successfully to this situation are not well defined. The behavioral steps discussed earlier for younger males also seem reasonable for reducing risk in this population.

You must educate those who work shifts. Although many shift workers are not in a position to change or affect their fundamental work situations, they and their families may benefit from information about risks associated with driving and effective countermeasures.

Some ways to maximize the chances of achieving quality sleep during the day include the following:

- Minimize light or wear a sleep mask.
- Use white noise, such as a fan, to block out disruptive noises; turn off the phone; and turn the answering machine volume all the way down.
- Lower room temperature.
- Create an association with sleep by maintaining bedtime routines and using the bedroom for sleep only.
- Post a "Day Sleeper" sign on the door.
- Exercise moderately every day (but not within 3 hours of sleep).
- Do not drink caffeine within 5 hours of bedtime.
- Get the support of family and friends.

The following is a simple truth, according to the National Sleep Foundation (NSF, 2009): The average adult requires 7 to 9 hours of good-quality sleep per night. A few people can sleep less, sometimes as little as 5 hours per night, without a problem. Whatever an individual's actual sleep needs are, regularly overextending oneself is not wise. It will catch up with you eventually.

Acute and chronic illness, chronic pain, irritability, poor judgment, and diminished decision-making abilities are evidence of a sleep-deprived lifestyle. These are not ingredients for a healthful, enjoyable life (or consistently compassionate prehospital care). One could even postulate that this country's collectively sleep-deprived population can count this phenomenon as one underlying reason for many of society's ills.

Clearly, this topic holds important consequences both for the emergency care world and the people EMS serves. For example, a very frightening and all-too-evident problem related to sleep deprivation is what the NSF calls drowsy driving. A 2009 National Sleep Foundation poll found 54% of drivers admitted driving a vehicle while feeling drowsy in the past year. The U.S. National Highway Traffic Safety Administration (n.d.) estimates that 100,000 crashes per year involve drowsiness or fatigue as principal causes. NHTSA estimates conservatively that drowsy driving may cause 4% of all traffic crash fatalities. Emergency providers could possibly help prevent some of these fatal grinders by teaching people—especially themselves—not to drive while drowsy. Here is a sampling of what emergency personnel need to know:

- Drowsy drivers are susceptible to a phenomenon called micro sleep. Micro sleep is a brief episode of unintentional sleep experienced by a person who is so tired that he cannot resist it. Microsleep may last from a split second to 20 or 30 seconds, certainly long enough to cause harm or death when driving, especially at high speed.
- Know the high-risk groups: shift workers (EMS!), commercial drivers, youths, people with undiagnosed sleep disorders, and business travelers.
- Sleepy times of day, according to research: midnight to 6:00 a.m. and 1:00 p.m. to 4:00 p.m.
- Research shows that opening windows, playing loud radios or CD players, chewing gum, and other "tricks" fail to keep sleepy drivers alert.
- Caffeine works only on people who do not drink it constantly, and not until about 30 minutes after ingestion.
- The only safe short-term solution to driving while drowsy is to pull over and take a nap (being careful to stop in a safe location).
- The only long-term solution for driving while drowsy is prevention, such as a good night's sleep before driving.

People who are tired and try to drive are a hazard to both themselves and others. One study funded by the American Automobile Association Foundation for Traffic Safety took an in-depth look at the driving habits of 1400 people (Stutts, Wilkins, and Vaughn, 1999). It found that "drivers in sleep crashes were nearly twice as likely to work at more than one job and their primary job was more likely to involve an atypical schedule. Fourteen percent of employed drivers in sleep crashes and 24 percent of employed drivers in fatigue crashes worked the night shift. Working the night shift increased the odds of a sleep-related (versus non-sleep-related) crash by nearly six times. Working more than 60 hours a week increased the odds by 40 percent" (p. 50).

Here are some ideas for emergency vehicle drivers:

- Make getting enough rest a priority. Altering a lifestyle is a personal choice. Drivers should exercise it.
- Drivers should do whatever it takes to wring a few more hours out of each day for sleeping, such as turning off the TV and going to bed when the kids do.
- Drivers should say "no" to overtime.

- Drivers should not drink caffeine as a habit so that it will work on occasions when they really need something to assist them in staying awake.
- Drivers should work with the agency to eliminate destructive practices, such as mandatory overtime and poor shift structures.

Continuing Physical and Mental Fitness

Good drivers will be aware of their own physical limitations and will compensate appropriately (e.g., wearing corrective lenses) or will avoid driving entirely when fatigued. A driver can do a number of things to improve his own physical abilities. They include obtaining a doctor's approval to do some stretching exercises and start a walking program. He can walk around the block or in a mall, or check health clubs, YMCAs, and colleges for fitness programs. He can get examined by a doctor if he has pain or swelling in his feet. If he has pain or stiffness in the arms, legs, or neck, a doctor may prescribe medication and/or physical therapy. He can eliminate the driver's-side blind spot by re-aiming the side mirror. First, he should lean his head against the window, then adjust the mirror outward so that when he looks at the inside edge, he can barely see the side of the vehicle. If he uses a wide-angle mirror, he should get lots of practice judging distances to other cars before using it in traffic. He should keep alert to sounds outside the vehicle and limit passenger conversation and background noises from the radio and stereo. He should sit at least 10 inches from the steering wheel to reduce the chances of an injury from the air bag. And he should remember to always wear a seatbelt (Figure 6.8).

Keep in mind that driving also is affected by the individual's state of mind. For example, if the driver is worried about a sick family member, money problems, or problems concerning children, he may be distracted and not perform at his best. Anger also can distract a driver. He may lose patience and take risks he normally would not consider. If a driver's attitude has been affected negatively, then he should not drive until he is calm.

A driver must consider his attitude, as well as his physical and mental condition, every time he is about to respond to an incident. This habit will help to ensure his safety and the safety of the crew and patients. Having a good attitude and being mentally and physically fit are the best influences on doing a good job.

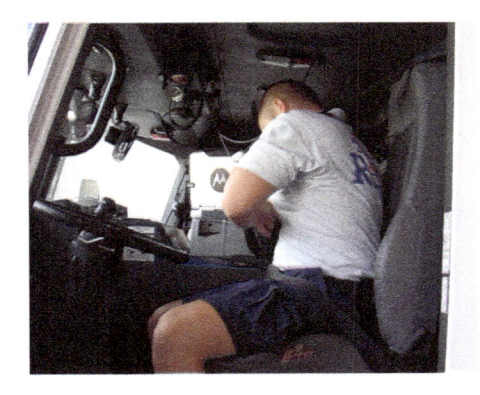

FIGURE 6.8 The driver's seat should be adjusted properly. *Courtesy of Jeffrey T. Lindsey, Ph.D.*

MAINTENANCE

Each year a percentage of EMS injuries and deaths are the result of mechanical problems and vehicle failure. In these cases, the public and legal systems are increasingly inclined to look to the organization's adherence to maintenance standards. In an ongoing attempt to minimize risks and fatalities, several groups have been working together to establish and implement standards, training and education, and certification programs supporting the safety of emergency vehicle equipment. You need to make sure your vehicle program is in conformance with the standards.

TABLE 6.1 ■ Emergency Vehicle Technician Ambulance Certifications

Ambulance Technician Level Requirements

ASE Exams	EVT Exams
Level I	
Ambulance Technician Level Requirements	E-1 Design and Performance and Preventive Maintenance of Ambulances
A-4 Automobile, Suspension, and Steering	
A-5 Automobile, Brakes	
A-6 Automobile, Electrical Systems	
A-8 Automobile, Engine Performance	
Level II	
A-1 Automobile, Engine Repair	E-2 Ambulance Electrical Systems
A-3 Automobile, Manual Drive Train, and Axle	E-3 Ambulance Heating, Air-Conditioning, and Ventilation
A-7 Automobile, Heating and Air Conditioning	
T-2 Truck, Diesel Engines	
Master Level III	
A-2 Automobile, Automatic Transmission and Transaxle	E-4 Ambulance Cab, Chassis, and Body
T-4 Truck, Brakes	
T-5 Truck, Suspension and Steering	

In August of 2000, NFPA 1071, Standard for Emergency Vehicle Technician Professional Qualifications (NFPA, 2011) was issued. This standard establishes a set of professional qualifications that can be used to develop educational requirements and corresponding certifications for **emergency vehicle technicians (EVTs)** and mechanics. These standards can and should be used whether you are a fire-based EMS service or a stand-alone EMS service.

In an ongoing effort to ensure vehicle safety, the Emergency Vehicle Technician (EVT) Certification Commission was established to write and administer tests that would demonstrate proficiency in established standards. The tests resemble those used by the Automotive Service Excellence (ASE) organization, with its "Blue Seal of Excellence." A technician who receives all of the EVT and ASE certifications is recognized as a Master EVT Certified Technician.

The EVT certification program presently has two certification tracks, one for technicians who service and maintain fire apparatus and another for technicians who service and maintain ambulances. The levels of ambulance certification are shown in Table 6.1.

Today, there are approximately 60,000 EVTs and mechanics in the United States (Figure 6.9). It is a common belief that increasing the number of certified EVTs will assist in reducing the number of emergency worker injuries and fatalities related to equipment failure. Ensuring that quality educational opportunities are readily available is central to increasing the number of certified EVTs.

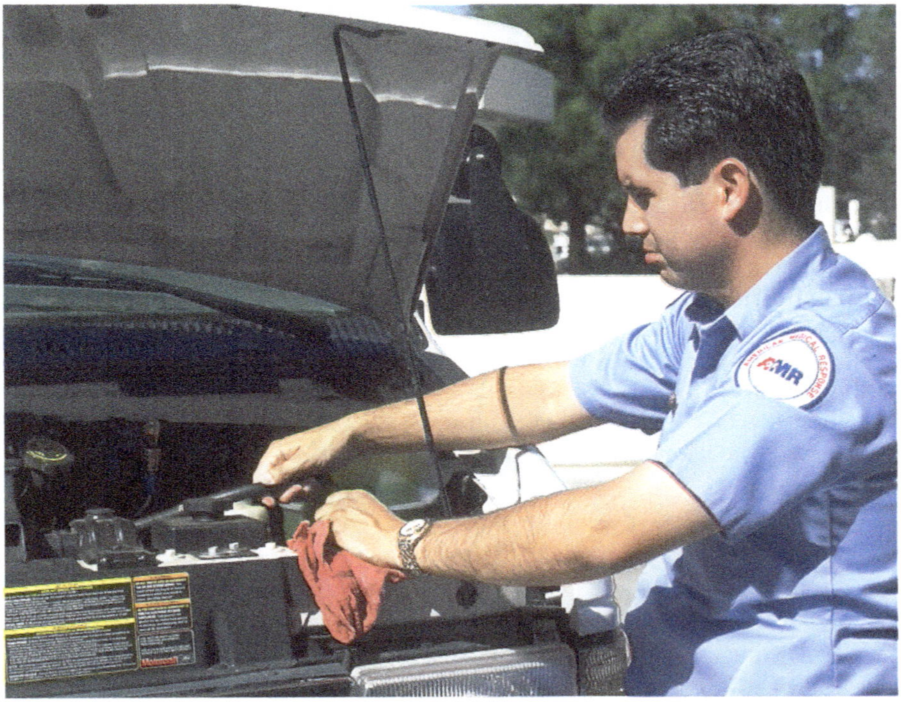

FIGURE 6.9 ■ Emergency vehicle technicians are becoming more prevalent in the EMS industry. *Courtesy of Richard W. Patrick. (All rights reserved.)*

TIRES

A number of mechanical features should be checked frequently. One area that the EMS safety officer should focus personnel's attention on is the tires of the vehicle. The tires are a critical element of the operation of the vehicle, yet tires are one of the last areas personnel pay attention to and are least educated to inspect.

Tread Wear

The tread-wear grade is a comparative rating based on the wear rate of the tire when tested under controlled conditions on a specified government test course. For example, a tire graded 150 would wear one and a half times as well on the government course as a tire graded 100. The relative performance of tires depends on the actual conditions of their use, however, and may depart significantly from the norm due to variations in driving habits, service practices, and differences in road characteristics and climate.

Traction

Traction grades from highest to lowest are AA, A, B, and C and represent the tire's ability to stop on wet pavement as measured under controlled conditions on specified government test surfaces of asphalt and concrete. A tire marked C may have poor traction performance.

Warning: The traction grade assigned to a tire is based on braking (straight ahead) traction tests and does not include cornering (turning) traction.

128 CHAPTER 6 *Vehicle Driving and Fleet Maintenance*

Temperature

The temperature grades are A (the highest), B, and C, representing the tire's resistance to the generation of heat and its ability to dissipate heat when tested under controlled conditions on a specified indoor laboratory test wheel. Sustained high temperature can cause the material of the tire to degenerate and reduce tire life, and excessive temperature can lead to sudden tire failure. The grade C corresponds to a level of performance that all passenger car tires must meet under Federal Motor Vehicle Safety Standard No. 109. Grades A and B represent higher levels of performance on the laboratory test wheel than the minimum required by law.

Warning: The temperature grade is established for a tire that is properly inflated and not overloaded. Excessive speed, underinflation, or excessive loading, either separately or in combination, can cause heat buildup and possible tire failure.

Tire Pressure and Loading

Tire information placards and vehicle certification labels contain information on tires and load limits. These labels indicate the vehicle manufacturer's information (Figure 6.10), including the following:

- Recommended tire size
- Recommended tire inflation pressure (usually given in PSI cold)
- Gross vehicle weight rating (GVWR)

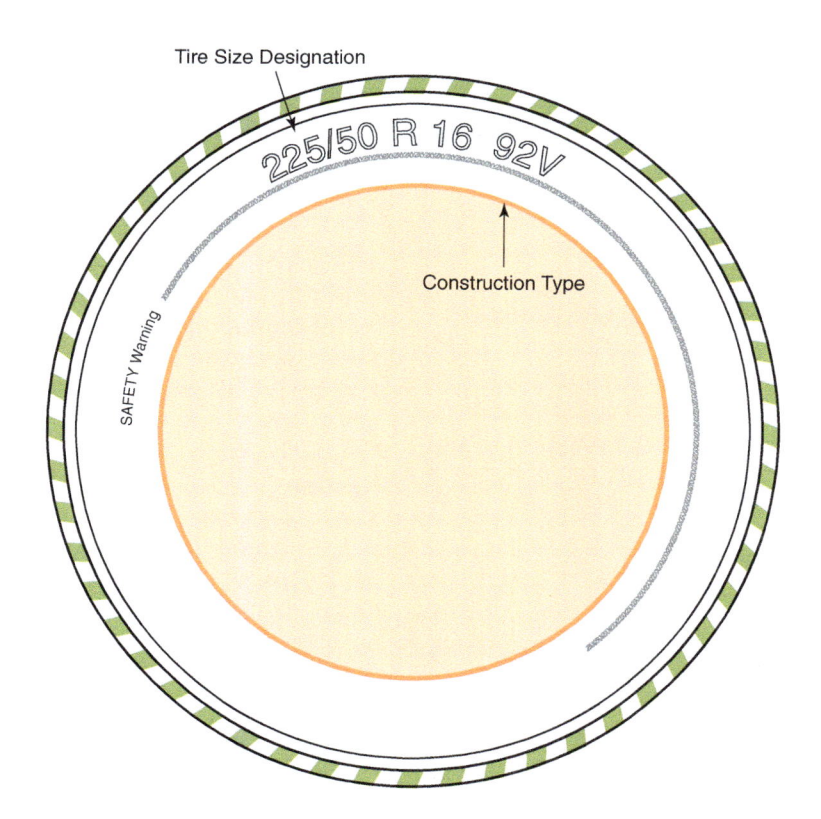

FIGURE 6.10 ■ Manufacturer's information can be found on the labeling on a tire.

CHAPTER 6 *Vehicle Driving and Fleet Maintenance* **129**

- Maximum occupant and cargo weight a vehicle is designed to carry
- Gross axle weight ratings (GAWR) for front and rear axles
- Maximum weight the axle systems are designed to carry
- Recommended tire pressure and load limit for the vehicle in the vehicle owner's manual

Tire inflation pressure is the level of air in the tire that provides it with load-carrying capacity and affects the overall performance of the vehicle. The tire inflation pressure is a number that indicates the amount of air pressure—measured in pounds per square inch (psi)—a tire requires to be properly inflated. This number also may be found on the vehicle information placard expressed in kilopascals (kPa), which is the metric measure used internationally.

Remember, the correct pressure for tires is what the vehicle manufacturer has listed on the placard, *not* what is listed on the tire itself. Because tires are designed to be used on more than one type of vehicle, tire manufacturers list the "maximum permissible inflation pressure" on the tire sidewall. This number is the greatest amount of air pressure that should ever be put in the tire under normal driving conditions.

Checking Tire Pressure

It is important to have personnel check the vehicle's tire pressure at least once a month for the following reasons:

- Most tires may naturally lose air over time.
- Tires can lose air suddenly if driven over a pothole or other object or if they strike the curb.
- With radial tires, it is usually not possible to determine underinflation by visual inspection.

A tire pressure gauge should be kept in the vehicle. Gauges can be purchased at tire dealerships, auto supply stores, and other retail outlets. The recommended tire inflation pressure that vehicle manufacturers provide reflects the proper psi when a tire is cold. The term *cold* does not relate to the outside temperature. Rather, a cold tire is one that has not been driven on for at least 3 hours. When driving, tires get warmer, causing the air pressure within them to increase. Therefore, to get an accurate tire pressure reading, tire pressure should be measured when the tires are cold; otherwise, one must compensate for the extra pressure in warm tires (Table 6.2).

If after driving the vehicle, the tire feels underinflated, they should be filled to the recommended cold inflation pressure indicated

TABLE 6.2 ■ Steps for Maintaining Proper Tire Pressure

Step 1	Locate the recommended tire pressure on the vehicle's tire information placard, certification label, or in the owner's manual.
Step 2	Record the tire pressure of all tires.
Step 3	If the tire pressure is too high in any of the tires, slowly release air by gently pressing on the tire valve stem with the edge of your tire gauge until you get to the correct pressure.
Step 4	If the tire pressure is too low, note the difference between the measured tire pressure and the correct tire pressure. These "missing" pounds of pressure are what will need to be added.
Step 5	Add the missing pounds of air pressure to each tire that is underinflated.
Step 6	Check all the tires to make sure they have the same air pressure (except in cases in which the front and rear tires are supposed to have different amounts of pressure).

on the vehicle's tire information placard or certification label. Although the tire may still be slightly underinflated due to the extra pounds of pressure in the warm tire, it is safer to drive with air pressure that is slightly lower than the vehicle manufacturer's recommended cold inflation pressure than to drive with a significantly underinflated tire. Since this is a temporary fix, the driver should not forget to recheck and adjust the tire's pressure when he can obtain a cold reading.

The tire tread provides the gripping action and traction that prevent the vehicle from slipping or sliding, especially when the road is wet or icy. In general, tires are not safe and should be replaced when the tread is worn down to 1/16 inch. Tires have built-in tread-wear indicators that let a driver know when it is time to replace the tires. These indicators are raised sections spaced intermittently in the bottom of the tread grooves. When they appear "even" with the outside of the tread, it is time to replace the tires.

Another method for checking tread depth is to place a penny in the tread with Lincoln's head upside down and facing you. If the top of Lincoln's head can be seen, the vehicle is ready for new tires (Figure 6.11).

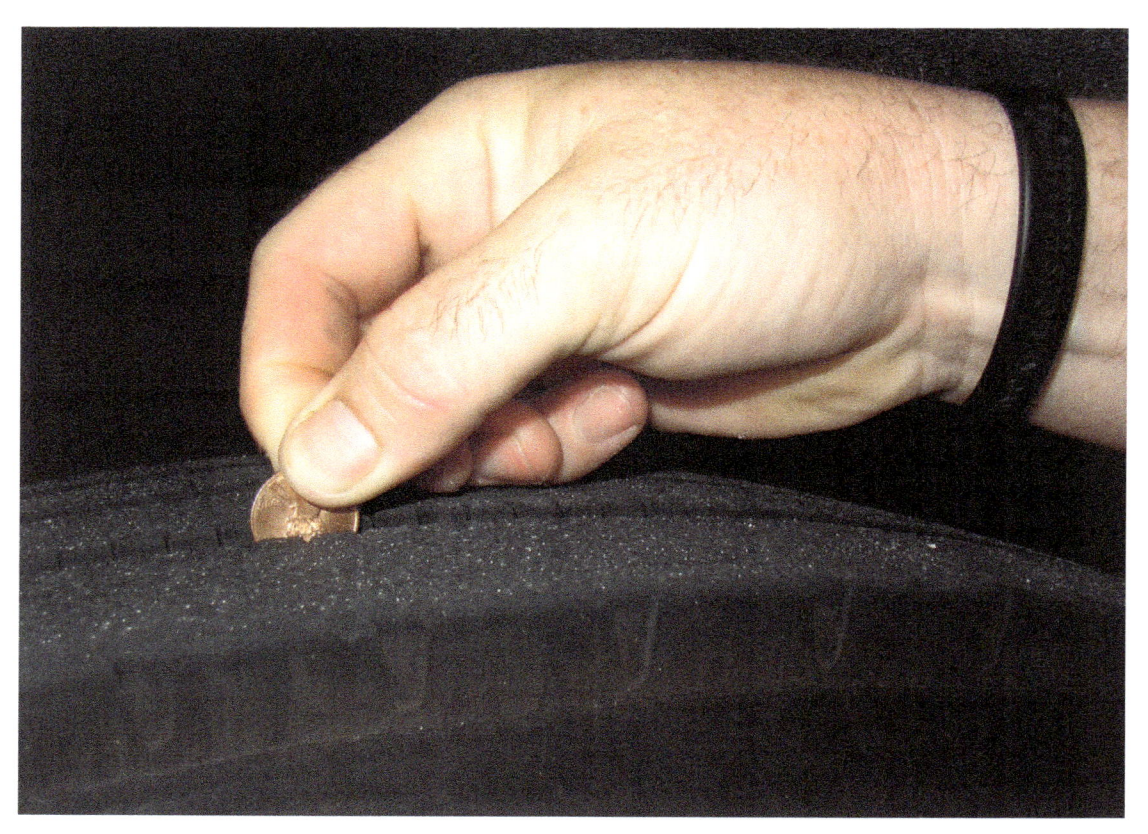

FIGURE 6.11 ■ Using a penny is one method to check the depth of the tread in a tire. *Courtesy of Jeffrey T. Lindsey, Ph.D.*

SUPPORT EQUIPMENT

All ambulances contain basic medical support equipment installed by the manufacturer. Each organization may customize its vehicle with additional equipment, often outfitting vehicles to meet specific requirements. Thus, not all vehicles will carry the same equipment.

When the typical ambulance leaves the factory, it is designed to carry a driver and an EMT at 175 pounds each, two patients at 175 pounds each, and the following medical support equipment:

- Main and portable oxygen bottles
- Stretchers, cots, and patient handling equipment
- Portable, removable medical devices
- Durable and disposable medical items
- Optional vehicle equipment such as battery charger, inverter, or auxiliary power unit
- Communications equipment
- Extrication and rescue equipment

The driver should be responsible for inspecting the vehicle and for properly operating the mechanical systems. The driver may also be responsible for providing routine servicing and preventive maintenance for each system and its components.

VEHICLE INSPECTION

The most important way to check the operating condition of the vehicle is to inspect it regularly and to document the results of those inspections. The inspection forms should be reviewed from time to time as a quality assurance process.

Systematic Inspections

By conducting regular, systematic vehicle inspections, the driver is able to:

- Find and report problems that need to be fixed.
- Keep track of preventive maintenance requirements.
- Document the overall condition of the vehicle.

The driver should evaluate the results of the inspection before deciding whether or not to place the vehicle into service.

Inspection Methodology

To ensure that vehicle inspections are consistent, thorough, and accurate, each EMS organization should develop specific vehicle inspection procedures and checklists to meet its needs. The completed checklists should then be kept on file and used to document the condition of the vehicles. Examples of these procedures and checklists will be discussed later in this chapter.

Importance of Maintaining Records

If an emergency vehicle is involved in a crash, and there is the possibility that a mechanical malfunction was the cause, the courts would be very interested in reviewing the maintenance records of the emergency vehicle. If the operating organization knew in advance of the malfunction and continued to operate the vehicle, it may be found negligent and held liable for all damages resulting from the crash.

Maintenance organizations must be able to document in writing the servicing, maintenance, and repair of the vehicles and equipment (Figure 6.12). A good general guideline for documenting inspections and maintenance actions is "If it's not in writing, it did not happen."

INSPECTION SCHEDULE

To maintain good records, personnel must conduct vehicle inspections. The following schedule is a recommendation and may be different from the one used in your organization. Whether the vehicle is inspected based on number of runs per week, hours of operation, or specific days of the week, the important thing is that the vehicle is inspected according to strict adherence to a specific schedule.

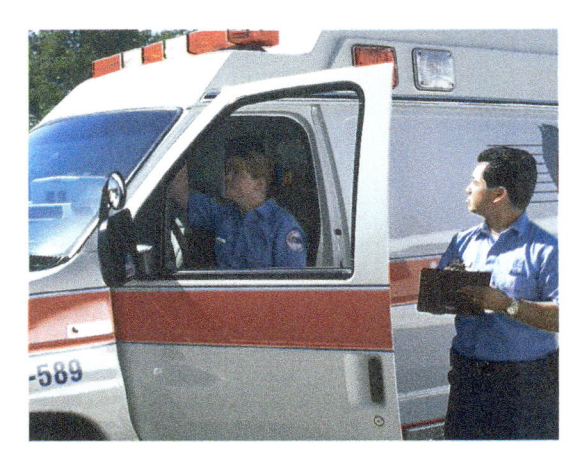

FIGURE 6.12 ■ Documentation is important for maintenance of vehicles.

An organization's inspection schedule should be determined by a number of factors, including vehicle age and mileage, insurance requirements, and past experience.

Inspection Types

Two types of vehicle inspections are recommended for emergency vehicles: The **quick check inspection** covers those systems that should be checked most often. The **full check inspection** covers all vehicle systems that can be checked without special equipment or facilities.

Quick Check Inspection. One example of a checklist to be used for such an inspection is shown in Figure 6.13. Whatever checklist your organization uses, the first specifics that should be documented are the vehicle number, the station where it is located, and the date and time of the inspection. This information must be included because the form may be reviewed by someone outside of the driver's organization and at a much later date when the driver may not be present to explain the entries.

When a driver conducts a quick check inspection, he should inspect each item and place a check mark in the column to indicate "OK" if there are no problems. By checking off an item as OK, the driver verifies that he inspected it and found no problems with it. Any problems found should be fixed by the driver or other person who is capable and authorized to do so. Document that the work was done in the "Work Completed" block, or file a work request for the problems found. Decide whether or not to place the vehicle in service (any starred [*] problems must be fixed before the vehicle is placed in service). Then document the decision by circling the appropriate word in the printed statement above the signature. Sign and date the checklist.

Eight areas need to be addressed in the quick check inspection (Figure 6.14). The sequence of the inspection is designed so that the driver inspects all the listed items in one area before moving clockwise around the vehicle to the next area. This helps to ensure that no area or no item will be missed.

Before starting a quick check inspection, the driver should arrange for another crew member to be present to help check the lights. Then the driver should place wheel chocks where they can be quickly retrieved if required. Finally, he should get a blank checklist and fill out the administrative information.

The quick check inspection consists of the following:

1. *Overall appearance.* The overall appearance to the public as a professional organization is enhanced by a clean, well-maintained vehicle.
   * Check vehicle cleanliness.
   * Check general vehicle condition.
   * Is the vehicle sitting level?
   * Are there any puddles or other signs of visible fluid leaks?
   * Are there any signs of new, unreported body damage?
2. *Driver compartment.*
   * Check the vehicle log. (The most recently completed Full Check and Quick Check

VFIS

Vehicle Driver's Safety Check

Date Odometer Reading Unit No.

☐ Pre-Trip Inspection ☐ Post-Trip Inspection

Only Items Checked Require Attention

☐ Gauges - Ammeter, Oil Pressure, Fuel, Water Temperatures, Air Pressure or Vacuum
☐ Windshield Wipers
☐ Windshield & Windows
☐ Heater & Defroster
☐ Mirrors
☐ Brakes (Foot & Parking)
☐ Engine Noises
☐ Horn & Sirens
☐ Steering
☐ Vehicle Body
☐ Wheels, Tires, Lugs
☐ Fuel Tank and Cap
☐ Leaks — Water, Fuel, Oil
☐ Head Lights
☐ Tail Lights
☐ Stop Lights
☐ Turn Signals and 4-Way Flasher
☐ Reflectors
☐ Emergency Equipment
Other - If Applicable
☐ Clearance Lights
☐ Emergency Warning Lights
☐ Side Marker Lights
☐ Brake Hoses
☐ Compartment Door Locks
☐ Drain Air Tanks of Moisture
☐ Air Systems
☐ Mounted Equipment

Remarks (explain unsatisfactory items noted above)

Signature of Driver ______

To be Completed by Repair Shop

Mechanic's Report (If defects are noted)

Signature of Repair Shop Foreman or Mechanic ______ Date ______

(Use back of form for additional remarks.)

WP\WINWORD\VFIS\SAFETYKITFORMS\VEHDRIVE.DOC C10:006 – 7/02

VFIS

Vehicle Driver's Safety Check

Date Odometer Reading Unit No.

☐ Pre-Trip Inspection ☐ Post-Trip Inspection

Only Items Checked Require Attention

☐ Gauges - Ammeter, Oil Pressure, Fuel, Water Temperatures, Air Pressure or Vacuum
☐ Windshield Wipers
☐ Windshield & Windows
☐ Heater & Defroster
☐ Mirrors
☐ Brakes (Foot & Parking)
☐ Engine Noises
☐ Horn & Sirens
☐ Steering
☐ Vehicle Body
☐ Wheels, Tires, Lugs
☐ Fuel Tank and Cap
☐ Leaks — Water, Fuel, Oil
☐ Head Lights
☐ Tail Lights
☐ Stop Lights
☐ Turn Signals and 4-Way Flasher
☐ Reflectors
☐ Emergency Equipment
Other - If Applicable
☐ Clearance Lights
☐ Emergency Warning Lights
☐ Side Marker Lights
☐ Brake Hoses
☐ Compartment Door Locks
☐ Drain Air Tanks of Moisture
☐ Air Systems
☐ Mounted Equipment

Remarks (explain unsatisfactory items noted above)

Signature of Driver ______

To be Completed by Repair Shop

Mechanic's Report (If defects are noted)

Signature of Repair Shop Foreman or Mechanic ______ Date ______

(Use back of form for additional remarks.)

WP\WINWORD\VFIS\SAFETYKITFORMS\VEHDRIVE.DOC C10:006 – 7/02

FIGURE 6.13 Sample vehicle checklist. *Reprinted with permission of VFIS.*

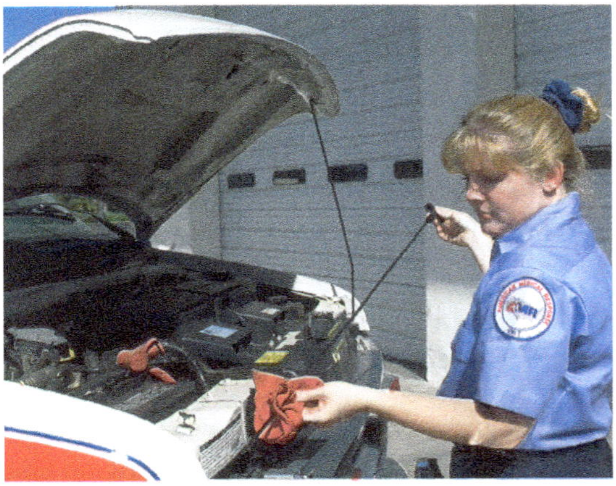

FIGURE 6.14 It is important to inspect vehicles according to a specific schedule.

checklists should be in the log, along with blank copies of the run report and a complete inventory list of installed equipment.)

- Check for stowage of items.
- Be sure switches for lights and communication equipment are in the off position.
- Adjust the seat, seat belt, and side view mirrors.
- Release the hood latch.
- Turn the key to the on position and check the fuel gauge.
- Each organization has specific procedures for refueling.
- An urban organization that makes several short runs each day may elect to refuel at the end of each day or when the quantity

drops below half full. A rural organization that only makes a few runs each week may refuel after each run because runs of 40 to 100 miles are common and fuel may not be readily available.
- Routine refueling should occur when the fuel level is between one-half and three-quarters empty. Follow the organization's procedures for refueling.

3. *Exterior walk-around on driver's side.*
   - Check left outside mirror bracket for general condition.
   - Check left-side window for general condition.
   - Check left side of windshield and left wiper for general condition.
   - Check the left front wheel and tire for general condition.
   - Check the tire for a properly inflated appearance, but do not check tire pressure.
   - Check left front fender for general condition.
   - Check the pump panel and run the pump, if equipped. (*Note:* More ambulances are becoming equipped with pumps to do immediate fire suppression. If this is the case, the pump must be inspected and serviced accordingly.)

4. *Exterior walk-around at front.*
   - Inspect the front of the vehicle and grill for general condition.
   - Remove any obstructions to the grill, radiator, or lights.
   - Visually check the condition of the headlights and turn signals.
   - Visually check the condition of the emergency lights from the front.

5. *Engine compartment.*
   - Open the hood and visually check the engine for signs of leaks.
   - Visually check the condition of all belts.
   - Visually check the condition of the batteries.
   - Check levels of engine oil, windshield washer fluid, and cooling system.
   - Check coolant level at overflow reservoir. Do not remove the radiator cap to check.
   - Replenish fluids according to your local organization's requirements.
   - Always replenish the engine oil when it is 1 quart low.
   - Close the hood and ensure that it is latched.

6. *Exterior walk-around at passenger's side.*
   - Check the right front fender for general condition.
   - Check the right front wheel and tire for general condition.
   - Check the tire for a properly inflated appearance, but do not check tire pressure.
   - Check the right side of windshield and right wiper for general condition.
   - Check the right-side window for general condition.
   - Check the right outside mirror bracket for general condition.
   - Check the right rear fender for general condition.
   - Check the right rear wheel and tire for general condition.
   - Check the tire for a properly inflated appearance, but do not check tire pressure.

7. *Patient compartment in ambulances.*
   - Open the rear doors and visually check the general condition of patient compartment.
   - Check that all equipment is properly secured.
   - Verify that no new equipment that may change vehicle weight has been added to the patient compartment.
   - Close the rear doors and ensure that they are properly latched.

8. *Exterior walk-around at rear.*
   - Visually check the condition of the emergency lights from the rear.
   - Visually check the condition of the rear lights and turn signals.
   - Visually check the condition of the external flood lights, if installed.
   - Check the left rear fender for general condition.
   - Check the left rear wheel and tire for general condition.
   - Check the tire for a properly inflated appearance, but do not check tire pressure.

When this inspection is completed, the driver must decide whether or not to place the vehicle into service, and then sign and date the form. Finally, the driver must place the completed checklist into the vehicle log.

Note: If the organization requires an operational check of the communications and emergency warning equipment, perform those checks after completing the visual inspection. To conduct an operational check, the driver must start the vehicle and drive it outdoors. He should check the communications equipment, following local procedures, operate and have another crew member check the emergency lights, and then check the siren. Finally, he should secure the communications and emergency equipment and return the vehicle to its parking space.

Full Check Inspection. The same eight areas identified for the quick check inspection are used for the full check inspection. More items are covered for the full check, some in greater detail.

Negligence Related to Inspection

A driver can be judged to be negligent with regard to vehicle inspection for two main reasons: for failing to inspect a vehicle thoroughly according to the organization's requirements, and for knowingly operating a vehicle with a problem that should have caused it to be taken out of service.

REFUSING TO DRIVE AN UNSAFE VEHICLE

The driver should never operate a vehicle that is not in safe operating condition. Although this seems like pretty basic information, when faced with an emergency some drivers might feel pressured to take an unsafe vehicle. A federal program, the Injury/Illness Prevention Program (IIP), supports a driver's right to refuse to drive an unsafe vehicle. Guidelines for this program are available from the Occupational Safety and Health Administration (OSHA).

COMPREHENSIVE MAINTENANCE PROGRAMS

There is a story that has been circulating among the emergency service community about a huge fire that is raging out of control. A number of units already on the scene making gallant efforts to extinguish the raging inferno. Over the crest of the hill a fire engine from a neighboring fire department comes speeding down the hill and into the fire. The firefighters jump off the vehicle and begin spraying water, and before you know it the fire is extinguished. The owner of the property is elated with the fire department and offers it a $10,000 reward for extinguishing the fire. The fire chief was interviewed and asked what the fire department would do with the money. Without hesitation the chief replied that the first thing he would do is get new brakes put on the fire engine.

Humor is always a vital element in shedding light on troubling issues. However, vehicle maintenance is one of those issues that must be taken seriously and not left to chance. Vehicle maintenance is an ongoing process. A comprehensive maintenance program anticipates the need for maintenance and completes it before a failure occurs and repairs are needed. In general, it has the following characteristics:

- It uses information from regular inspections to identify maintenance that may be needed.
- It uses regular inspections, including those performed by the operator, which can provide an indication that maintenance is needed.
- It requires documentation of all inspections, work requests, and work completed. Remember: "If it's not in writing, it did not happen."
- It includes preventive maintenance.

Vehicle maintenance is a critical part of an effective emergency response organization. If vehicles are not ready to respond to a service call, or if they break down during a run, the organization cannot mitigate the emergency effectively. It is every driver's responsibility to ensure that the vehicle being operated is functioning properly and safe to drive. It is the EMS safety officer's responsibility to ensure the drivers are aware of what to look for and that the vehicles are safe to operate.

Preventive Maintenance

Preventive maintenance focuses on preventing the most likely vehicle malfunctions by replacing parts or making adjustments before a failure occurs. It relies on fixing minor problems before they become major ones and has several important advantages over repairing equipment only when it breaks: It ensures safe, reliable vehicle operation; it reduces the total cost of repairs, and it minimizes major equipment failure.

Preventive maintenance takes the form of three different classifications. The classifications are typically referred to as **routine maintenance**, **scheduled maintenance**, and **crisis maintenance**. The last classification is not always avoidable, but efforts must be made to reduce the potential of crisis maintenance occurring. Each may be described as follows:

Routine maintenance. Routine maintenance is just what the name suggests. It involves areas such as replacing a burned-out light bulb or tightening a loose bolt.

Scheduled maintenance. Scheduled maintenance marks the regular times at which parts of a vehicle require attention. Oil changes, for example, are done every so many months or miles based on the manufacturer's recommendations. Some organizations establish a time frame, rather than a specific date, for units to automatically go through the maintenance process in order to keep units running at the highest possible efficiency.

Crisis maintenance. Crisis maintenance is—as the name suggests—maintenance or repairs that need to be made immediately. On the occasion of an air conditioner failing during a summer in Arizona, for example, where temperatures regularly soar above 100°F, the vehicle would have to be taken out of service and repaired immediately.

Driver Responsibility for Vehicle Maintenance

The driver is an important part of the maintenance program. The following are the primary responsibilities for maintenance:

- To document any needed maintenance a vehicle inspection may reveal
- To ensure that needed maintenance has been completed before the vehicle is placed in service
- To perform any maintenance for which the organization makes the driver responsible

The driver must document needed maintenance on the inspection checklist or other appropriate form as required by the organization. Before the driver places the vehicle in service, he must make sure needed maintenance has been completed following the organization's procedures.

Work Requests

A work request form tells maintenance what work is needed on a vehicle. When maintenance personnel finish the work, they record on the form the work performed, the tests run, and the results of their efforts. This work request covers those problems that the driver finds during an inspection as well as routine preventive maintenance. An organization may or may not use a work request to track maintenance and repairs.

Vehicle Maintenance Logs

Information from the inspection checklists and work requests are written into a vehicle maintenance log. The vehicle maintenance log is a vehicle's central record and is used as follows:

- Lists all maintenance needed and done, including routine maintenance and problems identified by inspections
- Supports the preventive maintenance program
- Documents that the vehicle has been properly maintained (Vehicle maintenance log pages are usually organized into binders and saved in an inspection file for use by a maintenance supervisor or manager.)

To determine whether or not the vehicle is in safe operating condition, the driver must know whether or not required maintenance has been performed. The driver must understand the organization's maintenance program in order to know the vehicle's maintenance status.

Driver's Responsibilities for Vehicle Repairs

The driver's primary responsibilities for repairs include documenting on a checklist or other appropriate form, as required by the organization, any needed repairs found during an inspection or a run. He must make sure needed repairs have been completed before placing the vehicle in service and according to the organization's procedures. He also must make any repairs for which he is responsible.

Making Repairs. In some organizations, drivers make a variety of repairs to the vehicles. In others, the driver is responsible for only minimal repairs. The driver should only perform repairs for which he is trained and authorized.

Malfunctions During a Run. There may be a time when, in spite of all precautions, the vehicle breaks down during a run. When this happens, the driver should think the situation through carefully before taking action. He also should use communications to ask for options (Table 6.3).

TABLE 6.3 ■ Decision Aid for Vehicle Malfunctions During a Run

Question	Decision
Is the driver trained and authorized to make the repair?	The driver should be both trained and authorized to make any repair. If the driver should not fix the problem, he should call for help.
Is a backup readily available?	The driver should use the communication system to inform dispatch of the situation and to determine if a backup is available. Develop a plan before starting any repair, in case the repair fails.
Am I outside my normal service area?	If operating outside the normal service area, the driver may need to coordinate with an organization based in that service area.
How quickly can the repair be made?	If it can be made in less time than it takes for the backup to arrive, then it should be repaired.
Can the vehicle's electrical system meet the demands made on it during the repair?	If a long stay at the scene has depleted the system, the driver may need a backup vehicle even if the driver can make the repair.

Note: This decision aid applies to any vehicle problem during a run. The organization's policies and procedures also may address what to do when a malfunction occurs.

Repairs During the Run. A driver is generally expected or allowed to make only the most minor repairs during a run. For example, he might change a flat tire or use duct tape to make temporary repairs to a broken radiator hose (usually the upper radiator hose).

Driving a Vehicle with Problems Safely. The driver may find himself in a situation where the vehicle has malfunctioned but is still drivable. For example, an ambulance with a steering belt failure can be driven carefully with compensation for the lack of power steering. The driver's decision about whether or not to continue to drive the vehicle should be based on the organization's policies and procedures. The driver may be required to inform a supervisor of the situation instead of making the decision himself.

CHAPTER REVIEW

Summary

Emergency vehicle drivers are selected based on their qualifications to perform the duties required of them. A driving record check and license check is a precondition to hiring. A medical evaluation should be required to determine physical ability to perform the job under all conditions.

The emergency vehicle driver has an important job to do—driving an emergency vehicle—and taking a training course will offer the emergency vehicle driver the training designed for all aspects of that job. The driver should pass the emergency vehicle driver course written test and driving test, and then pass the on-the-job driving evaluation. The driver is expected to be mentally and physically fit for every response.

Training should be presented in the classroom, behind the wheel, and on the job. When a driver has successfully completed all three modules, met all local and state requirements and recommendations made by the supervisor, the driver should be considered a qualified emergency vehicle driver. The EMS safety officer should also play a role in training and selecting drivers.

The driver should inspect his vehicle to decide whether it is in safe operating condition or whether it should not be driven. The driver may be found negligent for driving a vehicle that is not in safe operating condition. When the driver places his vehicle in service, he should indicate that the vehicle is in safe operating condition. To determine whether the vehicle is in safe operating condition, the driver must know whether or not required maintenance has been performed. The driver must understand his organization's maintenance program in order to know his vehicle's maintenance status. The driver is responsible for documenting any needed repairs he finds during an inspection or during a run. Before the driver places a vehicle in service, he must make sure that needed repairs have been completed. The driver and his organization should have a strategy for dealing with vehicle malfunctions during a run.

CHAPTER 6 Vehicle Driving and Fleet Maintenance 139

WHAT WOULD YOU DO? Reflection

You have taken the training officer's questions into consideration and prepared a report for her in regard to each of the questions. What qualifications should the driver possess? A driver should possess a number of qualifications. He should have a valid driver's license with a clean or driving record that does not have major driving offenses on his record. He should have the knowledge, both mental and physical, to be able to drive an emergency vehicle. In addition, the driver should have a positive attitude and ability to handle the vehicle. The driver candidate also should be able to pass the testing process to drive an ambulance.

What type of training should the driver go through that demonstrates a safe approach to driving? A formal comprehensive driving program must be implemented. A number of driver training programs are available. Regardless, the candidate should take a written exam, drive through a competency course, and then successfully drive an over-the-highway test. After the successful completion of testing, the driver should be assigned with an experienced, competent driver to drive so many responses during the day and during the night before being formally assigned as an official driver for the organization.

Should the safety officer serve on the driver selection committee? Yes, he should. Based on past experiences and understanding what happens when there is an incident with a vehicle, the safety officer provides a perspective that others may not be able to offer.

Review Questions

1. Describe some of the causes of ambulance crashes and the injuries and deaths that result from crashes.
2. Describe the three principles of safe operations.
3. Describe the four major considerations of a driver selection program.
4. List the concepts of a comprehensive defensive driving course that introduce and reinforce driving skills.
5. Outline the minimum education and training qualifications for emergency vehicle drivers.
6. What are the eight specific areas that you need to check during the quick check inspection? Include details of each of the specific areas.
7. Explain why record keeping and vehicle maintenance play a significant role in ambulance crashes.

References

AAA Foundation for Traffic Safety. (1999, November/December). "Multiple Jobs, Long Hours Implicated in Sleep Crashes." *Progress Report*, 6(6), 1–2. (See the organization website.)

Auerbach, P. S., J. A. Morris Jr., J. B. Phillips Jr., S. R. Redlinger, and W. K. Vaughn. (1987, September 18). "An Analysis of Ambulance Accidents in Tennessee." *Journal of the American Medical Association (JAMA)* 258(11), 1487–1490.

Biggers, W. A., B. S. Zachariah, and P. E. Pepe. (1996, July–September). "Emergency Medical Vehicle Collisions in an Urban System." *Prehospital and Disaster Medicine 11*(3), 195–201.

Canaan, S. (2000). "Sleep Deprivation, Shift Work, and Sweet Dreams."

Cook Jr., R. T., S. A. Meador, B. D. Buckingham, and L. V. Groff. (1991). "Opportunity for Seatbelt Usage by ALS Providers." *Prehospital and Disaster Medicine 6*(4), 469–471.

Fahy, R. F., P. R. LeBlanc, and J. L. Molis. (2009, July). "Firefighter Fatalities in the United States—2008." Quincy, MA: National Fire Protection Association. (See the organization website.)

Gershon, R. R., D. Vlahov, G. Kelen, B. Conrad, and L. Murphy. (1995, January–March). "Review of Accidents/Injuries Among Emergency Medical Services Workers in Baltimore, Maryland." *Prehospital and Disaster Medicine 10*(1), 14–18.

Gold, D. R., S. Rogacz, N. Bock, T. D. Tosteson, T. M. Baum, et al. (1992, July). "Rotating Shift Work, Sleep, and Accidents Related to Sleepiness in Hospital Nurses." *American Journal of Public Health* (7), 1011–1014.

Harma, M. (1993). "Individual Differences in Tolerance to Shift Work: A Review." *Ergonomics 36*(1–3), 101–109.

Kahn, C. A., R. G. Pirrallo, and E. M. Kuhn. (2001, July–September). "Characteristics of Fatal Ambulance Crashes in the United States: An 11-Year Retrospective Analysis." *Prehospital Emergency Care 5*(3), 261–269.

Land Transport Safety Authority. (2003, November). "Fatigue: Staying Alert While You're Driving." (See the organization website.)

Larmon, B., T. F. LeGassick, and D. L. Schriger. (1993, November). "Differential Front and Back Seat Safety Belt Use by Prehospital Care Providers." *American Journal of Emergency Medicine 11*(6), 595–599.

Lindsey, J. T., and R. W. Patrick. (2007). *Emergency Vehicle Operations.* Upper Saddle River, NJ: Prentice Hall.

Marcus, C. L., and G. M. Loughlin. (1996, December). "Sleepiness and Safety: Effect of Sleep Deprivation on Driving Safety in Housestaff." *Sleep 19*(10), 763–766.

Minors, D., and J. Waterhouse. (1981). "Anchor Sleep as a Synchronizer of Rhythms on Abnormal Routines." *International Journal of Chronobiology 7*, 165–188.

National Center on Sleep Disorders Research and NHTSA. "Drowsy Driving and Automobile Crashes: NCSDR/NHTSA Expert Panel on Driver Fatigue and Sleepiness." (n.d.). (See the organization website.)

National Fire Protection Association. (2011). "NFPA Standard 1071: Standard for Emergency Vehicle Technician Professional Qualifications." (See the organization website.)

National Highway Traffic and Safety Administration. "Tires." (See the organization website.)

National Sleep Foundation. (2009). "How Much Sleep Do We Really Need?" (See the organization website.)

National Sleep Foundation. (2011). "Drowsy Driving." (See the organization website.)

Nice, K. (2004) "How Anti-lock Brakes Work." HowStuffWorks, A Discovery Company. (See the organization website.)

Novak, R. D., and S. E. Auvil-Novak. (1996). "Focus Group Evaluation of Night Nurse Shiftwork Difficulties and Coping Strategies." *Chronobiology International 13*(6), 457–463.

Pirrallo, R. G., and R. A. Swor. (1994, April–June). "Characteristics of Fatal Ambulance Crashes During Emergency and Non-emergency Operation." *Prehospital and Disaster Medicine 9*(2), 125–132.

Rosa, R. (1990). "Editorial: Factors for promoting adjustment to night and shift work." *Work & Stress 4*, 201–202.

Stutts, J. C., J. W. Wilkins, and B. V. Vaughn. (1999). "Why Do People Have Drowsy Driving Crashes? Input from Drivers Who Just Did." Washington, DC: AAA Foundation for Traffic Safety.

U.S. National Highway Traffic Safety Administration (NHTSA). (n.d.). "Drowsy Driving and Automobile Crashes: NCSDR/NHTSA Expert Panel on Driver Fatigue and Sleepiness." (See the organization website.)

Key Terms

acquired abilities The abilities by which each individual coordinates and handles a vehicle based on a number of driving characteristics that he has acquired from the time he began to drive.

crisis maintenance Maintenance needed to be performed immediately; typically, the vehicle is placed out of service until completely repaired.

driver proficiency The demonstration of the ability to perform in all the varying components of driving emergency vehicles.

driver selection The process of choosing an individual to drive an emergency vehicle.

driver training A comprehensive program to teach an individual how to drive an emergency vehicle; the program should include both written and practical testing.

emergency vehicle technician (EVT) A person certified through a testing process who can mechanically work on emergency vehicles.

full check inspection An evaluation of all vehicle systems that can be checked without special equipment or facilities.

human aspects Factors that can promote a change in human activity to produce the safest possible emergency vehicle driver.

personnel records Those files that document the member's training, performance, and other demographic information.

preventive maintenance Maintenance that focuses on preventing the most likely vehicle malfunctions by replacing parts or making adjustments before a failure occurs.

quick check inspection An evaluation of all those vehicle systems that should be checked most often.

routine maintenance Maintenance performed as needed; does not usually affect the performance of the vehicle.

scheduled maintenance Maintenance performed at regular intervals, usually based on manufacturer's recommendations; planned times at which parts of a vehicle require attention.

vehicle characteristics The capabilities and limitations of a vehicle, such as speed, road conditions, auxiliary braking systems, and weight transfer.

Scene Operations

7 CHAPTER

Objectives

After reading this chapter, the student should be able to:

7.1 Identify and assess safety needs for both emergency and nonemergency situations.

7.2 Identify and analyze the major causes involved in line-of-duty deaths related to health, wellness, fitness, and vehicle operations.

Overview

This title on EMS safety and risk management has been written to assist EMS providers in the reduction of line-of-duty injuries, illnesses, and fatalities. It provides a framework for developing programs that will create an appropriate margin of health and safety for providers during the performance of EMS duties.

Key Terms

ANSI/ISEA Standard 207-2006
backlight
bloodborne pathogens
buffer zone
Class III safety vest
concealment
contaminated sharps
cover
decontamination
epidemiology
ergonomics
exposure incident
forecasting
Manual on Uniform Traffic Control Devices (MUTCD) for Streets and Highways
reduced profile
retroreflectorized
retroreflective material

WHAT WOULD YOU DO?

You have been assigned as the EMS safety officer. This is the first time in your organization that anyone has been assigned to this role. The EMS crews are circulating rumors that you will be responding to every incident and causing them all kinds of grief. It is the typical rumor that occurs any time something new occurs. So that the fears of the troops will be calmed, the EMS chief has asked you to create guidelines that identify the incidents to which you think you should respond. You set off to determine what type of calls should be included on your list.

Questions

1. What types of incidents would you include in your list?
2. What is the most important aspect of being a safety officer?
3. To what other situations would you respond?

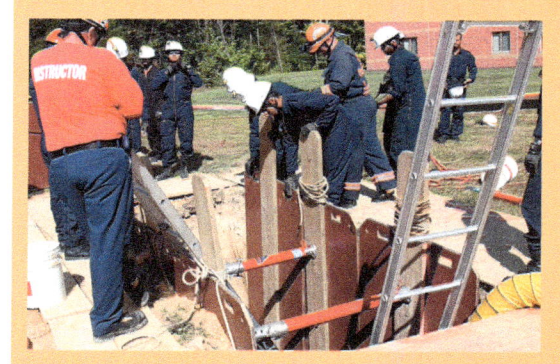

It is best to develop general guidelines that identify the types of incidents to which the safety officer will likely respond. Courtesy of MFRI Archives.

INTRODUCTION

This chapter covers many of the topics with which an EMS safety officer will be concerned. However, it is by no means all inclusive. Any incident can result in safety compromise, and care should be taken to ensure scene safety every time. Note that safety officers generally go to major incidents only, so every person in your organization must be thoroughly trained in safety.

STREET AND ROADWAY SCENES

Other than medical calls at homes, street and roadway incidents are one type of incident to which EMS personnel respond on a frequent basis. In most cases such incidents are the most dangerous working environments for the EMS responder.

MANUAL ON UNIFORM TRAFFIC CONTROL DEVICES FOR STREETS AND HIGHWAYS

The **Manual on Uniform Traffic Control Devices (MUTCD) for Streets and Highways** (2003) addresses virtually every component of highway safety. The MUTCD is published by the Federal Highway Administration (FHWA) under 23 Code of Federal Regulations (CFR), Part 655, Subpart F. The MUTCD is the national standard for all traffic control devices installed on any street, highway, or bicycle trail open to public travel. The MUTCD defines the purpose of traffic control devices, as well as the principles for their use, and promotes highway safety and efficiency by providing for the orderly movement of all road users on streets and highways throughout the nation. Traffic control devices notify road users of regulations and provide warning and guidance needed for the reasonably safe, uniform, and efficient operation of all elements of the traffic stream.

THE CHALLENGE

The number of firefighters struck and killed by motor vehicles has dramatically increased within recent years. During the 5-year period between 1995 and 1999, 17 firefighters were struck and killed by motorists. This represents an 89% increase in the number of line-of-duty deaths over the previous 5-year period (between 1990 and 1994), when 9 firefighters were struck and killed by motor vehicles (National Institute for Occupational Safety and Health [NIOSH], 2001). Struck-by incidents, where passing motorists hit responders, are on the rise. In 2005, NIOSH reported 390 workers of all kinds were killed in struck-by incidents, up from 278 in 2004. That year, struck-by incidents accounted for 7% of the total number of occupational injuries (NTIM, 2005).

This may be because of more traffic or inattentiveness of other drivers due to eating, drinking, smoking, reading, cell-phone use, radio or stereos blaring, applying makeup, and even using a computer. Perhaps it could be the inattentiveness of the emergency responders who are focused solely on the incident, lost in the potential crisis, sidetracked by other thoughts, or not thinking about the big picture. Maybe other drivers cannot even see EMS personnel. The long and short of this is that the cause is most likely a combination of all of these issues.

Safe positioning while operating in or near moving traffic is essential to responder safety. It should be the policy of the EMS organization to have emergency vehicle (EV) drivers position EVs at a vehicle-related incident on any street, road, highway, or expressway in a manner that best protects the incident scene and the work area. Such positioning must afford protection from the hazards of working in or near moving traffic to EMS personnel, fire service personnel, law enforcement officers, tow service operators, and the motoring public.

Always consider moving vehicles a threat to personnel safety. At every vehicle-related emergency scene, responders are exposed to passing motorists of varying driving abilities. Approaching vehicles may be driven at speeds from a creeping pace to well beyond the posted speed limit. Some of these vehicle operators may be vision impaired, under the influence of alcohol and/or drugs, or have a medical condition that affects their judgment or abilities. In addition, motorists may be completely oblivious to EMS presence due to distractions caused by cell phone use, loud music, conversation, inclement weather, and terrain or building obstructions. Approaching motorists often will be looking at the scene and not the roadway in front of them. Assume that all approaching traffic is out to get emergency responders until proven otherwise.

Nighttime incidents requiring personnel to work in or near moving traffic are particularly hazardous. Visibility is reduced and driver reaction time to hazards in the roadway is slowed.

SAFETY

All emergency personnel are at great risk of injury or death while operating in or near moving traffic. Remember to follow the specific tactical procedures that should be taken to protect all crew members who approach and arrive on scene. The following are guidelines for safe parking of EVs when operating in or near moving traffic:

- Always position first-arriving apparatus to protect the scene, patients, and emergency personnel.
- Initial apparatus placement should provide a work area protected from traffic approaching in at least one direction.

- Angle apparatus on the roadway with a "block to the left" or a "block to the right" to create a physical barrier between the crash scene and approaching traffic.
- Allow apparatus placement to slow approaching motorists and redirect them around the scene.
- Use fire apparatus, if available, to block at least one additional traffic lane more than that already obstructed by the crashed vehicle(s).

Positioning of large apparatus must create a safe parking area for EMS units and other EVs. Operating personnel, equipment, and patients should be kept at all times within the "shadow" created by the blocking apparatus.

When blocking with apparatus to protect the emergency scene, establish a work zone of sufficient size that includes all damaged vehicles, roadway debris, patient triage and treatment area, extrication work area, personnel and tool staging area, and ambulance loading zone.

Ambulances should be positioned within the protected work area with their rear patient loading door area angled away from the nearest lanes of moving traffic.

Unneeded EVs should be staged off the roadway or should be returned to service whenever possible.

At all intersections or where the incident may be near the middle lane of the roadway, two or more sides of the incident must be protected.
- *Traffic control.* Consider requesting police response. Provide specific directions to the police dispatch as to exactly what the traffic control needs are.
- *Police vehicles.* These must be strategically positioned to expand the initial safe work zone for traffic approaching from opposing directions. The goal is to effectively block all exposed sides of the work zone. The blocking of the work zone must be prioritized, from the most critical or highest traffic volume flow to the least critical traffic direction.
- *Fire engine or truck companies.* For vehicles arriving first where a charged hose line may be needed, block so that the pump panel is downstream—that is, on the opposite side of oncoming traffic. This will protect the pump operator.

Traffic cones must be deployed from the rear of the blocking apparatus toward approaching traffic to increase the advance warning provided for approaching motorists. Cones identify and only suggest the transition and tapering actions that are required of the approaching motorist.

Personnel shall place cones and flares and retrieve cones while facing oncoming traffic.

Traffic cones must be deployed at 15-foot intervals upstream of the blocking apparatus with the farthest traffic cone approximately 75 feet upstream to allow adequate advance warning to drivers.

Additional traffic cones, when available, can in many instances be retrieved from police units to extend the advance warning area for approaching motorists.

COMMAND AND CONTROL

After the first arriving supervisor and/or the incident commander have ensured that EVs are parked safely (as described above), he is to continue to act as the EMS safety officer until this assignment has been delegated to the EMS safety officer who arrives on the scene. Then the next steps are to ensure a safe and protected work environment for all EMS personnel, their patients, and of course the ambulance:

Assign a parking location for all ambulances as well as later-arriving apparatus.
- Directions "right" and "left" must be identified as from the approaching motorist's point of view.

- Lanes of traffic must be identified numerically as Lane 1, Lane 2, and so on, beginning from the right to the left when right and left are considered from the approaching motorist's point of view. Typically, vehicles travel a lower speed in the lower numbered lanes.
- Instruct the driver of the ambulance to "block to the right" or "block to the left" as it is parked at the scene to position the rear patient loading area away from the closest lane of moving traffic.

Ensure that all ambulances on scene are placed within the protected work area (shadow) of the larger apparatus.

Ensure that loading of all patients into EMS units is done from within the protected work zone.

If the vehicle is equipped with an Opticom strobe system, be sure it is turned OFF and that other emergency lighting remains ON.

At residential medical emergencies, ambulances must park at the curb nearest to the residence for safe patient loading whenever possible.

PERSONNEL FUNCTIONS

The following are guidelines for safe actions for individual personnel when operating in or near moving vehicle traffic:

- Always maintain an acute awareness of the high risk of working in or near moving traffic.
- Personnel should always look before they move!
- Never trust moving traffic. Keep an eye on it. That means personnel should never turn their back on traffic!
- Personnel arriving in crew cabs of apparatus should exit and enter the apparatus from the protected shadow side, away from moving traffic if at all possible.
- Supervisors, vehicle operators, and all ambulance personnel must exit and enter their units with extreme caution, remaining alert to moving traffic at all times.
- Protective clothing, a **Class III safety vest**, and a helmet must be donned prior to exiting the EV—during normal daylight conditions, dusk-to-dawn operations, and when ambient lighting is reduced due to inclement weather.
- Always look before opening doors and stepping out of an EV into any areas of moving traffic. When walking around the EV, personnel must be alert to the proximity of moving traffic.
  - Stop at the corner of the unit, check for traffic, and then proceed along the unit, remaining as close to the EV as possible.
  - Maintain a **reduced profile** when moving through any area where a minimum **buffer zone** exists.
- Law enforcement personnel may place traffic cones or flares at the scene to direct traffic. This action builds on initial ambulance cone deployment and can be expanded, if needed, as more police officers arrive. Always place and retrieve cones while facing oncoming traffic.
- Placing flares, where safe to do so, adjacent to and in combination with traffic cones for nighttime operations, greatly enhances scene safety. Where safe and appropriate to do so, place warning flares to slow and direct approaching traffic.

LIMITED ACCESS HIGHWAY OPERATIONS

Limited access highways include the expressways, tollways, and multilane roadways within the response area. Law enforcement and the Department of Transportation (DOT) have a desire to keep the traffic moving on these high-volume thoroughfares. When in the judgment of command it becomes essential for the safety of operating personnel and patients involved, any or all lanes, shoulders, and entry/exit ramps of these limited-access highways may be completely shut down. This, however, should occur rarely and should be for as short a period of time as practical.

Best Practices

One emergency-service insurance company has identified ten specific areas to which emergency responders should pay particular attention when operating on roadway/highway incidents.

Ten Cones of Highway Incident Safety

- There is no substitute for training.
- Multiagency coordination and communications are a must. A unified incident command is essential.
- Limit your exposure, limit your time.
- Give traffic plenty of warning.
- Protect the scene with apparatus.
- Always work away from the traffic.
- Be prepared to shut down the roadway.
- Be seen and not hurt.
- Dress for the occasion.
- Accountability matters.

Source: VFIS, 2004.

TRAFFIC CONES

Cones must be predominantly orange and made of a material that can be struck without causing damage to the impacting vehicle. The MUTCD outlines cone applications with details (FHWA, 2012):

- For daytime and low-speed roadways, cones should be no smaller than 450 mm (18 inches) in height (Figure 7.1).
- For freeways and other high-speed roads or at night on all highways or when more conspicuous guidance is needed, cones should be a minimum of 700 mm (28 inches) in height.
- For nighttime use, cones should be **retroreflectorized** or equipped with lighting devices for maximum visibility.

Retroreflectorization of 700 mm (28 inches) or larger cones should be provided by a white band 150 mm (6 inches) wide, located 75 to 100 mm (3 to 4 inches) from the top of the cone, with an additional 100 mm (4 inches) wide white band approximately 50 mm (2 inches) below the 150 mm (6 inches) band.

Cone tapering is also referenced by the MUTCD (FHWA, 2012): "One lane taper should have a 100-foot taper with cones placed at 10–20 feet apart. Downstream tapers should have 100 feet per lane with cones placed at 10–20 feet apart."

According to the MUTCD, an advanced warning sign should be placed 4 to 8 times the speed limit in miles per hour (mph) on

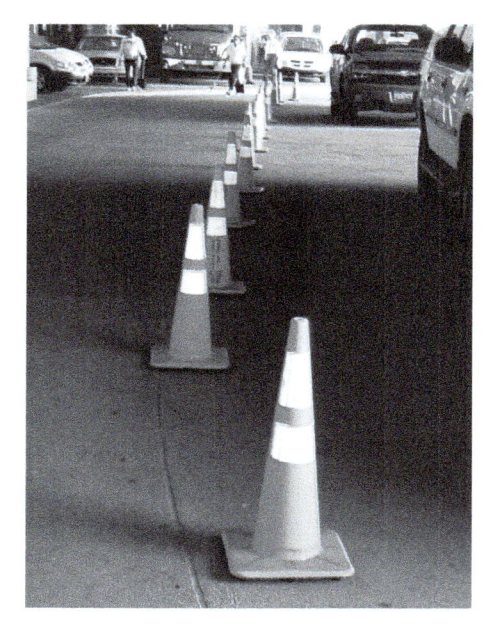

FIGURE 7.1 ■ Traffic cones should be set up to establish a safety zone at highway incidents.
Courtesy of Richard W. Patrick. (All rights reserved.)

TABLE 7.1 ■ Suggested Advance Warning Sign Spacing

	Distance Between Signs**		
	A	B	C
Road Type	Meters (feet)	Meters (feet)	Meters (feet)
Urban (low speed)*	30 (100)	30 (100)	30 (100)
Urban (high speed)*	100 (350)	100 (350)	100 (350)
Rural	150 (500)	150 (500)	150 (500)
Expressway/Freeway	300 (1,000)	450 (1,500)	800 (2,640)

* Speed category to be determined by highway agency.

** The A dimension is the distance from the transition or point of restriction to the first sign. The B dimension is the distance between the first and second signs. The C dimension is the distance between the second and third signs. (The third sign is the first one in a three-sign series encountered by a driver approaching a temporary traffic control [TTC] zone.)

Source: FHWA, 2012, Chapter 6C.

expressways and freeways at 0.5 mile, and 8 to 12 times the speed limit in mph in rural areas (Table 7.1). The second advanced warning sign should be placed at 100 feet in low-speed urban areas, 350 feet in high-speed urban areas, 1,500 feet on expressways and freeways, and 500 feet in rural areas.

Buffer areas should consist of 30 mph, 625 feet; 40 mph, 825 feet; 50 mph, 1,000 feet; 60 mph, 1,300 feet; and 70 mph, 1,450 feet.

PERSONAL PROTECTIVE EQUIPMENT

ANSI/ISEA Standard 207-2006 specifies the minimum amount of fabric and reflective materials to be placed on safety garments that are worn by personnel near vehicular traffic. This standard is now the most commonly used standard associated with safety vests.

Personnel visibility is critical during highway operations, especially at night. Dawn, dusk, and inclement weather compromises visibility and increases the risk of personnel being struck. It is imperative that personnel be visible as an individual among the flashing lights and other apparatus. Properly donned apparel is essential for provider safety. The MUTCD identifies specific reflective vest requirements, which represent the most visible attributes.

Use reflective vests to increase personnel visibility, regardless of the use of personal protective equipment (PPE). The reflective vests used by emergency personnel should have both retroreflective and fluorescent properties. **Retroreflective material** returns the majority of light from the light source back to the observer. Fluorescent material absorbs UV light of a certain wavelength and regenerates it into visual energy. The apparel background (outer) material should be either fluorescent orange-red or fluorescent yellow-green as defined in the ANSI/ISEA Standard 207-2006. The retroreflective material color should be orange, yellow, white, silver, and yellow-green, or a fluorescent version of any of these colors, and must be visible at a minimum distance of 300 meters (1,000 feet). The retroreflective safety apparel must be designed to clearly identify the wearer as a person.

SCENE LIGHTING

According to the FEMA-USFA Emergency Vehicle Safety Initiative (FEMA-USFA, 2004), emergency-vehicle lighting, although important, provides warning only and provides no effective traffic control. It is often confusing to road users, especially at night. In fact, road users approaching the traffic incident from the opposite direction on a divided facility are often distracted by emergency-vehicle lighting and slow their vehicles to look at the traffic incident, which poses a hazard to themselves and others traveling in the same direction.

Scene lighting should be directed at illuminating the functioning portion of the incident. Ideally, high-level lighting directed down on the operation is best. When traffic around the scene is considered secure, forward-facing headlights should be turned off. Limiting the number of flashing red lights is also recommended. This reduction of emergency lighting can be helpful, as strobes and red flashing lights can blind, attract, or confuse the public. The use of amber lights, arrow boards, arrow sticks, message boards, and police vehicles is generally effective in slowing traffic. The use of overhead lighting to illuminate the scene is preferable when visibility is limited.

Always expect the unexpected. When the incident is mitigated, the incident commander or EMS crew chief must limit time on scene. Incident termination can be as dangerous as any component of the operation. Limiting scene time reduces exposure. Emergency responders should be accounted for and then placed in available status as soon as possible. Cones and signage should be removed in the reverse order of how they were set up. Start at the incident scene and work in reverse until the last warning device is secured. This is a very dangerous task, and traffic must remain under control until the last cone is picked up and all emergency responders have left the scene.

Several emergency service organizations (ESOs) use directional arrows on the rear light bar of vehicles and then turn off headlights while leaving rotators and flashing beacons on while operating at highway incidents. When floodlights are used, they are raised to a height that allows light to be directed down on the scene.

The MUTCD policy for highway marking distances for a working incident zone (300 feet when light, 500 feet when dark) is based on vision and distance changes at night. The policy also identifies the minimum requirements for the work zone. The incident commander or EMS safety officer can adjust these distances, request additional units for protection, and block the entire road as dictated by existing conditions.

The "best" light color(s) and lighting pattern for highway operations is still being debated. Dr. Stephen Solomon, an ophthalmologist who has studied EV colors and lighting, notes that the philosophy has been to attract as much attention as possible through a combination of lights and light colors with varying degrees of reflection and flashes. Strong stimuli hold central gaze and drivers tend to steer in the direction of gaze. If fatigue, alcohol, or drugs impair the driver, the potential and degree of drift increase. He suggests this practice actually makes the vehicle a "visual magnetic target." He recommends reducing the time span of looking toward a complex flashing light display by reducing the number; brightness and array of color; revolving strobe; and reflecting lights during emergency travel, and using either filament bulbs in one or two amber flashers (mounted on the upper level of the vehicle on each corner) blinking in tandem or revolving beacons when the vehicle is parked along the road or at a curb and clear of all active traffic lanes (Solomon and King, 1995).

Drivers should extinguish forward-facing EV lighting. This is very important on divided roadways. This will help reduce distractions and glare for oncoming drivers. The headlights on the EV can temporarily blind approaching drivers, resulting in the problem of glare recovery. It takes at least 6 seconds, going from light to dark, and 3 seconds from dark to light for vision to recover.

CHAPTER 7 Scene Operations **151**

Responders should consider as much as possible the reduction of lighting at the scene. Establish good traffic control, including placement of advance warning signs and traffic control devices to divert or detour traffic. This will allow responders to reduce EV lighting. This is especially true for major traffic incidents that might involve a number of EVs.

Multiple EMS studies have shown, with the exception of a few conditions, no statistically significant difference in patient outcomes with emergency driving on ambulances versus nonemergency driving. The St. Louis Fire Department found responding without lights and sirens to calls that did not involve risk of property or life reduced by 62% its crash rate and by 81% the number of injuries (Ludwig, 2002). Commercial dispatch programs are available for priority dispatching, such as the National Academies of Emergency Dispatch (NAEMD) and the Association of Public-Safety Communications Officials (APCO), to help in the reduction of lights and siren responses.

EMERGENCY VEHICLE MARKINGS

Striping the rear of ambulances and EVs with fluorescent material in a herringbone pattern improves driver recognition while the apparatus is on the roadways. Vehicles should have high visibility. Contrasting colors can add to this effect. These factors are not highly dependent on driver behavior.

BUILDING FIRES

The EMS safety officer may not be responsible for the overall safety at the scene of a building fire (Figure 7.2). In most fire departments an assigned individual is the safety officer.

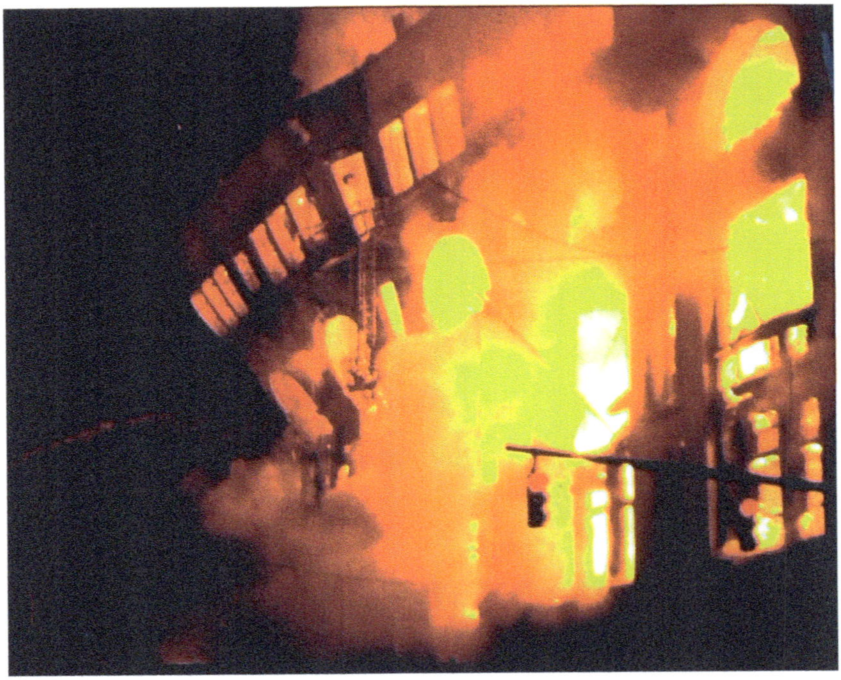

FIGURE 7.2 ■ EMS safety officers may have a variety of responsibilities at the scene of a building fire. *Courtesy of MFRI Archives.*

Depending on the circumstances, the designated safety officer for fire-related events may not arrive on the scene initially or may have a delayed response. EMS personnel may not have any responsibilities on the scene of a building fire; however, there may be instances when they may call on personnel to assist. Regardless, it is always good to know a little about the scene of a building fire and what is happening. In many instances, EMS personnel may have firefighting experience that will aid if ever called on to serve in this capacity.

FORECASTING TOOLS

Certain tools can assist in **forecasting** what may happen at the scene of a building fire. This ability is developed from a well-rounded education, training on building fires, and experience.

Features of the Fire Building

The fire building has a number of features that must be taken into consideration. These include means of access to the interior, floor plans, and utilities (Figure 7.3). There is

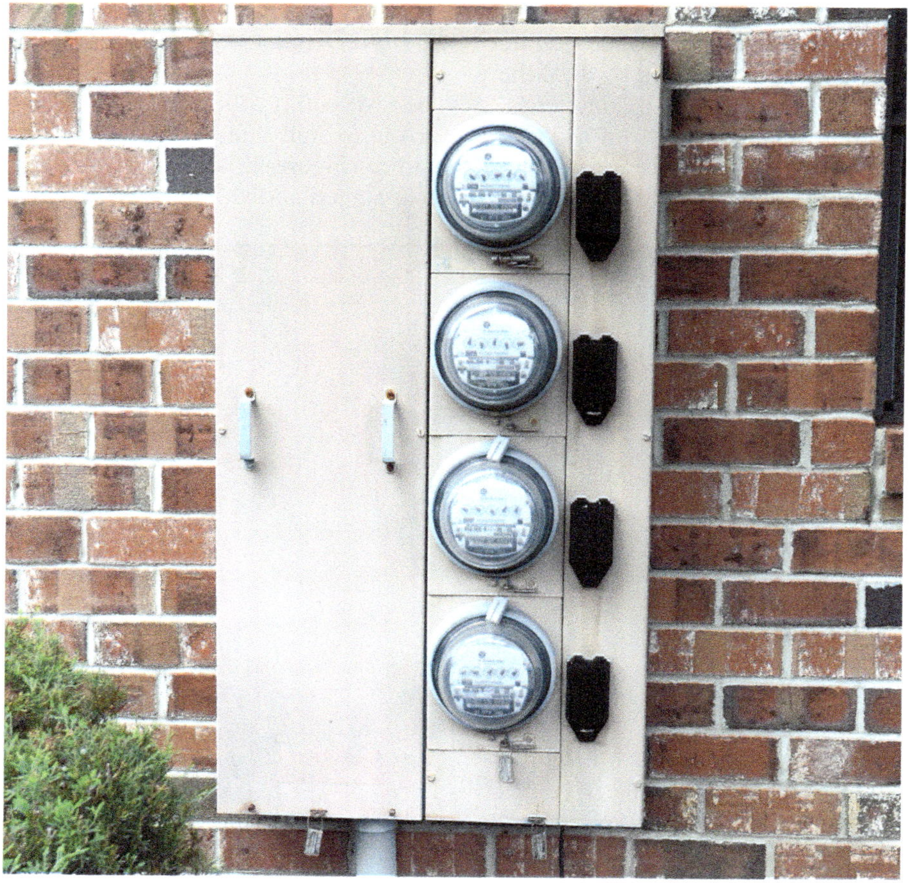

FIGURE 7.3 ■ It is a good idea to establish where the utilities come into a building. Although personnel should never pull an electric meter, shutting off the utilities to the building is a good practice. *Courtesy of Damian Moosang.*

a large proportion of EMS calls compared to fire calls, so EMS personnel probably access buildings more frequently than other emergency personnel. Therefore, EMS responders are more apt to be familiar with the inside of a building. This may include alternative means of entry, how to find one's way through a mazelike interior, and the location(s) of utility shutoff valves and switches. If your personnel are familiar with the interior layout of the fire building, they should convey this to the incident commander.

Access for Crews

Access to the building may be an issue for emergency personnel. Depending on the size and the occupancy of the building, access may be limited or may have numerous access points. In either case, it can present issues for personnel and their safety. As the EMS safety officer, it is important to recognize which entry points emergency service personnel access. It also may be critical to understand optional access points should crews need them. As noted previously, EMS may have an advantage in knowing access points that may not be readily visible or recognized by others.

Egress for Crews

Firefighters may enter a building and get disoriented. A fire on the 22nd floor of the 38-story Meridian Bank Building, also known as One Meridian Plaza, was reported to the Philadelphia Fire Department on February 23, 1991, at approximately 2040 hours. It burned for more than 19 hours. The fire caused three firefighter fatalities and injuries to 24 firefighters. The 12 alarms brought 51 engine companies, 15 ladder companies, 11 specialized units, and over 300 firefighters to the scene. It was the largest high-rise office building fire in modern U.S. history—completely consuming eight floors of the building—and was controlled only when it reached a floor that was protected by automatic sprinklers. Rescue crews were airlifted to the roof via a medical helicopter to assist with the rescue of the lost firefighters. When conditions reached the point that the mission had to be stopped, a medical helicopter was used to search the exterior of the building.

EMS personnel may be called to assist in many ways at the scene of a building fire. They must understand the procedures and inherent dangers when so called.

Construction Type

There are a variety of ways to build a structure. EMS personnel do not necessarily need to know every type of building construction. However, a basic understanding may be beneficial. Whether working at the scene of a building fire or operating at other incidents involving a structure, knowing the construction type may actually save a life. It takes time to learn the various types of construction, and entire courses and texts are devoted to construction types. It is recommended that EMS safety officers take a building construction course and provide the training to EMS personnel so they have a baseline understanding of building construction. This class will also be of benefit in gaining an understanding of the safety issues related to structure collapses.

Age of the Building

Another useful tool in forecasting fire behavior at a building fire is the age of the building. An older building may not have as many egresses as a newer building and may show signs of structural weakness prior to the fire. However, a new building can collapse as quickly as an old one. The construction of older buildings tends to be much different than in newer buildings. For example, newer buildings tend to have been constructed with lighter-weight materials.

Four Attributes of Smoke

The four attributes of smoke are color, thickness, pressure, and amount. It is good idea for the EMS safety officer to understand all four and how they relate to what is occurring on the fireground. Entire classes are devoted to reading smoke and the information about fire it can provide. Here is a very brief overview of what the attributes can tell you:

Color. The color of the smoke denotes the stage of burning. A black or dark smoke typically indicates that the fire is burning without any impingement. When water is applied to the fire, typically the smoke becomes lighter in color to almost a white hue. Various chemicals and chemical components may emit a colorful smoke. Smoke will also depict the location of the fire.

Thickness. The thickness of the smoke is the most important attribute. It illustrates the quality of burning. It also denotes the continuity of what is burning. If the smoke is dense, it typically illustrates an abundant source of materials available to burn.

Pressure. The pressure or force with which the smoke is emitting from the building will indicate the volume or heat associated with the fire. It also helps to determine the intensity of the fire. Typically the greatest pressure will be where the fire is most intense.

Amount. The volume of smoke typically indicates how much fuel is burning. If there is a heavy fire load or a buildup of smoke prior to its release, you will typically see a large volume of smoke.

FUNCTIONING AT BUILDING FIRES

EMS personnel may have limited roles at the scene of a building fire. Typically, it depends on the relationship the EMS agency has with the fire department. In some instances, EMS may be an integral part of the fire department and have a more active role. In other instances, this will not be the case. Regardless, the more EMS personnel understand about the happenings at the scene of a building fire, the better chance they have of assisting effectively and safely for everyone.

The fire service has adopted the slogan "Everyone Goes Home." EMS should embrace the same slogan and work together with all agencies to make sure everyone goes home at the end of their shift.

WILDLAND FIRE OPERATIONS

EMS personnel may be called to stand by at wildland fires, which have become more prevalent and have grown in magnitude in the western states. The southern states also have seen an increase in wildland fires. With the increase of fires and the urban-wildland interface growing, the potential for medical incidents at these incidents has also increased.

Over the past several years, there have been incidents and near misses in various parts of the country involving wildland fire personnel and equipment. They include serious injuries sustained by firefighters during a fire burnover in Nevada; two fire shelter deployment incidents in California, with one including the loss of vehicles; an entrapment situation in Montana involving three vehicles and seven people, without injuries; one air tanker, two single-engine air tankers (SEATs), and one helicopter being damaged while working on fires, without fatalities.

We know what kills firefighters on wildland fire operations; the causes of death do not change over time, just the numbers of people. We also know the mitigations for these hazards:

- Aviation operations
- Vehicular incidents
- Heart attacks

- Burnovers
- Human factors

There have not been any studies or data to show any injuries or deaths to EMS personnel at the scene of wildland fires. Regardless, EMS personnel must heed the causes of firefighter death because both specialties work at wildland fire incidents. EMS personnel must function within the incident command system (ICS) like any other incident. When at a large wildland incident, you may find there will be multiple agencies involved (Figure 7.4). An individual from the forestry service or other agency may be assigned to the EMS sector to serve in a variety of capacities. For example, he may be assigned as the logistic person for EMS.

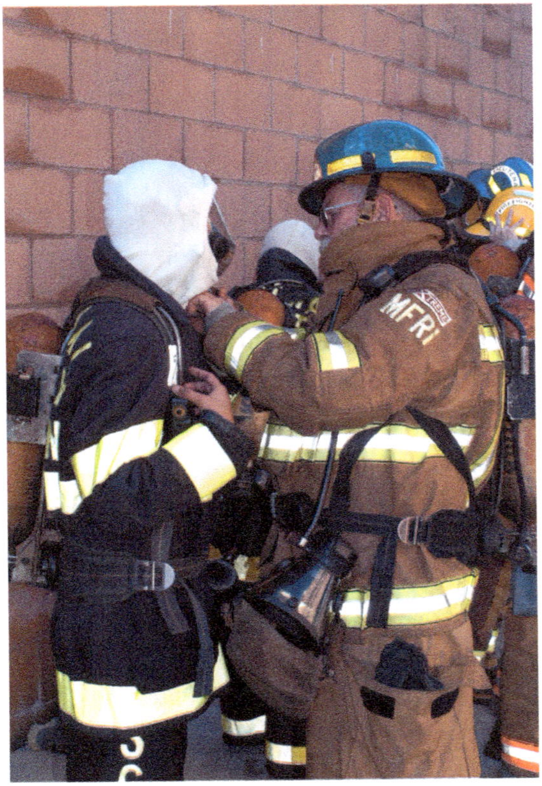

INFECTIOUS DISEASE

Infectious diseases are a universal issue and can be discussed in great length. Depending on the size of the organization, the EMS safety officer of the organization may also act as the infectious disease officer. In many instances this is a common practice.

OSHA created Bloodborne Standard 1910.1030 to provide guidance to implementing an infectious disease program. As part of the safety of all personnel, this standard should be followed by all EMS organizations. OSHA standard 1910.1030 is looked on as the standard in the industry for **bloodborne pathogens**. The first step is to create an exposure control plan, an often neglected component of the standard among EMS organizations.

EXPOSURE CONTROL PLAN

Each EMS organization must establish a written exposure control plan designed to eliminate or minimize personnel exposure. The exposure control plan should contain at minimum all of the following elements:

- Exposure determination
- Methods of compliance
- Hepatitis B vaccination policy and procedures for evaluation of follow-up of exposure incidents
- Employee training
- Record-keeping procedures

The plan must be made available and accessible to all members of the organization. The exposure control plan must be reviewed and updated at least annually and whenever necessary to reflect new or modified tasks and procedures that affect occupational exposure and new or revised personnel tasks and positions. The review and update of such plans

FIGURE 7.4 ■ EMS may take on different roles at the scene of the fire, depending on the relationship with the fire department. *Courtesy of MFRI Archives.*

should also reflect changes in technology that eliminate or reduce exposure to bloodborne pathogens. The plan also should require annual documentation of the consideration and implementation of appropriate commercially available, effective, and safer medical devices designed to eliminate or minimize occupational exposure.

Input regarding the identification, evaluation, and selection of effective engineering and work practice controls should be solicited from nonmanagerial personnel responsible for direct patient care who are potentially exposed to injuries from **contaminated sharps**. This must be documented in the exposure control plan.

Exposure Determination

Each EMS organization must prepare an exposure determination, which should contain the following:

- A list of all job classifications in which all personnel in those job classifications have occupational exposure
- A list of job classifications in which some personnel have occupational exposure
- A list of all tasks and procedures or groups of closely related tasks and procedures in which occupational exposure occurs

Any and all exposures should be counted, even those in which EMS personnel are wearing PPE to protect them from contact with pathogens.

Methods of Compliance

Universal precautions are to be observed to prevent contact with blood or other potentially infectious materials. Under circumstances in which differentiation of body fluid types is difficult or impossible, all body fluids are to be considered potentially infectious materials. There are a variety of ways to prevent contact, including the use of engineering and work practice controls, PPE, housekeeping practices, and regulated waste disposal.

Engineering and Work Practice Controls.

Engineering and work practice controls should be used to eliminate or minimize personnel exposure. Where exposure remains after these controls have been implemented, PPE also should be used. Engineering controls must be examined and maintained or replaced on a regular schedule to ensure their effectiveness.

EMS organizations should provide handwashing facilities that are readily accessible to all personnel. When that is not feasible, either an appropriate antiseptic hand cleanser in conjunction with clean cloth or paper towels, or antiseptic towelettes, should be provided. Note that when antiseptic hand cleansers or towelettes are used, hands also must be washed with soap and running water as soon as feasible.

EMS personnel should always wash their hands immediately or as soon as possible after removal of gloves or other PPE. In addition, they must wash their hands and any other skin with soap and water, or flush mucous membranes with water immediately or as soon as feasible following contact with blood or other potentially infectious materials.

Shearing or breaking of contaminated needles is prohibited. Contaminated needles and other contaminated sharps are not be bent, recapped, or removed unless the EMS organization can demonstrate that no alternative is feasible or that such action is required by a specific medical procedure. According to OSHA Bloodborne Standard 1910.1030, such bending, recapping, or needle removal must be accomplished through the use of a mechanical device or a one-handed technique that the standard provides.

Immediately or as soon as possible after use, contaminated reusable sharps are to be placed in appropriate containers until properly reprocessed. These containers are to be puncture resistant, labeled or color-coded in accordance with this standard, leakproof on the sides and bottom, and in accordance with the requirements set forth by OSHA Bloodborne Standard 1910.1030 for reusable sharps.

Eating, drinking, smoking, applying cosmetics or lip balm, and handling contact lenses all are prohibited in work areas where there is a reasonable likelihood of occupational exposure. Most agencies have adapted to this portion of the standard by prohibiting such actions in the back of the ambulance. Depending on the type of ambulance, these may be done in the cab of the ambulance. Make sure there is a clear delineation of the expectation defined in OSHA Bloodborne Standard 1910.1030. Food and drink are not to be kept in refrigerators, freezers, shelves, cabinets, or on countertops or benchtops where blood or other potentially infectious materials are present. This means that there must be a clear separation in EMS stations.

A separate area also should be designated for cleaning of equipment and medical equipment that has been potentially covered with infectious materials. This is not allowed in any part of the living quarters.

All procedures involving blood or other potentially infectious materials are to be performed in such a manner as to minimize splashing, spraying, spattering, and generation of droplets of these substances. Mouth pipetting/suctioning of blood or other potentially infectious materials is prohibited.

Personal Protective Equipment. When there is occupational exposure, the EMS organization must provide, at no cost to personnel, appropriate PPE, such as but not limited to gloves, gowns, laboratory coats, face shields or masks and eye protection, mouthpieces, resuscitation bags, pocket masks, or other ventilation devices. PPE is considered appropriate only if it does not permit blood or other potentially infectious materials to pass through or reach the responder's clothes, street clothes, undergarments, skin, eyes, mouth, or other mucous membranes under normal conditions of use and for the time during which the PPE will be used.

All personnel must use appropriate PPE unless the organization shows that someone temporarily and briefly declined to use PPE when, under rare and extraordinary circumstances, it was the EMS provider's professional judgment that in the specific instance its use would have prevented the delivery of health care or public safety services or would have posed an increased hazard to the safety of the worker or co-worker. When the provider makes this judgment, the circumstances are to be investigated and documented in order to determine whether or not changes can be instituted to prevent such occurrences in the future.

The EMS organization must ensure that appropriate PPE in the appropriate sizes is readily accessible at the worksite or is issued to members. Hypoallergenic gloves, glove liners, powderless gloves, or other similar alternatives are to be readily accessible to those who are allergic to the gloves normally provided. The EMS organization is to clean, launder, and dispose of PPE at no cost to personnel, and to repair or replace PPE as needed to maintain its effectiveness, at no cost to personnel.

Gloves are to be worn when it can be reasonably anticipated that personnel may have hand contact with blood, other potentially infectious materials, mucous membranes, and nonintact skin; when performing vascular access procedures; and when handling or touching contaminated items or surfaces. This part of the standard has drawn some controversy. When OSHA Bloodborne Standard 1910.1030 was implemented, it was difficult to get personnel to wear gloves. Many

EMS organizations implemented a policy that stated personnel would wear gloves on all calls. The standard was never intended for personnel to wear gloves on every patient contact, but rather only on those calls that had or had a potential of infectious materials. Kathy West (West, 2009), a leading expert in infectious diseases, encourages EMS organizations to reevaluate the use of gloves and comply with the standard.

Masks in combination with eye protection devices, such as goggles or glasses with solid side shields or chin-length face shields, are to be worn whenever splashes, spray, spatter, or droplets of blood or other potentially infectious materials may be generated and eye, nose, or mouth contamination can be reasonably anticipated.

Appropriate protective clothing such as, but not limited to, gowns, aprons, lab coats, clinic jackets, shoe coverings, or similar outer garments are to be worn in occupational exposure situations. The type and characteristics will depend on the task and degree of exposure anticipated.

Housekeeping. As the EMS safety officer, you should ensure that the station and ambulances are maintained in a clean and sanitary condition by personnel. Determine and implement an appropriate written schedule for cleaning and method of **decontamination** based on the location within the facility, type of surface to be cleaned, type of soil present, and tasks or procedures being performed in the area. All equipment and environmental and working surfaces are to be cleaned and decontaminated after contact with blood or other potentially infectious materials.

According to OSHA Bloodborne Standard 1910.1030, contaminated work surfaces are to be decontaminated with an appropriate disinfectant after completion of procedures; immediately or as soon as feasible when surfaces are overtly contaminated or after any spill of blood or other potentially infectious materials; and at the end of the shift if the surface may have become contaminated since the last cleaning.

Protective coverings, such as plastic wrap, aluminum foil, or imperviously backed absorbent paper used to cover equipment and environmental surfaces are to be removed and replaced as soon as feasible when they become overtly contaminated or at the end of the shift if they may have become contaminated during the shift.

All bins, pails, cans, and similar receptacles intended for reuse and that have a reasonable likelihood for becoming contaminated with blood or other potentially infectious materials are to be inspected and decontaminated on a regularly scheduled basis and cleaned and decontaminated immediately or as soon as feasible upon visible contamination.

Regulated Waste. Contaminated sharps are to be discarded immediately or as soon as feasible in containers that are closable, puncture resistant, leakproof on sides and bottom, and labeled or color coded per OSHA Bloodborne Standard 1910.1030. During use, containers for contaminated sharps are to be easily accessible to personnel and located as close as is feasible to the immediate area where sharps are used or can be reasonably anticipated to be found, maintained upright throughout use, and replaced routinely and not allowed to overfill.

Disposal of all regulated waste must be in accordance with applicable regulations of the United States, states and territories, and political subdivisions of states and territories. Check with a local biohazard waste hauler for your area.

Hepatitis B Vaccination and Post-exposure Evaluation and Follow-up

According to OSHA Bloodborne Standard 1910.1030, the hepatitis B vaccine and vaccination series must be made available at no cost to all personnel who have occupational exposure. Post-exposure evaluation and follow-up also should be available at no cost to all personnel who have had an **exposure incident**. The EMS organization must ensure that all medical evaluations and procedures, including prophylaxis, are made available at no cost and at a reasonable time and place. They must be performed by or under the supervision of a licensed physician or by or under the supervision of another licensed healthcare professional, and provided according to recommendations of the U.S. Public Health Service current at the time the evaluations and procedures take place. The organization also must ensure that all laboratory tests are conducted by an accredited laboratory at no cost to personnel.

Hepatitis B Vaccination. The hepatitis B vaccination is to be made available after personnel have received the training required in OSHA Bloodborne Standard 1910.1030 and within 10 working days of initial assignment to all who have occupational exposure unless the individual previously received the complete hepatitis B vaccination series, antibody testing revealed that the individual is immune, or the vaccine is contraindicated for medical reasons. The organization is not to make participation in a prescreening program a prerequisite for receiving the hepatitis B vaccination.

If anyone in the organization initially declines the hepatitis B vaccination but at a later date decides to accept it, the organization has to make the vaccination available at that time. The organization must ensure that individuals who decline to accept the hepatitis B vaccination sign a declination statement.

Post-exposure Evaluation and Follow-up. OSHA Bloodborne Standard 1910.1030 requires that following a report of an exposure incident, you make immediately available to the exposed personnel a confidential medical evaluation and follow-up, including at least the following elements:

- Documentation of the route(s) of exposure, and the circumstances under which the exposure incident occurred
- Identification and documentation of the source individual, unless the organization can establish that identification is infeasible or prohibited by state or local law
- Testing of the source individual's blood as soon as feasible and after consent is obtained in order to determine HBV and HIV infectivity (If consent is not obtained, the organization must establish that legally required consent cannot be obtained. When the source individual's consent is not required by law, the source individual's blood, if available, is to be tested and the results documented. When the source individual is already known to be infected with HBV or HIV, testing for the source individual's known HBV or HIV status need not be repeated.)
- Results of the source individual's testing made available to the exposed personnel of the organization, and that personnel informed of applicable laws and regulations concerning disclosure of the identity and infectious status of the source individual
- If the individual consents to baseline blood collection, but does not give consent at that time for HIV serologic testing, the sample is to be preserved for at least 90 days. If, within 90 days of the exposure incident, the individual elects to have the baseline sample tested, such testing is to be done as soon as feasible.
- Post-exposure prophylaxis, when medically indicated, as recommended by the U.S. Public Health Service
- Counseling
- Evaluation of reported illnesses to determine if there are any connections with the exposure

Immunizations

Personnel should be offered other immunizations, including the annual influenza vaccine, and the 10-year pneumonia vaccine. In addition, the surge of new strains of influenza or other communicable diseases, such as H1N1, should be offered to personnel in order to provide the maximum protection to them. This will help reduce loss time from personnel being unavailable to function as an EMS provider. The EMS safety officer should stay current with the available vaccinations and encourage personnel to be immunized.

INFORMATION AND TRAINING

The EMS organization should make sure that all personnel with occupational exposure participate in a training program that must be provided at no cost to them during working hours (Figure 7.5). Training should be provided at the time of initial assignment to tasks where occupational exposure may take place and annually (beginning 1 year after previous training) thereafter. The EMS organization is to provide additional training for any change in the responsibilities of its personnel and when new tasks or procedures affect the occupational exposure of personnel.

Not only should the training program be accompanied by material appropriate in content and vocabulary to the educational level, literacy, and language of personnel; it must also contain at a minimum the following elements per OSHA Bloodborne Standard 1910.1030:

- An accessible copy of the regulatory text of this standard and an explanation of its contents
- A general explanation of the **epidemiology** and symptoms of bloodborne diseases

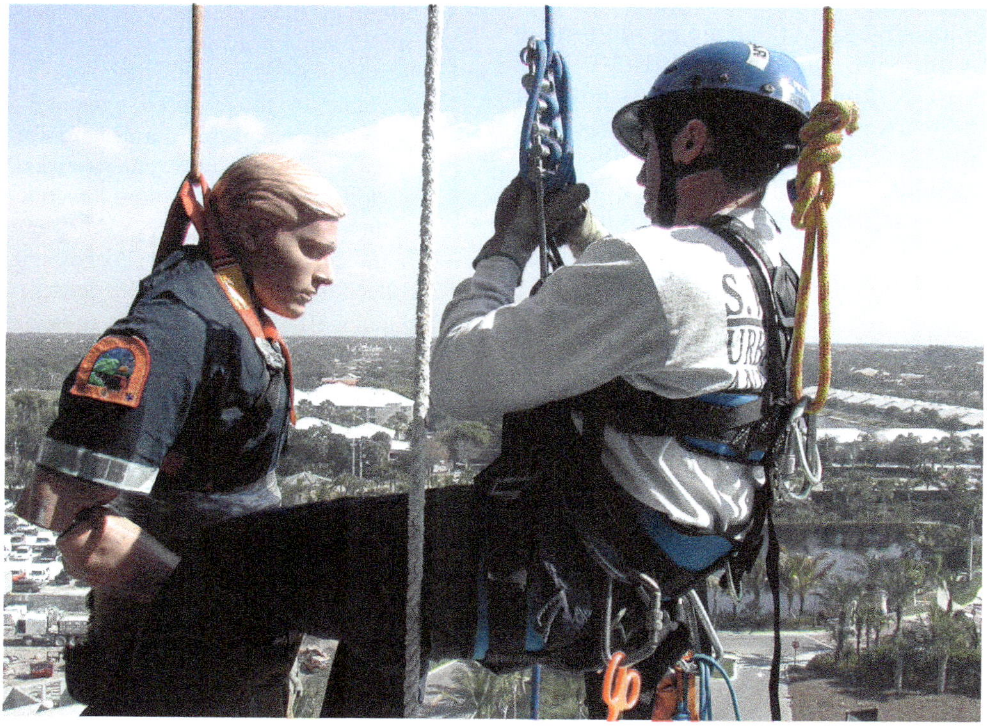

FIGURE 7.5 ■ Training must be provided to all members at no cost during working hours. *Courtesy of Estero Fire Rescue.*

- An explanation of the modes of transmission of bloodborne pathogens
- An explanation of the EMS organization's exposure control plan and the means by which personnel can obtain a copy of the written plan
- An explanation of the appropriate methods for recognizing tasks and other activities that may involve exposure to blood and other potentially infectious materials
- An explanation of the use and limitations of methods that will prevent or reduce exposure, including appropriate engineering controls, work practices, and PPE
- Information on the types, proper use, location, removal, handling, decontamination, and disposal of PPE
- An explanation of the basis for selection of PPE
- Information on the hepatitis B vaccine, including its efficacy, safety, method of administration, the benefits of being vaccinated, and that both the vaccine and vaccination are offered free of charge
- Information on the appropriate actions to take and persons to contact in an emergency involving blood or other potentially infectious materials
- An explanation of the procedure to follow if an exposure incident occurs, including the method of reporting the incident and the medical follow-up that will be made available
- Information on the post-exposure evaluation and follow-up that the organization is required to provide to personnel after an exposure incident
- An explanation of the signs and labels and/or color coding of biohazardous waste
- An opportunity for interactive questions and answers with the person conducting the training session

The person conducting the training must be knowledgeable in the subject matter covered by the elements contained in the training program as it relates to the environment that the training will address.

Stay current on the latest in infectious diseases. The Ryan White Act, Part G, is a provision for EMS personnel to be notified by hospitals or by other agencies when a patient was transported to their location with any of a variety of infectious diseases. Your designated officer for the organization should be familiar with this law.

Record keeping is not discussed in this chapter, although it is required. You can find the information regarding record keeping in Chapter 9.

PATIENT HANDLING

EMS work requires personnel to be able to lift patients. It is also one of the most frequent work events that causes injury. The well-being and fitness of EMS personnel is paramount. Emphasis must be placed on physical fitness and the ability to carry heavy bags or cases, suction units, ECG monitor-defibrillators, and other heavy and bulky equipment, in addition to lifting and moving patients of all sizes and shapes.

There also has been a dramatic increase in obesity in the United States. The implications of this trend for EMS are twofold: (1) heavier patients are often more difficult to lift safely; and (2) a growing trend of obesity in the United States suggests the possibility of a greater number of relatively immobile patients requiring EMS assistance.

Many different lifting and moving devices are used in EMS to get the patient from the location where they are found to their destination. These devices can present challenges in and of themselves, especially when going up or down steps, climbing or descending embankments, stepping off or up curbs, and traveling down narrow hallways (Figure 7.6).

Back strain leads the list of injuries sustained by EMS personnel. One group of researchers looked retrospectively at 254 injuries that occurred in 3½ years in a busy urban EMS system with a strict policy of job-related

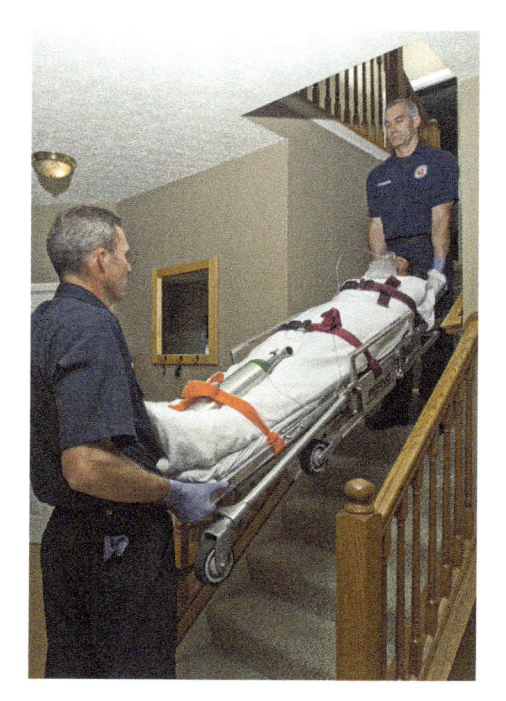

FIGURE 7.6 ■ EMS personnel face many different obstacles when carrying a patient from the scene.

injury reporting. An overwhelming majority, 36%, of injuries were back strains, all due to lifting. (The next most common injuries were nonspecific contusions at 7%, toxic effects of gases at 6%, and ankle sprains at 5%.) Back injury rates were significantly higher both in women and in EMT-Basics. Of 481 days for which compensation was paid, 375 (78%) were due to low back strain (Hogya and Ellis, 1990).

Another issue related to patient handling is dropping the patient. An estimated 28 million ambulance calls are received in the United States annually. Out of these, an estimated 42,000 patients are dropped. That equals 115 patients dropped every day, or one every 12 minutes. The frequency is actually relatively low; however, the severity of patient drops is rather significant according to one insurance company. On a 3-year average of insurance claims, for every 100 claims there were approximately 8 insurance claims involving a patient drop, in contrast with for every $100 of claims being paid out, $13 was paid for patient drops. This is considered a high frequency with a low severity rate (Lindsey, 2000).

CAUSES OF PATIENT DROPS

Causes of patient drops that are relevant to EMS include the following:

- Improper use of equipment
- Inadequate balance/strength
- Improper maintenance of equipment
- Equipment failure or malfunction
- Provider haste

Improper Use of Equipment

It was not too long ago that EMS used one type of stretcher from one manufacturer. Now, there are just about as many models of stretchers (and vendors) as there are models of cars. In addition, there are many types of lifting and moving devices for virtually every situation, yet there continues to be issues with patient drops and provider injuries. The most fundamental precaution is the proper training of personnel on the use of equipment. In some instances, personnel use the wrong piece of equipment for the situation. In other instances, the piece of equipment is the proper piece of equipment, but it is not used correctly.

Personnel should be trained on every piece of equipment. Before new equipment is placed into service, all personnel should be properly trained on how and when to use the device.

Improper Balance/Strength

Take a look around. Every individual is different. EMS crew members, too, are of different height, weight, and strength. Patients also vary in height and weight, and scene conditions can vary widely. There is no ideal situation. Part of the uniqueness of EMS is the challenges

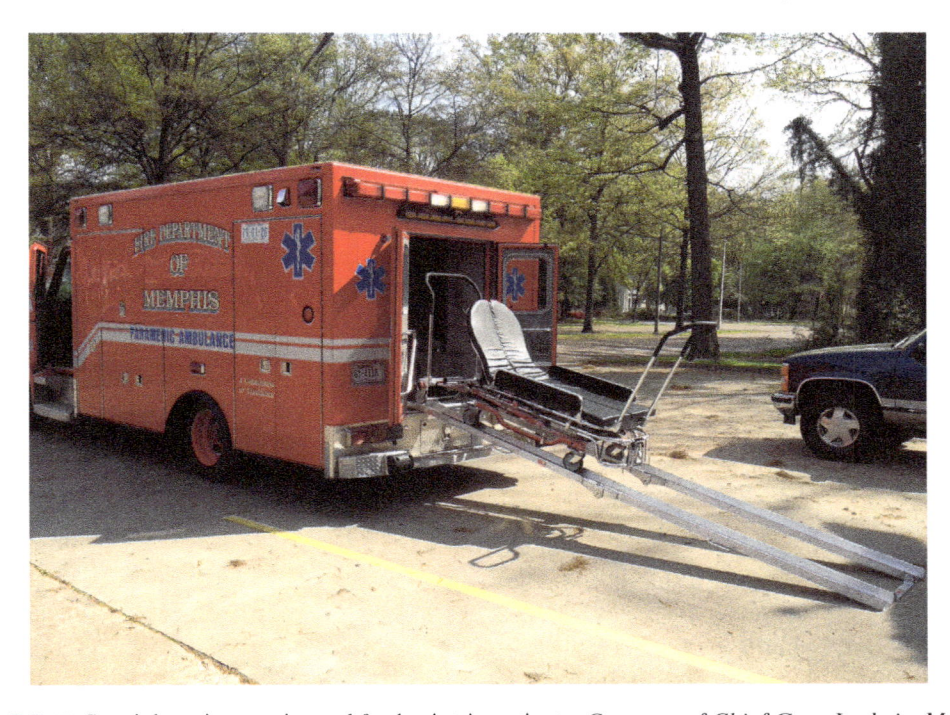

FIGURE 7.7 ■ Special equipment is used for bariatric patients. *Courtesy of Chief Gary Ludwig, Memphis Fire Department.*

it presents on virtually every call. However, every challenge can be overcome. When assigning crews, personnel should be matched to equal the team out as closely as possible. Team members should have compatible strength, height, and weight; this will allow for proper balancing and lifting of patient moving devices. However, the ideal match is not often possible. In these cases, personnel must understand how to offset the incompatibilities. In other words, if two individuals are of unequal height, and you are moving a patient down a set of stairs on a stair chair, you would want the taller person on the foot end of the stair chair to help offset the difference.

Another area of concern is, of course, the patient. Every patient is different. Equipment is designed for a set weight limit and can safely accommodate certain heights. Many agencies provide bariatric services and related equipment (Figure 7.7) for markedly obese patients. If a piece of equipment is used for a patient who it is not designed to handle, the EMS organization and personnel could be assuming liability. Personnel could also be subjected to serious injury. It is appropriate for personnel to call for additional lifting assistance when needed.

The other issue with balance is the type of terrain. Patients are never in an ideal location. They may be down an embankment, for example. You may have to cross over ice or terrain that is rocky.

It is essential that personnel use caution when carrying a patient regardless of the conditions. Use of the proper equipment with the proper treatment and the right number of personnel is a combination that will help reduce the chances of anything detrimental occurring.

IMPROPER MAINTENANCE

Equipment typically comes with a user manual. It will describe the proper use of the equipment, warranty information, parts and components, and the maintenance for the device. If you walk into virtually any EMS organization and ask where the user manuals are located, in many instances no one will know, and if they do, the cellophane wrapper is still on and covered in dust. User manuals are not the easiest thing to read, but they should be reviewed and made available for reference.

It is good practice to designate an individual in the organization as the person responsible for equipment. This person should have a good understanding of the proper maintenance for each piece of equipment. This does not mean this person is the one who actually does the maintenance, because many pieces of equipment require trained and certified individuals to work on them. One thing to remember is that EMS equipment is medical equipment, which takes on a new level of liability if an unqualified individual works on it and the device later fails. A qualified individual is someone who is trained and authorized by the manufacturer to perform maintenance on the device or equipment.

A number of simple things can be done to maintain your equipment; however, you must make sure that the proper materials are used. For example, one manufacturer recommends the only lubricant to be used on its products' moving parts should either be 30W motor oil or lithium grease. The manufacturer further states that using the wrong lubricant may cause damage to the product. Pay attention to detailed instructions such as this.

Personnel tend to want to alter equipment. However, if a device is altered in any way, any warranty or manufacturer's liability will likely be negated. Wheeled ambulance stretchers are probably one of the most altered pieces of equipment. For example, there is a three-point harness that comes on virtually every stretcher to secure the patient's upper torso. In many instances, these are removed or tucked behind the mattress. This is an alteration to the design of the stretcher and can put the patient at risk for injury. In addition, it can place the organization at risk and may negate any warranty or manufacturer's liability.

Equipment maintenance is an essential element of the organization's risk control program. Using a contracted service is a means of risk control to eliminate any potential liability by performing the maintenance in-house. Qualified companies that perform maintenance offer services such as these:

> *Preventive maintenance.* Cleaning, inspection, and lubrication.
>
> *Equipment tune-up.* Hardware tightening and alignment adjustments.
>
> *Equipment evaluation.* Reveal needed repairs and detect potential problems.
>
> *Usage evaluation and training.* Reveals improper usage.
>
> *Report.* Documentation of preventive maintenance.

Equipment Failure/Malfunction

The lack of equipment maintenance and inspections may lead to equipment failure/malfunction as well as to litigation. If this is the case, the organization must prove that the failure or the malfunction was not a result of its negligence and show the training records to demonstrate that personnel were properly trained in the use of the device.

One mistake organizations typically make is not immediately removing from service a device that has malfunctioned or failed. It must be properly inspected, and any malfunctions or defects must be documented, identified, and corrected.

Documentation is critical in these scenarios. Equipment logs should be maintained that contain the maintenance schedule, when maintenance was actually performed, and the results of tests carried out in accordance with manufacturer's specifications. The quality assurance program, which should be in place, must identify any specific manufacturer's areas that are recommended for inspection, such as straps, wheels, frames, and other features of a device.

The Food & Drug Administration (FDA) requires EMS agencies to report any medical device that malfunctions. The statutory authority for the medical device reporting (MDR) regulation is section 519(a) of the Federal Food Drug and Cosmetic (FFD&C) Act as amended by the Safe Medical Devices Act (SMDA) of 1990. The SMDA requires user facilities to report the following:

- Device-related deaths to the FDA and the device manufacturer
- Device-related serious injuries to the manufacturer, or to FDA if the manufacturer is not known
- An annual summary to FDA of all reports submitted during that period

Provider Haste

Providers run call after call. Soon, it becomes commonplace to do so, and the provider begins to take shortcuts or use objects for purposes for which they were not designed. The crew may decide to carry the patient out of the house on the patient's dining room chair rather than getting their stair chair; the chair breaks, and the patient falls. First, the dining room chair is not designed to carry a patient. Second, the crew members have now subjected themselves to injury and further injury to the patient. Third, the patient now has an issue with a broken chair. This is a bad situation that can be easily avoided. Equipment should be used as it is designed to be used. EMS personnel must take a few extra minutes and do the job the right way with the right equipment.

EMS providers are often in a hurry. Whether it is from an adrenaline rush or from being pushed to move quicker on a call, hurrying on the scene of an incident can cause detrimental effects for the crew and the patient. Mistakes will be made more often. As one adage goes, "Haste makes waste." Providers should stop, take a breath, and plan the move. A few extra seconds may make all the difference in the outcome of the call.

INJURY PREVENTION

The study of the relationship between a worker and the workplace is known as **ergonomics**. Essentially, three work hazards can be identified in relation to patient movement:

- Moving patients from multistory buildings or homes using stairways, up and over embankments or inclines, and down sloping terrains
- Moving patients on and off stretchers or moving devices, and loading and unloading stretchers from ambulances
- Moving patients in any other situation

Other areas of concern should be taken into account when planning to avoid provider back injury. One is ambulance seats. Office workers know the value of a chair that fits properly to the body. Those who routinely sit in an EMS unit between calls also deserve properly fitted lumbar supports. Another area of concern is the amount of time spent driving. People who spend more than half their working hours driving are said to be three times more likely to develop back problems than the average worker, due to prolonged sitting that is followed immediately by physical exertion. Evidence suggests that the vibration of movement over roadways causes accelerated muscle and disk fatigue, which can result in degeneration of back strength. Worth scrutiny is the increasingly common practice of system status management of EMS units in which crews rove among different districts of the service area and sit in their units at designated posts. Unnecessary shifting of crews from one place to another may contribute to the deterioration of back health among field personnel. One preventive physical strategy is to do frequent pelvic tilts by tightening the gluteal and abdominal muscles to flatten the lower back against the seat (or better, the floor, if a place to lie down can be found).

EMS is very physical and not everyone is able to do the work. The organization must implement a physical examination and physical agility test to assist in identifying those individuals who are not physically able to do the job. Keep in mind that medical examinations and back X-rays alone have not been shown to be effective screening tests. A screening program must test physical fitness and flexibility. To pass the Equal Employment Opportunity Commissions standards (EEOC, 2008), it must be safe, reliable, practical, and relevant to the job. Once members are with the organization, another preventive measure is periodic physical strength and agility testing. Personnel should expect to have to achieve and maintain a certain standard of conditioning.

Various programs that deal specifically with preventing back injuries are available. A few programs are specific to EMS and, since back injuries are not unique to EMS, there are a variety of preventing back injury programs in general. It is also a good idea to seek advice from physical therapists or occupational therapists to give a class to personnel; a physical fitness coach may also be helpful. Regardless, it is important for the individual to understand the characteristics of EMS and the inherent risks.

Consider having responders use a back support belt. Different back support devices are intended to help reduce back injury, but differences of opinion remain about how effective back support belts actually are. Back support belts do not necessarily prevent back injuries. They are more of a reminder to lift properly. In some instances, back support belts are actually more detrimental in that they give the user a false sense of protection from a back injury. Nothing works better than being in good physical condition and lifting in a proper manner.

PROPER LIFTING DYNAMICS

Every situation is unique. Applying the basic principles of lifting in each lifting situation will result in more consistently safe lifts. Attention to this detail is a vital self-care habit. Proper lifting dynamics include the following:

- Think through the situation.
- Anticipate and troubleshoot tight corners, stairs, and small elevators, and evaluate better alternative routes.
- Determine which partner will lead.
- Communicate with helpers.
- Check for adequate footing.
- Stay balanced.
- Use your legs, not your back, to lift.
- Exhale during exertion.
- Keep the weight as close to the body as possible.
- Know your limits.

Lifting is one of the most recurrent tasks an EMS provider faces. Many do it for years, on thousands of EMS calls, without a problem. For others, back injury becomes a limiting factor in their ability to pursue a calling they enjoy.

Good strategies for minimizing the chances of back injury have been described. Backs are not inherently weak. They can be strengthened. Back pain is not inevitable, provided a person understands how to avoid it and then pursues an appropriate prevention program. Dropping patients has a low frequency of occurrence; however, it has a high severity rate. Lifting and moving patients safely are important considerations for EMS providers.

VIOLENT SITUATIONS

EMS personnel are called to the scene of violent situations. Whether an EMS agency is a rural or an urban provider, violence makes no exceptions, so EMS personnel must take precautions at every scene. *Remember:* The number one priority is scene safety. EMS personnel must remember to look out for themselves first, the other crew members second, and the patient third.

VIOLENCE TO EMS

According to a 2004 report by the RAND Corporation (RAND, 2004), an average of 19 EMS personnel are killed in the line of duty each year. A 2005 study (Maguire et al.) indicates that EMS practitioners have a rate of 34.6 injuries per 100,000 workers.

Violence toward EMS is becoming more prevalent (Suyama et al., 2009). EMS personnel are being assaulted on the scene of incidents and in some cases in the station. There are essentially two categories of assaults. One is the assault that takes place on the scene of an incident. The second is workplace violence.

Violence On Scene

The study of violence in the context of prehospital occupational injury is rather new. One of the earliest accounts of EMS workforce exposure to violence is a review conducted by Tintinalli (1993) of EMS run reports in North Carolina. The study reported that approximately 1% of a small sample of EMS patient care records indicated violence. The situations included cases involving weapons on the scene, but also included patients who were recorded as having been aggressive secondary to hypoglycemia. No on-duty injuries to EMS personnel were reported as a consequence of these emergency responses. In a prospective observational field study, 5% of EMS calls were classified as involving physical and/or verbal aggression (Mock, Wrenn, Wright, Eustis, and Slovis, 1998). A further 14% of EMS runs occurred in response to a violent event. The authors estimated a frequency for EMS providers of exposure to one violent episode every four 12-hour shifts, or every 19 runs. Another prospective study examined 4,102 consecutive EMS calls over a 1-month period in a southern Californian metropolitan area (Grange and Corbett, 2002). Some type of violence was identified in 8.5% of the calls.

Risk factors for violence at the scene of an emergency, and in EMS facilities, are offered in OSHA's 2004 guidelines (OSHA, 2004). They include the following:

- The carrying of handguns and other weapons by patients, their families, or friends
- The use of EMS by police and the criminal justice system for the care and transport of acutely disturbed, violent individuals
- The increasing number of acute and chronically mentally ill patients being released from hospitals without follow-up care, who now have the right to refuse medicine, and who can no longer be hospitalized involuntarily unless they pose an immediate threat to themselves or others
- The availability of drugs in EMS units and drugs or money at hospitals
- Lack of training of staff in recognizing and managing escalating hostile and assaultive behavior

Violence in the Workplace

If personnel ever have concerns about a situation that may turn violent, they should alert their supervisor immediately and follow the specific reporting procedures provided by the organization. It is better to err on the side of safety than to risk having a situation escalate.

The following are warning indicators of potential workplace violence:

- Intimidating, harassing, bullying, belligerent, or other inappropriate and aggressive behavior
- Numerous conflicts with customers, co-workers, or supervisors

- Bringing a weapon to the workplace (unless necessary for the job), making inappropriate references to guns, or making idle threats about using a weapon to harm someone
- Statements showing fascination with incidents of workplace violence, statements indicating approval of the use of violence to resolve a problem, or statements indicating identification with perpetrators of workplace homicides
- Statements indicating desperation (over family, financial, and other personal problems) to the point of contemplating suicide
- Direct or veiled threats of harm
- Substance abuse
- Extreme changes in normal behaviors

If personnel notice others showing any signs of these indicators, they should take the following steps:

- If they see these indicators in other members of the organization, they should notify their supervisor immediately of their observations.
- If it is the public, they should notify their supervisor immediately.
- If it is their subordinate, they should evaluate the situation by taking into consideration what may be causing the individual's problems.
- If it is their supervisor, they should notify that person's supervisor.

It is very important for personnel to respond appropriately (i.e., not to overreact but also not to ignore a situation). Sometimes that may be difficult to determine. Supervisors should discuss the situation with expert resource staff to get help in determining how best to handle the situation.

Recommendations for reducing violence include the following (OSHA, 2004):

- Adopting a written violence-prevention program, communicating it to all personnel.
- Advising all patients in EMS units and visitors to EMS stations and facilities that violence, verbal and nonverbal threats, and related behavior will not be tolerated.
- Encouraging personnel to promptly report incidents to the appropriate person designated per SOG and to suggest ways to reduce or eliminate risks to management.
- Reviewing workplace layout to find existing or potential hazards; installing and maintaining alarm systems and other security devices such as panic buttons, handheld alarms or noise devices, cellular phones, and private channel radios where risk is apparent or may be anticipated; and arranging for a reliable response system when an alarm is triggered.
- Providing medical and psychological counseling and debriefing for personnel experiencing or witnessing assaults and other violent incidents.

The team designated to form an effective workplace violence strategy should consider the following important principles (OSHA, 2004):

- There must be support from the top. If an organization's senior management are not truly committed to a preventive program, it is unlikely to be effectively implemented.
- There is no one-size-fits-all strategy. Effective plans may share a number of features, but a good plan must be tailored to the needs, resources, and circumstances of a particular organization and a particular group of personnel.
- A plan should be proactive, not reactive.
- A plan should take into account the organization's culture: atmosphere, relationships, traditional management styles, and so on. If there are elements in that culture that appear to foster a toxic climate—tolerance of bullying or intimidation; lack of trust among personnel and/or between personnel and management; high levels of stress, frustration, and anger; poor communication; inconsistent discipline; and erratic enforcement of organization policies—these should be called to the attention of top management for remedial action.

- Planning for and responding to workplace violence calls for expertise from a number of perspectives including law enforcement and social workers. A workplace violence prevention plan will be most effective if it is based on a multidisciplinary team approach. Managers should take an active role in communicating the workplace violence policy to personnel. Personnel must be alert to warning signs, the violence prevention plan and response, and must seek advice and assistance when there are indications of a problem.
- Practice your plan! No matter how thorough or well-conceived, preparation will not do any good if an emergency happens and no one remembers or carries out what was planned. Training exercises must include all personnel, including management, who will be making decisions during a real incident.
- Exercises must be followed by careful, clear-eyed evaluation and changes to fix whatever weaknesses have been revealed. Reevaluate, rethink, and revise. Policies and practices should not be set in concrete. Personnel, work environments, business conditions, and society all change. A prevention program must change with them.

The components of a workplace violence prevention program should include the following (OSHA 2004):

- A statement of the organization's no threats or violence policy and complementary policies such as those regulating harassment and drug and alcohol use
- A physical security survey and assessment of premises
- Procedures for addressing threats and threatening behavior
- Access to outside resources, such as threat assessment professionals and trainers for different management and personnel groups
- Crisis response measures
- Consistent enforcement of behavioral standards, including effective disciplinary procedures

UNIFORMS

EMS personnel are part of public safety. In many organizations across the country EMS personnel uniforms resemble those of law enforcement personnel. They should not. Wearing a badge, for example, is one of the distinct similarities between the two. For this reason, many EMS organizations have changed their dress code so that the public will be able to distinguish them from law enforcement (Figure 7.8). In addition, the various devices and equipment can be controversial in many organizations. These include body armor, Maglite clubs, mace and pepper spray, and handguns. As the EMS safety officer, you should ensure that the organization conveys in policy its stance on these items and ensure that personnel are trained on the organization's policy. There is not necessary a right or wrong policy; rather, it is more about the organization having a policy on these items.

HIGHWAY SAFETY

As stated earlier in this chapter, highway incidents have become one of the greatest threats to EMS personnel. Extra effort should be paid to

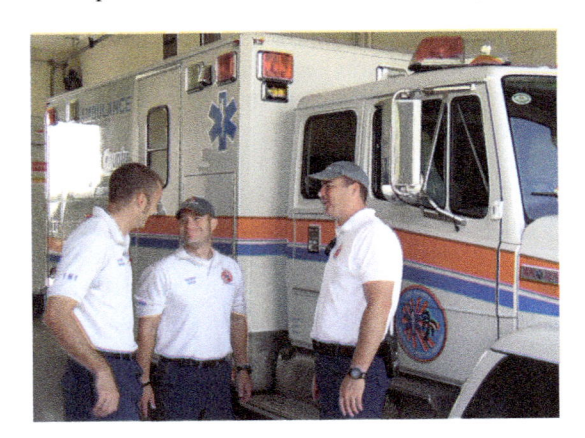

FIGURE 7.8 ■ Many EMS organizations are changing their uniforms to distinguish EMS from law enforcement personnel. *Courtesy of Jeffrey T. Lindsey, Ph.D.*

safety at the scene on a highway. In addition, to moving vehicles as a threat, there are a number of other considerations. You may be called to an incident where the vehicle is disabled, "Man slumped over wheel" calls, or motor vehicle crashes. In any of these calls, occupants may be intoxicated or drugged. The patient or individuals involved in the incident may be armed and dangerous. They may have been involved in committing a crime, feel threatened when EMS arrives, and react in a violent manner. The crew must pay particular attention to anything that looks suspicious. If it looks suspicious, then there is probably something potentially dangerous going on. The crew must retreat to a safe area until law enforcement can clear the scene.

Scene Observation

Some things to look for at the scene include individuals grabbing or hiding items in the vehicle. This should increase the level of suspicion, and caution should be taken. Never approach a potentially violent situation. Another scenario would be the occupants arguing or fighting. This is not a safe environment, and crews should retreat immediately. This is not a place for EMS to intervene; most EMS personnel are not trained to deal with such situations and would be placing themselves and possibly those involved in the altercation in jeopardy.

Increase your level of suspicion if you notice a lack of activity where you would expect it to be. Never take any chances. Things happen in a split second, and it is nearly impossible to reverse a bad situation.

Another situation to be aware of is open or unlatched trunks. In many cases, people hide in trunks and may create an unsafe hazard for EMS personnel. If you arrive on scene and notice the trunk is open or unlatched and you can safely shut it, do so.

Approaching the Vehicle

When approaching the vehicle, personnel should use caution. It is best if one provider approaches while the driver remains near or in the ambulance. Personnel should be instructed to call for law enforcement and wait for them to clear the scene if there is any indication the scene is not safe. This provides personnel with further opportunity to survey the scene and notify others if the situation does not look right. If the incident occurs at night, use the lights from the ambulance to illuminate the vehicle. It also is a good practice to notify dispatch of the situation, location, and license plate number and state of issue.

It is good practice to approach the vehicle on the passenger side of the vehicle (Figure 7.9). This protects you from passing traffic and typically gives you a place to escape. In most instances, the police approach on the driver's side; therefore, it is usually not expected by the occupant in the vehicle.

It is best not to walk between the ambulance and the other vehicle. If the individual in the vehicle decides to ram the ambulance with his car or the vehicle is in gear, you may be pinned or seriously injured as a result of being stuck between the two vehicles. As you approach the vehicle, consider that posts (a, b, c) provide best ballistic protection. Do not stand directly in

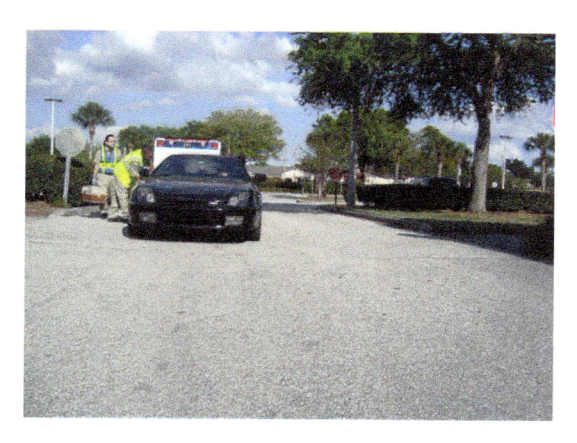

FIGURE 7.9 Personnel should use caution when approaching a vehicle. Approaching on the passenger's side is safer than approaching from the driver's side. *Courtesy of Jeffrey T. Lindsey, Ph.D.*

front of the windows. Observe the rear seat; do not move forward of "c" post unless there are no threats in the back seat. Observe the front seat from behind "b" post. Move forward only after ensuring safety. Retreat at the first sign of violence or problem.

EMS providers must be vigilant at all times. They should never assume the scene is safe, regardless of the nature of the call or the location of the incident. Safety is paramount.

RESIDENCES

Many EMS calls are made at a residence. Personnel should pay particular attention when arriving on the scene. As with any call, scene safety begins the moment a call is received. EMS responders should take into consideration past calls to the residence or location. What type of calls have come from the residence, and who lives there? If the house is known as a drug house or for domestic violence, take this into consideration. Many dispatch centers are able to retrieve past information about incidents, including law enforcement responses. Personnel should be instructed to use this information as a means to protect them and their crew from harm. As responders approach the scene, they should be scanning the area for anything unusual. If the house is completely dark, particular attention should be paid to a careful approach. Personnel may be better off calling for law enforcement and letting them ensure the scene is safe.

Scene safety begins as soon as the unit is dispatched. The crew must listen to the dispatch information, which may provide key words or conditions that alert personnel to a possible unsafe environment. Dispatchers should be trained to gather information that can aid EMS crews in determining whether a scene may or may not be safe. In many systems, a law enforcement agency is dispatched along with EMS, either on every incident or incidents where the scene may be unsafe. Crews who know of past incidents at the call address should increase their level of suspicion or call for appropriate assistance. Regardless of the situation, if the scene is not safe, personnel must immediately retreat to a safe location.

EMS personnel are assaulted at times and, in some cases, murdered. EMS organizations must make sure appropriate precautions are included in their protocols and SOPs. Personnel must be aware of these protocols and SOPs and follow them. As the safety officer, you should be part of developing these protocols and SOPs.

Personnel should begin to make observations several blocks from the scene. The use of red lights and sirens should be used minimally because they draw curious bystanders and those who might cause harm on the EMS provider. If personnel are working in a roadway area, lights will help to assist with providing a safer scene.

Scene safety is not just about individuals doing harm, but also being vigilant for other safety concerns. There may be hazardous materials, power lines, or dangerous animals or pets. There are more and more exotic animals being kept in homes. These animals, as well as more typical pets, may be very dangerous, and EMS personnel should never try and intervene with them. Meth labs are found virtually everywhere in the United States. Whether you are an urban provider or rural provider there is no difference. These labs can be very dangerous and EMS personnel should not enter such locations until the scene has been secured by law enforcement and deemed safe.

As the call progresses, personnel should never let their guard down. People come and go. Scenes can change. EMS crews have encountered many situations during the treatment of a patient. If the crowd or individuals in the crowd do not think EMS is handling the call properly or taking too much time on the scene, they may assault EMS personnel. Scene safety must be considered at all times. Personnel should never be complacent even if law enforcement is present. Violence still may break out, and EMS personnel must always be alert.

No call is ever a routine response. Every call should be handled with the same level of caution. Scene safety is emphasized in the certification courses from EMS first responder to paramedic and must be emphasized on a regular basis. From the time crews receive the dispatch until the patient is transferred to another party, safety of the scene should be considered. As personnel arrive on the scene, they should begin to look for clues of any warning signs that could result in an unsafe scene. Some warning signs of danger could include:

- Past history of problems or violence
- Known drug or gang area
- Loud noises or items breaking
- Seeing or hearing fighting
- Intoxication or drug use
- Evidence of dangerous pets (droppings, barking, signs)
- Unusual silence or darkened residence

If personnel arrive on an unsafe scene or a scene that presents a threat, a tactical approach that matches the situation should be undertaken. If actual danger is present, all crews should retreat and call for police immediately. When requesting police, make sure the dispatcher understands the nature of the situation. Crews must not broadcast their approach with lights or sirens. The stealth mode is the best method. No time will be lost by approaching a scene without lights and sirens. In virtually every case, shutting down and running cold into the actual scene provides more benefit.

When exiting the ambulance and heading toward the house, use a foot approach and take an unconventional path (not the sidewalk or the regular path of travel), in case someone is lying in wait. Crews must not **backlight** themselves (getting between the rig and the residence). This sets the person up as an easy target.

When approaching the door, EMS personnel should be to the side of it, preferably on the doorknob side. The reason for this is to avoid having a thrown-open door knocking them off balance or to the ground. They should never stand in front of a door or window either, which would make them perfect targets. When arriving at the door, EMS responders should listen for signs of danger before announcing their presence. Upon determining the scene to be safe, they should announce their arrival, making sure to identify themselves as "Emergency Medical Service" personnel so as not to be confused with law enforcement.

VIOLENT GROUPS AND SITUATIONS

EMS personnel should be aware of street gangs in their response areas and use caution when responding into areas unfamiliar to them. Well-known group names include the Crips, Bloods, Latin Kinds (Almighty Latin King Nation), Hell's Angels, Outlaws, Pagans, and Banditos. A number of other gangs may not be widely recognized and are considered local variations.

Gang Characteristics

Clothing defines a gang. A specific group will wear clothing unique to its members. The clothing not only identifies the affiliation with a particular group, but may also identify the rank within the group. If the clothing is disfigured or if the gang colors are disrespected, violence may ensue.

Graffiti identifies gang presence (Figure 7.10). It also marks gang territory. EMS personnel should look daily for graffiti when out on responses in order to identify any areas where gangs may be present. This will assist in the future if ever called to that locale: Personnel will know that they are entering an area with possible gang presence.

Safety Issues

It goes without saying that if crews respond into an area with known gangs, the potential for violence is prevalent. EMS may appear to look like law enforcement and, therefore, extreme caution must be taken. If personnel cocaine HCl to base form. Other types of labs do tableting, extraction, and so on. It is not as important for EMS personnel to identify the type of lab, but rather it is important to be able to identify that it is a lab and to retreat from the scene immediately.

Hazards of Drug Labs
Toxic inhalation from clandestine drug labs is a real threat to EMS providers. Fires and explosions have occurred in these labs. Booby traps are very much a possibility. Those who operate the labs try to safeguard them from law enforcement and other individuals who may attempt to enter. EMS personnel must be constantly vigilant of their surroundings, especially during retreat. EMS personnel may encounter armed or otherwise violent occupants, so they must make sure the occupants know that they are EMS and not law enforcement.

Actions
If a lab is identified, EMS personnel should leave the area immediately and notify law enforcement, making sure they understand the situation. EMS personnel should initiate the incident command system and follow the hazardous materials procedures for their area. Additional resources must be called, including the local hazardous materials teams (fire services), the police, the Drug Enforcement Administration, and a chemist or chemistry specialists, who will be of great value on scene.

EMS Concerns
The area in which the clandestine drug lab is found may need to be evacuated. If this must be done, EMS responders should not wait for additional resources. They should begin immediately. They should notify the dispatcher of the situation and then their supervisor. Make sure crews do not touch anything; a lab can be a lethal environment, and any disruption can cause severe consequences. If EMS responders see any processes in place, they should never

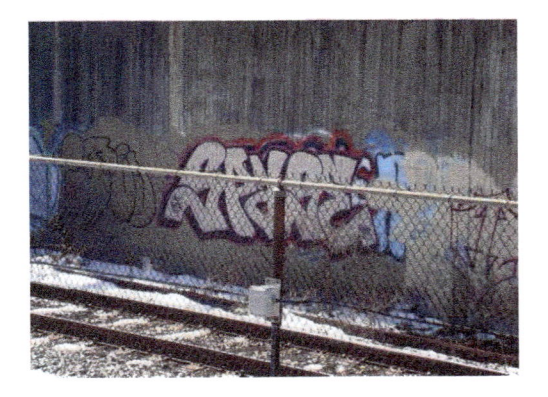

FIGURE 7.10 ■ Graffiti may define a gang's presence. *Courtesy of Jeffrey T. Lindsey, Ph.D.*

get into a situation where they are confronted with gangs, they should immediately retreat to the ambulance, leave the area, and wait until law enforcement clears the scene. Personnel should use methods similar to those described in this chapter for handling a scene with violent individuals.

CLANDESTINE DRUG LABS

Clandestine drug labs are appearing in virtually every demographic area of the country. They are more prevalent in some areas than others, but no area is immune from these dangerous locations. It is important to be able to identify these labs. EMS personnel should look for the following:

* Chemical odors
* Chemistry equipment, such as glassware, chemical containers, heating mantles, and burners
* Suspicious persons, activities, and deliveries
* An area that provides the needs of a clandestine drug lab: privacy, operational utilities, and good ventilation

Types of Drug Labs
There are various types of drug labs. A synthesis lab creates drugs from chemical precursors, such as LSD and methamphetamine. A conversion lab changes drug forms, such as

DOMESTIC VIOLENCE

The situation is considered domestic violence if there is violence between persons in a domestic relationship (spousal, boyfriend-girlfriend, or same sex). The victims may be male or female. Domestic violence may be physical, emotional, sexual, verbal, or economic. Here are some indicators:

- Apparent fear of household member
- Different or conflicting accounts by parties at the scene
- One party preventing another from speaking
- Patient reluctant to speak
- Injuries do not match reported mechanism of injury
- Unusual or unsanitary living conditions or hygiene

EMS personnel should treat the patient and not be judgmental about the situation. They should provide the phone number for a domestic violence hotline or shelter, and notify the appropriate authorities if this is consistent with the organization's policy and/or regulations. In many states, reporting may be mandatory. When personnel arrive at the emergency department, they should notify the appropriate staff of their concerns with discretion in protecting the patient's privacy. Personnel should be aware of the potential for violence to break out on the scene of a domestic violence incident. Personnel should not enter a scene of domestic violence unless law enforcement is present and the scene is considered safe.

OTHER TACTICS

A number of responses to violent situations have been discussed in this chapter, most of which are consistent with basic training for EMS personnel. The following covers other tactics for which EMS personnel should be trained to be able to optimize safety at the scene of a violent situation.

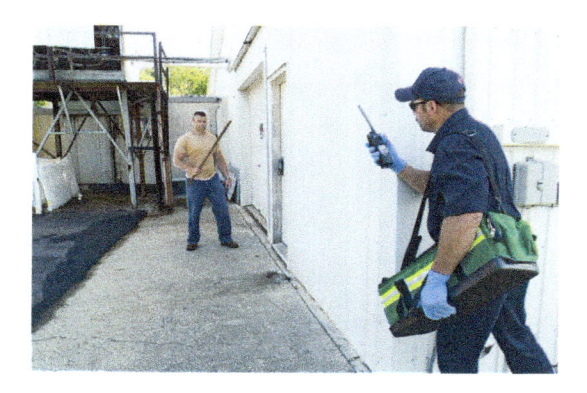

FIGURE 7.11 Concealment hides your body, but typically does not offer any ballistic protection.

Cover and Concealment

There are two methods of responding to violent situations that should be considered: concealment and cover. **Concealment** hides your body from view, but it does not offer any ballistic protection. Some examples of concealment would be hiding behind a bush, a wallboard, or vehicle door (Figure 7.11). **Cover** also hides your body from view, but it also offers at least some ballistic protection. Some examples of cover would include the trunk of a large tree, a telephone pole, or a vehicle engine block.

EMS personnel should always be aware of their surroundings. Cover and/or concealment should be integrated in retreat from danger as well as when hemmed in and unable to retreat to a safe location. It should be stressed to personnel that cover and/or concealment must be used properly. The responder should place as much of his body as possible behind the cover. Personnel should be constantly looking to improve their protection and location and be conscious of reflective clothing that may make them stand out.

Distraction and Evasive Tactics

Other distractions and evasive tactics can be used in response to violence. The use of equipment can be effective. For example, an EMS responder can wedge a stretcher in a doorway to block an aggressor. This action is similar to what the airline industry has instituted in the air. When a pilot or individual from the cockpit must enter the main fuselage, the flight attendants block the entrance with the beverage carts and stand guard. This places something between the aggressor and the target. *Remember:* Personal safety is number one; equipment can be replaced.

Personnel also can throw equipment to trip or slow the aggressor. However, consideration must be given to the fact that the aggressor could throw it back.

Evasion is always the best when it can be done effectively and safely. It includes such things as anticipating the moves of the aggressor by taking an unconventional path while retreating and not running in a straight line to try to throw off the aggressor.

Tactical EMS

Tactical EMS has become a popular service provided by a number of EMS agencies. Tactical EMS provides emergency medical care in violent or tactically "hot" zones requiring special training and authorization from local and, in some cases, state law enforcement agencies. EMS personnel who are assigned to a tactical EMS team require special equipment, including body armor and a tactical uniform—*and an individual should never be sent into a hot zone without the proper equipment.* These situations put EMS personnel into circumstances that are of higher risk than typical responses. The EMS agency must be willing to support these individuals if they elect to provide this type of service and must support such a service by providing the appropriate equipment and training to personnel serving on the team.

Contact and Cover Tactics. Tactical EMS personnel have a number of techniques that could be used by all EMS personnel on any scene, if and when they have been trained to do so. For example, there are specific evasive techniques for threats of physical violence, firearms encounters, and edged weapons encounters. In these situations providers have preassigned roles, such as the "contact" provider. This individual initiates and provides direct patient care. He performs the patient assessment and handles most interpersonal scene contact. The "cover" provider, in a tactical context, "covers" or observes the scene for danger while the "contact" provider takes care of the patient. For a small crew, the "cover" provider is likely to have other functions, such as getting equipment.

Communication among the providers on scene is important. Crews should develop methods of alerting other providers to danger without alerting aggressors. For this, verbal and nonverbal signals are needed and should be determined, along with dispatch, prior to entering the scene. Some agencies use the term "Code RED" on the radio to notify dispatch there is trouble on scene. Some radios have an emergency button that can be activated by pushing it, which alerts the dispatch that assistance is needed. The safety officer should not be active in the hot zone unless he is properly trained and part of the team. The EMS safety officer should be cognizant of areas outside of the hot zone.

Body Armor. Body armor, also known as bulletproof vests, is commonplace among many EMS agencies in the country. Body armor offers protection from most handgun bullets and most knives, and reduces blunt trauma from such objects as a steering wheel in a motor-vehicle collision. It does not offer protection against high-velocity (rifle) bullets or thin or dual-edged weapons, such as an ice pick. It offers only reduced protection when it is wet. And it most definitely offers no protection at all if it is not worn.

Caution must be instilled on the wearer of body armor not to feel a false sense of security. Personnel should never do anything they would not do without body armor. Body armor does not cover all of a person's body. A number of critical points remain exposed.

EMS AT CRIME SCENES

Crime scenes are locations where any part of a criminal act occurred or where evidence relating to a crime may be found. There can be a lot of evidence at the scene of a crime, and EMS should be careful not to disturb it. Among that evidence is prints. There are two kinds of prints to be aware of at a crime scene: fingerprints and footprints.

A fingerprint is a set of ridge characteristics that are left behind on a surface with oils and moisture from skin. They are unique; no two people have identical fingerprints. Caution must be taken to avoid touching anything unless you positively need to. If a crew member touches anything, it should be so noted.

Footprints may contain blood and body fluids. They are important in establishing DNA and ABO blood typing. They also may denote blood spatter evidence. When entering and leaving the scene, be cautious to avoid walking in well-traveled areas or areas where it looks like others have traveled. Providers should make a mental note of where they are and how they travel on scene in order to be able to tell investigators and document that in the prehospital care report.

Other evidence includes particulate evidence, such as hair and carpet and clothing fibers. These may or may not be obvious on scene.

Preserving Evidence

The EMS crew's safety is the number-one priority, with patient care being the ultimate priority. Evidence protection is performed while caring for the patient and looking out for the safety of the crew. The crew should carry in only the necessary equipment.

The different evidence preservation techniques include the following:

- Being observant and reporting pertinent observations.
- Touching only what is required for patient care. If it is necessary to touch something, remember it and tell police.
- Wearing latex gloves. They will prevent EMS personnel from leaving their own fingerprints, and will provide infection protection. Note, however, that gloves will not prevent the smudging of other fingerprints.

Crime scenes can present many challenges for EMS providers. First and foremost must be the safety of all EMS personnel. Providing the appropriate patient care and scene preservation should follow.

HAZMAT SCENES

EMS may be called to stand by at a hazmat scene, so personnel must be able to assist with patients safely. The individual EMS agency will identify the extent to which personnel may get involved. There are three roles that personnel should be ready to assist with at the minimum on the hazmat scene. They are rehabilitation, medical surveillance, and medical emergencies.

The location of EMS personnel is an important element of safety at a hazmat scene. EMS personnel should remain in the cold zone, although in many instances EMS personnel may function in the hot zone as a medical rapid-intervention team. They also may perform predecontamination triage. EMS personnel who are properly trained may also work in the warm zone at a cut-out rescue/ambulatory treatment area. This area is designed for patients who are not ambulatory.

The cut-out rescue area is the decontamination lane where fire and EMS personnel who enter the hot zone in full protective gear go when they have a medical problem. The cut-out zone is designed to quickly decontaminate and remove the PPE from the provider to begin medical treatment.

Scene safety is first and foremost when managing the medical emergencies of hazmat victims. Scene safety is always the theme. In a hazmat situation it is critical. In addition to scene safety, you must consider substance identification, research, and nomenclature of the product. In addition, the route of exposure is important. Personnel also must look at hazmat incident evaluation and characteristics, scene and control zones, and the medical management of hazmat victims.

EMS personnel should be familiar with four standards in order to function safely at the scene of a hazmat incident. They are OSHA 29 CFR 1910.120, NFPA 471, NFPA 472, and NFPA 473.

OSHA 29 CFR 1910.120. This is the Superfund Amendments and Reauthorization Act (SARA) of 1986. It requires standards for hazmat emergencies and established the Hazardous Waste Operations and Emergency Response (HAZWOPER) requirements. It addresses PPE, medical surveillance, air monitoring, and pre-entry briefing. This standard should be reviewed by all personnel.

NFPA 471. This is a recommended practice for responding to hazmat incidents. It covers the minimum recommended tactical objectives, incident response planning, response levels, site safety, PPE, incident mitigation, decontamination, and medical monitoring for hazmat incidents.

NFPA 472. This standard addresses professional competency of responders to hazmat incidents. The competency levels are as follows:
- First Responder at Awareness Level, 8 to 16 training hours. These individuals are trained to recognize the presence of hazardous materials and how to protect oneself, secure the area, and call for help.
- First Responder at Operational Level, 24 to 40 training hours. These individuals are trained to assume a defensive posture at a safe distance, control release, and keep hazardous material from spreading.
- Hazardous Materials Technician, 160 to 180 training hours. These individuals are trained to use specialized protective clothing and control equipment, and operate within the hot zone, and they are given specialized training in hazardous materials chemistry, air monitoring equipment, and tools used within the hot zone.

NFPA 473. This standard applies to the competencies of EMS personnel responding to hazmat incidents. It identifies two levels of responders:
- EMS/HM Level I Responder, trained at First Responder at Awareness Level, provides patient care in the cold zone.
- EMS/HM Level II Responder, trained at First Responder at Operational Level, provides patient care in the warm zone.

AIR OPERATIONS

Side Bar

Advanced Hazmat Life Support

The University of Arizona developed a program designed for health care responders in relation to hazmat incidents. The program, Advanced Hazmat Life Support (AHLS) is a 2-day, 16-hour course. After completion of the course, participants are able to do a rapid assessment of a hazmat patient, recognize toxic syndromes, demonstrate the ability to medically manage hazmat patients, apply the poisoning treatment paradigm, and identify and administer specific antidotes. The program incorporates the various hazmat standards along with the best practices in hazmat medicine in the course. The EMS safety officer for the organization should consider attending the course in order to gain a better understanding of hazmat incidents.

According to the General Accounting Office (GAO) report on aviation safety, the air ambulance industry averaged 13 accidents per year from 1998 through 2008. The annual number of air ambulance accidents increased from 8 in 1998 to a high of 19 in 2003. Since 2003, the number of accidents has slightly declined, fluctuating between 11 and 15 accidents per year. Although the total number of air ambulance accidents peaked in 2003, the number of fatal accidents peaked in 2008, when 9 fatal accidents occurred. Of 141 accidents that occurred from 1998 to 2008, 48 of them resulted in the deaths of 128 people. From 1998 through 2007, the air ambulance industry averaged 10 fatalities per year. The number of overall fatalities increased sharply in 2008, however, to 29 (Dillingham, 2009). After a series of medical helicopter crashes, the Federal Aviation Administration (FAA) released a fact sheet on helicopter safety. The following is from that fact sheet, which provides a foundation for EMS helicopter safety (FAA, 2006):

> Helicopter Emergency Medical Service (HEMS) operations are unique due to the emergency nature of the mission. In August 2004, the FAA initiated a new government and industry partnership to improve the safety culture at EMS operators and recommend short- and long-term strategies for reducing accidents. While the FAA has not ruled out proposing new or changing existing rules, the agency has prompted significant short-term safety gains that do not require rulemaking. The FAA's immediate focus has been on:
> - Encouraging risk management training to flight crews so that they can make more analytical decisions about whether to launch on a mission.
> - Offering better training for night operations and responding to inadvertent flight into deteriorating weather conditions.
> - Promoting technology such as night vision goggles, terrain awareness and warning systems, and radar altimeters.
> - Providing airline-type FAA oversight for operators, and identifying regional FAA HEMS operations and maintenance inspectors to help certificate new operators and review the operations of existing companies.

BACKGROUND

There are approximately 750 EMS helicopters operating today, most of which operate under Part 135 rules. HEMS operators may ferry or reposition helicopters (without passengers/patients) under Part 91 (FAA, 2006).

The number of accidents nearly doubled between the mid-1990s and the HEMS industry's rapid growth period from 2000 to 2004. There were 9 accidents in 1998, compared with 15 in 2004. There were a total of 83 accidents from 1998 through mid-2004. The main causes were controlled flight into terrain (CFIT), inadvertent operation into instrument meteorological conditions, and pilot spatial disorientation/lack of situational awareness in night operations (FAA, 2006).

FAA OVERSIGHT

The FAA inspects HEMS operators, but is prompting changes beyond inspection and surveillance. Rather, the FAA is moving to a risk-based system that includes the initiatives outlined in the following sections, including weather, night vision goggles, flight data recorders, terrain awareness warning systems, and helicopter safety, which focus on the leading causes of the HEMS accidents (FAA, 2006).

Weather

In March 2006, the FAA and the University Corporation for Atmospheric Research hosted a weather summit in Boulder, Colorado, to identify the HEMS-specific issues related to weather products and services. Attendees explored possible regulatory improvements, weather product enhancements, and operational fixes specific to HEMS operations. Attendees included the National Weather Service, National Center for Atmospheric Research (NCAR), Helicopter Association International, American Helicopter Society International, Association of Air Medical

Services, National EMS Pilots Association, National Association of Air Medical Communications Specialists, manufacturers, and many operators.

As a result, the FAA funded the development and implementation of a graphical flight-planning tool for ceiling and visibility assessment along direct flights in areas with limited available surface observations capability. Its use improves the quality of go/no-go decisions for HEMS operators.

Night Vision Goggles
The FAA has a solid record of facilitating safety improvements and new technologies for EMS helicopters, including certification of night vision goggles (NVGs). Since 1994, the FAA has worked 28 projects or design approvals called Supplemental Type Certificates (STCs) for installation of NVGs on helicopters. This number includes EMS, law enforcement, and other types of helicopter operations. Of the 28 projects, the FAA has approved approximately 15 NVGs STCs for EMS helicopters. The FAA initiated and wrote (in coordination with Radio Technical Commission for Aeronautics [RTCA]) the minimum standards for NVGs/cockpit lighting (FAA, 2006).

Certification is just one step. The operator must also have an FAA-approved training program for using NVGs. The issue has been the lack of EMS helicopters being able to obtain the NVGs.

Flight Data Recorders
Flight data recorders (FDRs) are not required for HEMS operations. FDRs offer value in any accident investigation by providing information on aircraft system status, flight path, and attitude. The weight and cost of FDR systems are factors. Research and development are required to determine the appropriate standards for FDR data and survivability in the helicopter environment, which typically involves substantially lower speeds and altitudes than airplanes. Funds are currently best invested in preventive training.

However, the FAA is studying alternatives to expensive and heavy airliner-style FDRs, especially in light of the relatively low-impact forces in most helicopter accidents. By establishing a standard appropriate to the helicopter flight envelope, the FAA may be able to make meaningful future FDR rulemaking efforts.

Terrain Awareness Warning Systems
The FAA supports the voluntary implementation of terrain awareness warning systems (TAWS) and did consider the possibility of including rotorcraft in the TAWS rulemaking process. Through this process, however, the FAA concluded that a number of issues are unique to visual flight rules (VFR) helicopter operations that must be resolved before the FAA considers mandating the use of TAWS in this area, such as modification of the standards used for these systems. For example, helicopters typically operate at lower altitudes, so TAWS could potentially generate false alerts and warnings that could negatively impact the crew's response to a valid alert. TAWS application to HEMS would require study of TAWS interoperability within the lower-altitude HEMS environment, and possibly a modification of TAWS system standards.

Helicopter Safety
HEMS safety will continue to be a concern. Various precautions should be taken regardless of the situation. Most, if not all, operators have criteria they use for landing zones. Careflite from Grand Prairie, Texas, has developed safety guidelines for providers to establish a landing zone for medical operations.

Helicopter safety must be taken into serious consideration. Protocols must be specific on when to call for air transport. Incidents must be monitored to ensure that air transports are being used for those patients that truly need to be airlifted to a medical facility.

Best Practices

Landing Zone (LZ) Criteria
- 100 feet wide × 100 feet long
- Level with a firm surface
- Clear of sand, gravel, and other debris
- No power lines, trees, poles, buildings, or other overhead obstructions near or in the area
- No vehicles or people within the zone
- Avoid sloped areas

Marking the Landing Zone (LZ)
- Weighted construction cones
- Two vehicles with headlights crossed at the center of the LZ
- Smoke canisters during daylight operations
- Battery-operated strobe lights
- Cylume Chem-lite Sticks
- No use of markings such as barrier tape and flag tape

LZ Coordinator Responsibilities
- Command and secure the LZ.
- Establish radio contact with aircraft.
- Assist pilot in locating the LZ.
- Keep all bystanders 100 feet away from the LZ.
- Keep everyone away from the tail rotor.
- Contact pilot after landing to determine any safety issues.

Helicopter Safety
- Approach and depart the aircraft from the side only.
- Never walk around the tail rotor.
- Shield your eyes from rotor wash during landing and takeoff.
- Do not carry anything above your head.
- Do not approach the helicopter while the blades are turning unless instructed by the CareFlite crew.
- Do not run toward the aircraft. Approach in a calm, slow manner.
- No smoking anywhere in the vicinity of the aircraft.
- Pilot and/or medical crew control activity around the aircraft.
- Secure loose items such as hats, clothing, stretcher sheets, and any other object light enough to be blown into rotor blades.

Source: Careflite, n.d.

CHAPTER REVIEW

Summary

This chapter has covered many of the areas that pose a safety risk to EMS personnel as it relates mainly to scene safety. The EMS provider and staff also must be aware of safety concerns in the station and administrative facilities. Workplace violence is a safety issue that every member of the organization must be concerned about. The three main areas—highway incidents, violence, and patient handling—present some of the highest risks to EMS personnel in regard to safety at incidents. A continued effort must be made to improve the safety of all EMS providers. The EMS safety officer must ensure proper policy, training, and enforcement of safety in order to provide the safest environment for personnel.

WHAT WOULD YOU DO? Reflection

As the safety officer, you know your role is an important one. You cannot be on scene for every incident, but every incident must have a safety officer. So, the most important aspect of being the safety officer is to train all personnel of the organization to be a safety officer in practice. If you can get everyone to begin to think about safety, then during every incident you will be in the back of crew members' minds, looking out for the health and safety of every other crew member. You know that the chief also will want a list of items to include in the guidelines for those incidents to which you plan to personally respond. You advise the chief that when available you will respond to incidents at streets and roadways and that you will respond to all confirmed building fires and wildland fires that are considered of any magnitude. You will respond to potentially violent situations as needed. You will respond to confirmed hazmat incidents and to incidents when medical air operations are requested. You assure the chief that you will not be available for every one of these incidents, but will respond when available if nothing more than a quality assurance check is required. In addition to responding to the incidents, any time a patient is dropped or there is an infectious disease exposure, you will be notified and respond as necessary. You know that your job will be challenging.

Review Questions

1. Describe the purpose of the Manual on Uniform Traffic Control Devices for Streets and Highways.
2. What are the guidelines for safe parking when operating in or near moving traffic?
3. You arrive on the scene of a building fire. What forecasting tools would you use to evaluate the status of the building?
4. You are assigned to write an exposure control plan. What elements must you include in the plan to be in compliance?
5. Describe ways to decrease back injuries and patient drops when lifting and moving patients.
6. What are the components of a workplace violence prevention program?
7. Your chief asked you to put together a proposal for responding to hazmat scenes. She would like the personnel to be able to function in the hot zone. She would like for you to propose to her what training is needed so the EMS personnel can do this.
8. Discuss at least two recommendations the FAA has proposed to reduce medical helicopter crashes.
9. Review your organization's policies. Determine any areas where there is a lack of focus on safety. Make a proposal to your supervisor on how to increase the focus on safety.

References

Careflite. (n.d.). "Helicopter Landing Zone and Safety Procedures." Grand Prairie, TX: Author. (See the organization website.)

Dernocoeur, K. (1986, September). "Big Bodies: How to Deal with Them." *Journal of Emergency Medical Services 8*, 46.

Dillingham, G. L. (2009). "Aviation Safety: Potential Strategies to Address Air Ambulance Safety Concerns." GAO-09-627T. April 22, 2009, Testimony Before the Subcommittee on Aviation, Committee on Transportation and Infrastructure, House of Representatives. Washington, DC: Government Accounting Office. (See the organization website.)

Equal Employment Opportunity Commission (EEOC). (2008). "Employment Tests and Selection Procedures." (See the organization website.)

Federal Aviation Administration (FAA). (2006). "Fact Sheet: EMS Helicopter Safety." (See the organization website.)

National Highway Transportation and Safety Administration. (2007). "Feasibility for an EMS Workforce Safety and Health Surveillance System, Final Report." Washington, DC: Author.

Federal Highway Association (FHWA), U.S. Department of Transportation. (2012). (See the Manual on Uniform Traffic Control Devices (MUTCD) website.)

FEMA-USFA. (2004, August). "Emergency Vehicle Safety Initiative, FA-272." (See the organization website.)

Grange, J. T., and S. W. Corbett. (2002). "Violence Against Emergency Medical Services Personnel." *Prehospital Emergency Care*, 186–190.

Gurba R. M. (2004). *Highway Safety for Emergency Service Personnel.* York, PA: VFIS.

Hogya, P. T., and L. Ellis. (1990, July). "Evaluation of the Injury Profile of Personnel in a Busy Urban System." *American Journal of Emergency Medicine 8*.

Houser, A., Jackson, B., Bartis, J., Peterson, D. (March 2004). Emergency Responder Injuries and Fatalities: An Analysis of Surveillance Data, TR-100-NIOSH.

Jackson, B., J. Baker, S. Ridgely, J. Bartis, and H. Linn. (2004) Protecting Emergency Responders, Volume 3 Safety Management in Disaster and Terrorism Response." Santa Monica, CA: RAND Corporation.

Kahn, C. A., R. G. Pirrallo, and E. M. Kuhn. (2001). "Characteristics of Fatal Ambulance Crashes in the United States: An 11-Year Retrospective Analysis." *Prehospital Emergency Care 5*, 261–269.

Kipp, J. D., and M. E. Loflin. (1996). *Emergency Incident Risk Management: A Safety and Health Perspective.* New York: Van Nostrand Reinhold.

Lindsey, J. (2000). *Patient Handling: Lifting and Moving Done Right!* York, PA: VFIS.

Ludwig, G. (2002, June). "Emergency Medical Runs: Urgent Vs. Non-urgent." *Firehouse Magazine*. (See the organization website.)

Maguire, B., K. Hunting, T. Guidotti, and G. Smith. (2005). "Occupational Injuries Among Emergency Medical Services Personnel." *Prehospital Emergency Care* 9(4), 405–411.

Mitterer, D. M. (2000). *Risk Management for EMS and Ambulance Transportation Industry*. York, PA: VFIS.

Mock, E. F., K. D. Wrenn, S. W. Wright, T. C. Eustis, and C. M. Slovis. (1999). "Anxiety Levels in EMS Providers: Effects of Violence and Shifts Schedules." *The American Journal of Emergency Medicine* 17(6), 509–511.

National Fire Protection Association. (2000). *U.S. Fire Fighters Struck by Vehicles, 1977–1999*. Quincy, MA: National Fire Protection Association. Unpublished.

National Highway and Traffic Safety Administration. (2004). *Traveling on Federal Business?* Washington, DC: OSHA and National Highway Traffic Safety Administration.

National Institute for Occupational Safety and Health (NIOSH), Hazard ID, HID 12. (2001, June). "Traffic Hazards to Fire Fighters While Working Along Roadways." (See the organization website.)

National Safety Council. (1998). "Defensive Driving Course," 7th ed. Itasca, IL: Author.

National Traffic Incident Management Coalition (NTIMC). "Move Over/Slow Down Laws." (See the organization website.)

OSHA. (2004). "Guidelines for Preventing Workplace Violence for Health Care & Social Service Workers." OSHA 3148-01R 2004. (See the organization website.)

Patrick, R. W. (2005, May). "Follow the Cones: Highway Scenes and Your Protection." *Journal of Emergency Medical Services*.

Rugala, E. A. (2001). *Workplace Violence: Issues in Response*. Washington, DC: U.S. Department of Justice, Federal Bureau of Investigation.

Solomon, S., and J. King. (1995). "Influence of Color on Fire Vehicle Accidents." *Journal of Safety Research* 26(1), 41–48.

Suyama, J., J. Rittenberger, D. Patterson, and D. Hostler (2009). "Comparison of Public Safety Provider Injury Rates." *Prehospital Emergency Care* 13(4), 451–455.

Terribilini, C. (1992, August) "The Spinal Column: Nifty Ways to Love Your Lumbar." *Journal of Emergency Medical Services*.

Terribilini, C., and K. Dernocoeur. (1989, October). "Save Your Back: Injury Prevention for EMS Providers." *Journal of Emergency Medical Services*, pp. 34–41.

Tintinalli, J. E. (1993). "Violent Patients and the Prehospital Provider." *Annals of Emergency Medicine* 22, 1276–1279.

U.S. Department of Health and Human Services, National Institute for Occupational Safety and Health. (2001). "26-Year-Old Emergency Medical Technician Dies in Multiple Fatality Ambulance Crash." Kentucky. Pub. No. FACE-2001-11.

U.S. Department of Health and Human Services, Centers for Disease Control and Prevention. (2003, February 28). "Ambulance Crash-Related Injuries Among Emergency Medical Services Workers—United States, 1991–2002."

Morbidity Mortality Weekly Report 52(08), 154–156.

U.S. Department of Transportation, Federal Highway Administration. (2009). "Standards and Guides for Traffic Controls for Street and Highway Construction, Maintenance, Utility, and Incident Management Operations." Part VI of the *Manual on Uniform Traffic Control Devices for Streets and Highways.*

U.S. Food and Drug Administration. "Reporting Adverse Events." (See the organization website.)

Van Natter, C., J. Steffens, and J. Lindsey (2003). *Dynamics of Emergency Vehicle Response.* York, PA: VFIS.

VFIS. (2004). *Ten Cones of Highway Incident Safety Training Program.* York, PA: VFIS.

West, K. (2009). *Communicable Disease: Childhood & Travelers.* EMS Third Quarter Video Series. Eugene, OR: 24-7 EMS.

Wildland Fire Operations Risk Management Information Paper. (2007). (See the U.S. Fire Administration website.)

Key Terms

ANSI/ISEA Standard 207-2006 The American National Standards Institute and the International Safety Equipment Association standards for high-visibility public safety vests.

backlight The process of illuminating the subject from the back.

bloodborne pathogens Bacteria, viruses, or other microorganisms that can cause disease in humans, including but not limited to hepatitis B virus (HBV) and human immunodeficiency virus (HIV).

buffer zone A neutral area around an area of danger that serves to prevent a safe environment.

Class III safety vest A type of PPE that is required to be worn by all public safety personnel while on the scene of a highway or roadway incident.

concealment Hides a person's body from view, but does not offer any ballistic protection. Compare *cover*.

contaminated sharps Any object contaminated with blood or other potentially infectious material that can penetrate the skin, including but not limited to needles, scalpels, broken glass, broken capillary tubes, and exposed ends of dental wires.

cover Hides a person's body from sight and at the same time offers some ballistic protection.

decontamination The use of physical or chemical means to remove, inactivate, or destroy pathogens on a surface or item to the point where they are no longer capable of transmitting infectious particles and the surface or item is rendered safe for handling, use, or disposal.

epidemiology The study of the causes, distribution, and control of disease in populations.

ergonomics The study of the relationship between people and their workplaces.

exposure incident A specific eye, mouth, other mucous membrane, or nonintact skin contact with blood or other potentially infectious materials that results from the performance of an employee's duties.

forecasting Predicting or estimating; in the fire service this refers to determining what a fire in a building will do.

Manual on Uniform Traffic Control Devices (MUTCD) for Streets and Highways A document published by the Federal Highway Administration that addresses virtually every component of highway safety, including the national standard for all traffic control devices installed on any street, highway, or bicycle trail open to public travel.

reduced profile Making yourself less visible and less of a target in a dangerous or potentially dangerous environment.

retroreflective material Material made using tiny glass beads that reflect light directly back toward its source, from a much wider angle than reflective material.

retroreflectorized Reflects light or other radiation back to its source.

CHAPTER 8: Station, Office, and Facility Safety

Objectives

After reading this chapter, the student should be able to:

8.1 Evaluate methods of risk management and safety.
8.2 Identify and assess safety needs for nonemergency situations.
8.3 Identify the role of EMS personnel in risk management and safety.
8.4 Conduct a safety inspection of facilities.

Overview

This title on EMS safety and risk management has been written to assist EMS providers in the reduction of line-of-duty injuries, illnesses, and fatalities. It provides a framework for developing programs that will create an appropriate margin of health and safety for providers during the performance of EMS duties.

Key Terms

computer terminal hazards
electrical equipment hazards
exits and egress
fire hazards
handling and storage hazards
housekeeping
housekeeping hazards
illumination hazards
noise hazards
office furniture hazards
office machinery/tools hazards
physical layout
self-inspection
vehicle maintenance areas
ventilation hazards

CHAPTER 8 *Station, Office, and Facility Safety* **187**

WHAT WOULD YOU DO?

You have been reviewing your loss ratio with your workers' compensation insurance carrier and have noticed a lot of claims from the office staff. However, the claims don't seem to involve large dollar amounts. Regardless, you have been asked to find out why there are so many claims. You have never really considered office safety as an issue, let alone even something to focus on.

Questions

1. Where do you begin?
2. What are some of the things to take into consideration?
3. Are there items that could be improved in order to make the office environment a safer working area?

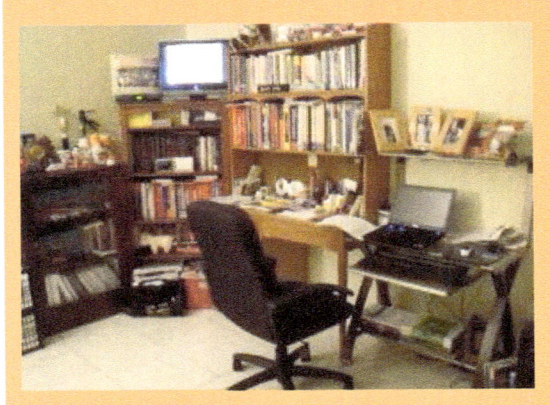

The office environment can create a variety of safety concerns. Courtesy of Jeffrey T. Lindsey, Ph.D.

■ INTRODUCTION

In many cases, EMS is strategically placed in static locations otherwise known as EMS stations. Depending on the type of organization, EMS might share facilities with the fire department, it might be based out of a hospital, or it might have a station that houses only EMS personnel. Regardless, safety at the station and other facilities occupied by EMS must be kept in mind when considering a safety program. This chapter considers EMS organizations of all sizes and dynamics.

■ ORGANIZE THE WORKPLACE

It is important to keep the workplace clean. According to OSHA, poor **housekeeping** contributes to low morale and sloppy work in general (OSHA, 2005). Most good safety action programs start with an intensive cleanup effort in all areas of the business. Get all personnel involved in the process, and emphasize exactly what must be done. For example, get rid of unnecessary items, provide proper waste containers, store flammables properly, make sure exits are not blocked, mark aisles and passageways properly, and ensure adequate lighting (Figure 8.1). Everyone should be involved and impressed upon to make the workplace safer, more healthful, and more efficient.

The most widely accepted way to identify hazards is to conduct safety and health inspections. The only way to be certain of an actual situation is to look at it directly from time to time. Begin a program of self-inspection in your own facilities. **Self-inspection** is essential if you are to know where probable hazards exist and whether they are under control. Checklists can give you some indication of where to begin taking action to make your organization safer and

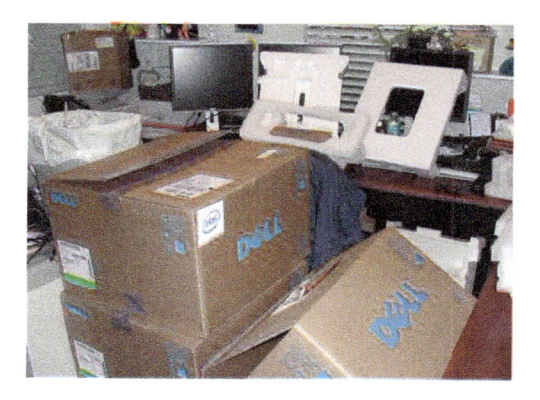

FIGURE 8.1 ■ Housekeeping is an important topic. Cluttered areas can be breeding grounds for injuries. *Courtesy of Estero Fire Rescue.*

more healthful for all of your members. You might want to start by selecting the areas that are most critical to your organization. Then expand your self-inspection checklists over time to cover all areas that pertain to your organization. Remember that a standard checklist is a tool to help, not a definitive statement of what is mandatory.

Do not spend time with items that have no application to your organization. Keep in mind that standard checklists are designed to encompass any organization's risk and may not be completely applicable to your organization. You can take a checklist and tailor it to your organization. Then make sure you or the person you designate with the task of conducting the inspection sees every item on the checklist. Never leave anything to memory or chance. Write down what you see or do not see and what you think should be done to fix or better the situation.

Add information from your completed checklists to injury information, personnel information, and process and equipment information to build a foundation to help you determine what problems exist. If you use OSHA standards in your problem-solving process, it will be easier for you to determine the actions needed to solve any problems you find. Once hazards have been identified, institute control procedures and establish the hierarchy of controls (four general strategies for managing hazards: engineering controls, management controls, personal protective equipment, and interim measures).

SELF-INSPECTION SCOPE

A self-inspection scope that will cover most EMS facilities includes the following:

- *Building and grounds conditions*—floors, walls, ceilings, exits, stairs, walkways, ramps, platforms, driveways, aisles
- *Housekeeping program*—waste disposal (including biomedical waste), tools, objects, materials, leakage and spillage, cleaning methods, schedules, work areas, remote areas, storage areas
- *Electricity*—equipment, switches, breakers, fuses, switchboxes, junctions, special fixtures, circuits, insulation, extensions, tools, motors, grounding, national electric code compliance
- *Lighting*—type, intensity, controls, conditions, diffusion, location, glare and shadow control
- *Heating and ventilation*—type, effectiveness, temperature, humidity, controls, natural and artificial ventilation, and exhausting
- *Machinery*—points of operation, flywheels, gears, shafts, pulleys, key ways, belts, couplings, sprockets, chains, frames, controls, lighting for tools and equipment, brakes, exhausting, feeding, oiling, adjusting, maintenance, lockout/tagout, grounding, work space, location, purchasing standards
- *Personnel*—training, including hazard identification training; experience; methods of checking machines before use; type of clothing; PPE; use of guards; tool storage; work practices; methods for cleaning, oiling, or adjusting machinery
- *Hand and power tools*—purchasing standards, inspection, storage, repair, types, maintenance, grounding, use, and handling
- *Chemicals*—storage, handling, transportation, spills, disposals, amounts used, labeling, toxicity

or other harmful effects, warning signs, supervision, training, protective clothing and equipment, hazard communication requirements
- *Fire prevention*—extinguishers, alarms, sprinklers, smoking rules, exits, personnel assigned, separation of flammable materials and dangerous operations, explosion-proof fixtures in hazardous locations, waste disposal, and training of personnel
- *Maintenance*—regular and preventive maintenance on all equipment used at the worksite, records of all work performed on the machinery
- *PPE*—type, size, maintenance, repair, age, storage, assignment of responsibility, purchasing methods, standards observed, training in care and use, rules of use, method of assignment
- *Transportation*—motor vehicle safety, seat belts, vehicle maintenance, safe driver programs
- *First aid program/supplies*—medical care locations, posted emergency phone numbers, accessible first aid kits for personnel (Keep in mind that not all personnel at an EMS facility will have medical training, such as office staff and maintenance personnel.)
- *Evacuation plan*—procedures for an emergency evacuation (e.g., fire, chemical/biological incidents, bomb threat, escape procedures and routes, critical plant operations, personnel accounting following an evacuation, rescue and medical duties and ways to report emergencies)

REQUIRED POSTINGS

A number of postings are required in each EMS facility. It is important that you make sure that those required are posted accordingly. The following are a few questions to assist you in making sure you are in compliance: Is the required OSHA Job Safety and Health Protection Poster displayed in a prominent location where all personnel are likely to see it? Are emergency telephone numbers posted where they can be readily found in case of emergency? Where personnel may be exposed to toxic substances or harmful physical agents, has appropriate information concerning personnel access to medical and exposure records and Material Safety Data Sheets (MSDS) been posted or otherwise made readily available to affected personnel? Are signs concerning exit routes; room capacities; floor loading; biohazards; exposures to X-rays, microwaves, or other harmful radiation or substances all posted where appropriate? Is the Summary of Work-Related Injuries and Illnesses (OSHA Form 300A) posted during the months of February, March, and April?

Some of the statutes and regulations enforced by agencies within the U.S. Department of Labor require that such notices be posted in the workplace. The Department of Labor provides electronic copies of such notices, some of which are available in languages other than English.

It is important to note that posting requirements vary by statute; that is, not all personnel are covered by each of the U.S. Department of Labor's statutes and thus may not be required to post a specific notice. For example, some small organizations may not be covered by the Family and Medical Leave Act and thus would not be subject to that act's posting requirements. Figures 8.2 through 8.9 offer a sampling of posters that you should post at each facility.

■ OFFICE, STATION, AND FACILITY—

Maintaining a healthy office environment requires attention to chemical hazards, equipment and work station design, physical environment (temperature, humidity, light, noise, ventilation, and space), task design, psychological factors (personal interactions, work pace, job control), and sometimes chemical or other environmental exposures.

A well-designed office allows personnel to work comfortably (correct ergonomic design) without needing to overreach, sit, or

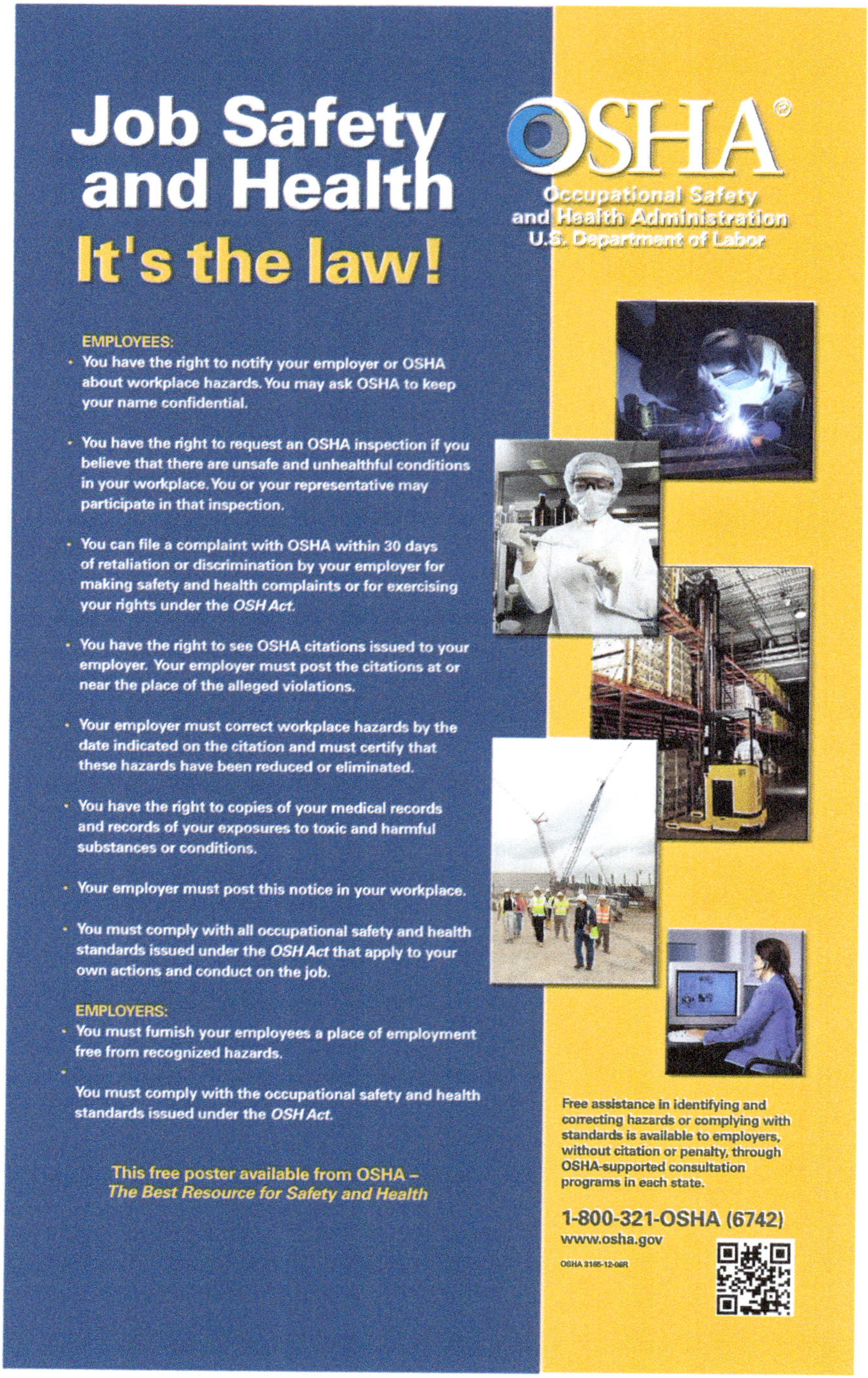

190 CHAPTER 8 *Station, Office, and Facility Safety*

FIGURE 8.2 ■ Job Safety and Health poster. *Source: U.S. Department of Labor.*

Equal Employment Opportunity is

THE LAW

Private Employers, State and Local Governments, Educational Institutions, Employment Agencies and Labor Organizations

Applicants to and employees of most private employers, state and local governments, educational institutions, employment agencies and labor organizations are protected under Federal law from discrimination on the following bases:

RACE, COLOR, RELIGION, SEX, NATIONAL ORIGIN
Title VII of the Civil Rights Act of 1964, as amended, protects applicants and employees from discrimination in hiring, promotion, discharge, pay, fringe benefits, job training, classification, referral, and other aspects of employment, on the basis of race, color, religion, sex (including pregnancy), or national origin. Religious discrimination includes failing to reasonably accommodate an employee's religious practices where the accommodation does not impose undue hardship.

DISABILITY
Title I and Title V of the Americans with Disabilities Act of 1990, as amended, protect qualified individuals from discrimination on the basis of disability in hiring, promotion, discharge, pay, fringe benefits, job training, classification, referral, and other aspects of employment. Disability discrimination includes not making reasonable accommodation to the known physical or mental limitations of an otherwise qualified individual with a disability who is an applicant or employee, barring undue hardship.

AGE
The Age Discrimination in Employment Act of 1967, as amended, protects applicants and employees 40 years of age or older from discrimination based on age in hiring, promotion, discharge, pay, fringe benefits, job training, classification, referral, and other aspects of employment.

SEX (WAGES)
In addition to sex discrimination prohibited by Title VII of the Civil Rights Act, as amended, the Equal Pay Act of 1963, as amended, prohibits sex discrimination in the payment of wages to women and men performing substantially equal work, in jobs that require equal skill, effort, and responsibility, under similar working conditions, in the same establishment.

GENETICS
Title II of the Genetic Information Nondiscrimination Act of 2008 protects applicants and employees from discrimination based on genetic information in hiring, promotion, discharge, pay, fringe benefits, job training, classification, referral, and other aspects of employment. GINA also restricts employers' acquisition of genetic information and strictly limits disclosure of genetic information. Genetic information includes information about genetic tests of applicants, employees, or their family members; the manifestation of diseases or disorders in family members (family medical history); and requests for or receipt of genetic services by applicants, employees, or their family members.

RETALIATION
All of these Federal laws prohibit covered entities from retaliating against a person who files a charge of discrimination, participates in a discrimination proceeding, or otherwise opposes an unlawful employment practice.

WHAT TO DO IF YOU BELIEVE DISCRIMINATION HAS OCCURRED
There are strict time limits for filing charges of employment discrimination. To preserve the ability of EEOC to act on your behalf and to protect your right to file a private lawsuit, should you ultimately need to, you should contact EEOC promptly when discrimination is suspected:
The U.S. Equal Employment Opportunity Commission (EEOC), 1-800-669-4000 (toll-free) or 1-800-669-6820 (toll-free TTY number for individuals with hearing impairments). EEOC field office information is available at www.eeoc.gov or in most telephone directories in the U.S. Government or Federal Government section. Additional information about EEOC, including information about charge filing, is available at www.eeoc.gov.

Employers Holding Federal Contracts or Subcontracts

Applicants to and employees of companies with a Federal government contract or subcontract are protected under Federal law from discrimination on the following bases:

RACE, COLOR, RELIGION, SEX, NATIONAL ORIGIN
Executive Order 11246, as amended, prohibits job discrimination on the basis of race, color, religion, sex or national origin, and requires affirmative action to ensure equality of opportunity in all aspects of employment.

INDIVIDUALS WITH DISABILITIES
Section 503 of the Rehabilitation Act of 1973, as amended, protects qualified individuals from discrimination on the basis of disability in hiring, promotion, discharge, pay, fringe benefits, job training, classification, referral, and other aspects of employment. Disability discrimination includes not making reasonable accommodation to the known physical or mental limitations of an otherwise qualified individual with a disability who is an applicant or employee, barring undue hardship. Section 503 also requires that Federal contractors take affirmative action to employ and advance in employment qualified individuals with disabilities at all levels of employment, including the executive level.

DISABLED, RECENTLY SEPARATED, OTHER PROTECTED, AND ARMED FORCES SERVICE MEDAL VETERANS
The Vietnam Era Veterans' Readjustment Assistance Act of 1974, as amended, 38 U.S.C. 4212, prohibits job discrimination and requires affirmative action to employ and advance in employment disabled veterans, recently separated veterans (within three years of discharge or release from active duty), other protected veterans (veterans who served during a war or in a campaign or expedition for which a campaign badge has been authorized), and Armed Forces service medal veterans (veterans who, while on active duty, participated in a U.S. military operation for which an Armed Forces service medal was awarded).

RETALIATION
Retaliation is prohibited against a person who files a complaint of discrimination, participates in an OFCCP proceeding, or otherwise opposes discrimination under these Federal laws.

Any person who believes a contractor has violated its nondiscrimination or affirmative action obligations under the authorities above should contact immediately:

The Office of Federal Contract Compliance Programs (OFCCP), U.S. Department of Labor, 200 Constitution Avenue, N.W., Washington, D.C. 20210, 1-800-397-6251 (toll-free) or (202) 693-1337 (TTY). OFCCP may also be contacted by e-mail at OFCCP-Public@dol.gov, or by calling an OFCCP regional or district office, listed in most telephone directories under U.S. Government, Department of Labor.

Programs or Activities Receiving Federal Financial Assistance

RACE, COLOR, NATIONAL ORIGIN, SEX
In addition to the protections of Title VII of the Civil Rights Act of 1964, as amended, Title VI of the Civil Rights Act of 1964, as amended, prohibits discrimination on the basis of race, color or national origin in programs or activities receiving Federal financial assistance. Employment discrimination is covered by Title VI if the primary objective of the financial assistance is provision of employment, or where employment discrimination causes or may cause discrimination in providing services under such programs. Title IX of the Education Amendments of 1972 prohibits employment discrimination on the basis of sex in educational programs or activities which receive Federal financial assistance.

INDIVIDUALS WITH DISABILITIES
Section 504 of the Rehabilitation Act of 1973, as amended, prohibits employment discrimination on the basis of disability in any program or activity which receives Federal financial assistance. Discrimination is prohibited in all aspects of employment against persons with disabilities who, with or without reasonable accommodation, can perform the essential functions of the job.

If you believe you have been discriminated against in a program of any institution which receives Federal financial assistance, you should immediately contact the Federal agency providing such assistance.

FIGURE 8.3 Equal Employment Opportunity Is the Law poster. *Source: U.S. Department of Labor.*

EMPLOYEE RIGHTS

UNDER THE FAIR LABOR STANDARDS ACT

THE UNITED STATES DEPARTMENT OF LABOR WAGE AND HOUR DIVISION

FEDERAL MINIMUM WAGE

$5.85 PER HOUR	$6.55 PER HOUR	$7.25 PER HOUR
BEGINNING JULY 24, 2007	BEGINNING JULY 24, 2008	BEGINNING JULY 24, 2009

STATE AND LOCAL GOVERNMENT EMPLOYEES

OVERTIME PAY

At least 1½ times your regular rate of pay for all hours worked over 40 in a workweek.

Law enforcement and fire protection personnel: You may be paid overtime on the basis of a "work period" of between 7 and 28 consecutive days in length, rather than on a 40-hour workweek basis.

COMPENSATORY TIME

Employees may receive compensatory time off instead of cash overtime pay, at a rate of not less than 1½ hours for each overtime hour worked, where provided pursuant to an agreement or understanding that meets the requirements of the Act.

EXEMPTIONS

The Act does not apply to persons who are not subject to the civil service laws of State or local governments and who are: elected public officials, certain immediate advisors to such officials, certain individuals appointed or selected by such officials to serve in various capacities, or employees of legislative branches of State and local governments. Employees of legislative libraries do not come within this exclusion and are thus covered by the Act.

Certain types of workers are exempt from the minimum wage and overtime pay provisions, including bona fide executive, administrative, and professional employees who meet regulatory requirements.

Any law enforcement or fire protection employee who in any workweek is employed by a public agency employing less than 5 employees in law enforcement or fire protection activities is exempt from the overtime pay provisions.

YOUTH EMPLOYMENT

16 years old is the minimum age for most occupations. An **18**-year old minimum applies to hazardous occupations. Minors **14** and **15** years old may work outside school hours under certain conditions. For more information, visit the YouthRules! Web site at **www.youthrules.dol.gov**.

ENFORCEMENT

The Department of Labor may recover back wages either administratively or through court action for the employees that have been underpaid in violation of the law. Violations may result in civil or criminal action.

Civil money penalties of up to $11,000 per violation may be assessed against employers who violate the youth employment provisions of the law and up to $1,100 per violation against employers who willfully or repeatedly violate the minimum wage or overtime pay provisions. This law prohibits discriminating against or discharging workers who file a complaint or participate in any proceedings under the Act.

ADDITIONAL INFORMATION

- Some state laws provide greater employee protections; employers must comply with both.
- Employees under 20 years of age may be paid a youth minimum wage of not less than $4.25 an hour during their first 90 consecutive calendar days after initial employment by an employer.
- Employers are required to display this poster where employees can readily see it.

For additional information:

1-866-4-USWAGE

WHD U.S. Wage and Hour Division

(1-866-487-9243) TTY: 1-877-889-5627

WWW.WAGEHOUR.DOL.GOV

U.S. Department of Labor | Employment Standards Administration | Wage and Hour Division

WH Publication 1385
(Revised July 2007)

FIGURE 8.4 Employee Rights Under the Fair Labor Standards Act poster. *Source: U.S. Department of Labor.*

EMPLOYEE RIGHTS AND RESPONSIBILITIES
UNDER THE FAMILY AND MEDICAL LEAVE ACT

Basic Leave Entitlement

FMLA requires covered employers to provide up to 12 weeks of unpaid, job-protected leave to eligible employees for the following reasons:

- For incapacity due to pregnancy, prenatal medical care or child birth;
- To care for the employee's child after birth, or placement for adoption or foster care;
- To care for the employee's spouse, son or daughter, or parent, who has a serious health condition; or
- For a serious health condition that makes the employee unable to perform the employee's job.

Military Family Leave Entitlements

Eligible employees with a spouse, son, daughter, or parent on active duty or call to active duty status in the National Guard or Reserves in support of a contingency operation may use their 12-week leave entitlement to address certain qualifying exigencies. Qualifying exigencies may include attending certain military events, arranging for alternative childcare, addressing certain financial and legal arrangements, attending certain counseling sessions, and attending post-deployment reintegration briefings.

FMLA also includes a special leave entitlement that permits eligible employees to take up to 26 weeks of leave to care for a covered servicemember during a single 12-month period. A covered servicemember is a current member of the Armed Forces, including a member of the National Guard or Reserves, who has a serious injury or illness incurred in the line of duty on active duty that may render the servicemember medically unfit to perform his or her duties for which the servicemember is undergoing medical treatment, recuperation, or therapy; or is in outpatient status; or is on the temporary disability retired list.

Benefits and Protections

During FMLA leave, the employer must maintain the employee's health coverage under any "group health plan" on the same terms as if the employee had continued to work. Upon return from FMLA leave, most employees must be restored to their original or equivalent positions with equivalent pay, benefits, and other employment terms.

Use of FMLA leave cannot result in the loss of any employment benefit that accrued prior to the start of an employee's leave.

Eligibility Requirements

Employees are eligible if they have worked for a covered employer for at least one year, for 1,250 hours over the previous 12 months, and if at least 50 employees are employed by the employer within 75 miles.

Definition of Serious Health Condition

A serious health condition is an illness, injury, impairment, or physical or mental condition that involves either an overnight stay in a medical care facility, or continuing treatment by a health care provider for a condition that either prevents the employee from performing the functions of the employee's job, or prevents the qualified family member from participating in school or other daily activities.

Subject to certain conditions, the continuing treatment requirement may be met by a period of incapacity of more than 3 consecutive calendar days combined with at least two visits to a health care provider or one visit and a regimen of continuing treatment, or incapacity due to pregnancy, or incapacity due to a chronic condition. Other conditions may meet the definition of continuing treatment.

Use of Leave

An employee does not need to use this leave entitlement in one block. Leave can be taken intermittently or on a reduced leave schedule when medically necessary. Employees must make reasonable efforts to schedule leave for planned medical treatment so as not to unduly disrupt the employer's operations. Leave due to qualifying exigencies may also be taken on an intermittent basis.

Substitution of Paid Leave for Unpaid Leave

Employees may choose or employers may require use of accrued paid leave while taking FMLA leave. In order to use paid leave for FMLA leave, employees must comply with the employer's normal paid leave policies.

Employee Responsibilities

Employees must provide 30 days advance notice of the need to take FMLA leave when the need is foreseeable. When 30 days notice is not possible, the employee must provide notice as soon as practicable and generally must comply with an employer's normal call-in procedures.

Employees must provide sufficient information for the employer to determine if the leave may qualify for FMLA protection and the anticipated timing and duration of the leave. Sufficient information may include that the employee is unable to perform job functions, the family member is unable to perform daily activities, the need for hospitalization or continuing treatment by a health care provider, or circumstances supporting the need for military family leave. Employees also must inform the employer if the requested leave is for a reason for which FMLA leave was previously taken or certified. Employees also may be required to provide a certification and periodic recertification supporting the need for leave.

Employer Responsibilities

Covered employers must inform employees requesting leave whether they are eligible under FMLA. If they are, the notice must specify any additional information required as well as the employees' rights and responsibilities. If they are not eligible, the employer must provide a reason for the ineligibility.

Covered employers must inform employees if leave will be designated as FMLA-protected and the amount of leave counted against the employee's leave entitlement. If the employer determines that the leave is not FMLA-protected, the employer must notify the employee.

Unlawful Acts by Employers

FMLA makes it unlawful for any employer to:

- Interfere with, restrain, or deny the exercise of any right provided under FMLA;
- Discharge or discriminate against any person for opposing any practice made unlawful by FMLA or for involvement in any proceeding under or relating to FMLA.

Enforcement

An employee may file a complaint with the U.S. Department of Labor or may bring a private lawsuit against an employer.

FMLA does not affect any Federal or State law prohibiting discrimination, or supersede any State or local law or collective bargaining agreement which provides greater family or medical leave rights.

FMLA section 109 (29 U.S.C. § 2619) requires FMLA covered employers to post the text of this notice. Regulations 29 C.F.R. § 825.300(a) may require additional disclosures.

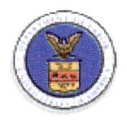

For additional information:
1-866-4US-WAGE (1-866-487-9243) TTY: 1-877-889-5627
WWW.WAGEHOUR.DOL.GOV

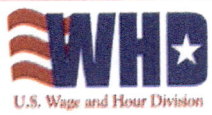

U.S. Department of Labor | Employment Standards Administration | Wage and Hour Division

WHD Publication 1420 Revised January 2009

FIGURE 8.5 Employee Rights and Responsibilities Under the Family and Medical Leave Act poster. *Source: U.S. Department of Labor.*

YOUR RIGHTS UNDER USERRA

THE UNIFORMED SERVICES EMPLOYMENT AND REEMPLOYMENT RIGHTS ACT

USERRA protects the job rights of individuals who voluntarily or involuntarily leave employment positions to undertake military service or certain types of service in the National Disaster Medical System. USERRA also prohibits employers from discriminating against past and present members of the uniformed services, and applicants to the uniformed services.

REEMPLOYMENT RIGHTS

You have the right to be reemployed in your civilian job if you leave that job to perform service in the uniformed service and:

- ☆ you ensure that your employer receives advance written or verbal notice of your service;
- ☆ you have five years or less of cumulative service in the uniformed services while with that particular employer;
- ☆ you return to work or apply for reemployment in a timely manner after conclusion of service; and
- ☆ you have not been separated from service with a disqualifying discharge or under other than honorable conditions.

If you are eligible to be reemployed, you must be restored to the job and benefits you would have attained if you had not been absent due to military service or, in some cases, a comparable job.

RIGHT TO BE FREE FROM DISCRIMINATION AND RETALIATION

If you:

- ☆ are a past or present member of the uniformed service;
- ☆ have applied for membership in the uniformed service; or
- ☆ are obligated to serve in the uniformed service;

then an employer may not deny you:

- ☆ initial employment;
- ☆ reemployment;
- ☆ retention in employment;
- ☆ promotion; or
- ☆ any benefit of employment

because of this status.

In addition, an employer may not retaliate against anyone assisting in the enforcement of USERRA rights, including testifying or making a statement in connection with a proceeding under USERRA, even if that person has no service connection.

HEALTH INSURANCE PROTECTION

- ☆ If you leave your job to perform military service, you have the right to elect to continue your existing employer-based health plan coverage for you and your dependents for up to 24 months while in the military.
- ☆ Even if you don't elect to continue coverage during your military service, you have the right to be reinstated in your employer's health plan when you are reemployed, generally without any waiting periods or exclusions (e.g., pre-existing condition exclusions) except for service-connected illnesses or injuries.

ENFORCEMENT

- ☆ The U.S. Department of Labor, Veterans Employment and Training Service (VETS) is authorized to investigate and resolve complaints of USERRA violations.
- ☆ For assistance in filing a complaint, or for any other information on USERRA, contact VETS at **1-866-4-USA-DOL** or visit its **website at http://www.dol.gov/vets**. An interactive online USERRA Advisor can be viewed at **http://www.dol.gov/elaws/userra.htm**.
- ☆ If you file a complaint with VETS and VETS is unable to resolve it, you may request that your case be referred to the Department of Justice or the Office of Special Counsel, as applicable, for representation.
- ☆ You may also bypass the VETS process and bring a civil action against an employer for violations of USERRA.

The rights listed here may vary depending on the circumstances. The text of this notice was prepared by VETS, and may be viewed on the internet at this address: http://www.dol.gov/vets/programs/userra/poster.htm. Federal law requires employers to notify employees of their rights under USERRA, and employers may meet this requirement by displaying the text of this notice where they customarily place notices for employees.

U.S. Department of Labor 1-866-487-2365 | **U.S. Department of Justice** | **Office of Special Counsel** | ESGR **1-800-336-4590**

Publication Date—October 2008

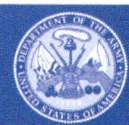

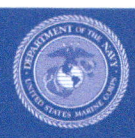

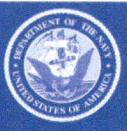

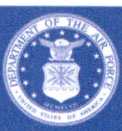

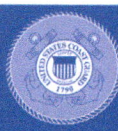

FIGURE 8.6 Your Rights Under USERRA: The Uniformed Services Employment and Reemployment Rights Act poster. *Source: U.S. Department of Labor.*

EMPLOYEE RIGHTS
ON GOVERNMENT CONTRACTS

THE UNITED STATES DEPARTMENT OF LABOR WAGE AND HOUR DIVISION

This establishment is performing Government contract work subject to (check one)

☐ **SERVICE CONTRACT ACT (SCA) or**

☐ **PUBLIC CONTRACTS ACT (PCA)**

MINIMUM WAGES Your rate must be no less than the Federal minimum wage established by the Fair Labor Standards Act (FLSA).

A higher rate may be required for SCA contracts if a wage determination applies. Such wage determination will be posted as an attachment to this Notice.

FRINGE BENEFITS SCA wage determinations may require fringe benefit payments (or a cash equivalent). PCA contracts do not require fringe benefits.

OVERTIME PAY You must be paid 1.5 times your basic rate of pay for all hours worked over 40 in a week. There are some exceptions.

CHILD LABOR No person under 16 years of age may be employed on a PCA contract.

SAFETY & HEALTH Work must be performed under conditions that are sanitary, and not hazardous or dangerous to employees' health and safety.

ENFORCEMENT Specific DOL agencies are responsible for the administration of these laws. To file a complaint or obtain information for: Contact the Wage and Hour Division by calling its toll-free help line at 1-866-4-USWAGE (1-866-487-9243), or visit its Web site at www.wagehour.dol.gov.

Contact the Occupational Safety and Health Administration (OSHA) by calling 1-800-321-OSHA (1-800-321-6742), or visit its Web site at www.osha.gov.

For additional information:

1-866-4-USWAGE **WHD** U.S. Wage and Hour Division

(1-866-487-9243) TTY: 1-877-889-5627

WWW.WAGEHOUR.DOL.GOV

U.S. Department of Labor | Employment Standards Administration | Wage and Hour Division

WHD Publication 1313 (Revised April 2009)
over ▶

FIGURE 8.7 ■ Employee Rights on Government Contracts poster. *Source: U.S. Department of Labor.*

FIGURE 8.8 Employee Polygraph Protection Act poster. *Source: U.S. Department of Labor.*

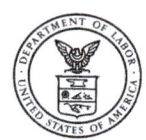

CHAPTER 8 Station, Office, and Facility Safety

This notice must be posted and maintained by the employer in one or more conspicuous places.

★ NOTICE ★
Your employer is subject to the Kansas Workers Compensation law which provides compensation for job-related injuries.
1-800-332-0353

WHAT TO DO IF AN INJURY OCCURS ON THE JOB
Notify your employer immediately. <u>**Your claim may be denied if you fail to tell your employer within 10 DAYS of the injury**</u>. For just cause you may have 75 days to tell the employer of your injury. Thereafter you **must** file a written claim within 200 days of the accident or last date benefits are paid. Submission of Employer's Report of Accident does not constitute a written claim.

MEDICAL BENEFITS
An employer is required to furnish all necessary medical treatment and has the right to designate the treating physician. If the employee seeks treatment from a doctor not authorized by the employer, the employer or its insurance carrier is only liable up to $500.00.

WEEKLY BENEFITS
Benefits are paid by the employer's insurance carrier or self-insurance program. Injured workers are not entitled to compensation for the first week they are off work unless they lose three consecutive weeks. The first compensation payment is normally due at the end of the 14th day of lost time. An injured employee is entitled to a weekly amount of 66 2/3% of his average weekly wage up to a maximum of 75% of the state's average weekly wage.

These benefits are subject to legislative changes and for the latest information on benefit levels, please contact the Division at the address and phone number below. If the injury results in permanent disability, the Kansas compensation law provides for additional benefits.

Helpful Information – Ombudsman

Contact the **Ombudsman/Claims Advisory Section** at the Division of Workers Compensation immediately if you do not receive compensation in a timely manner. The Division has full-time personnel who specialize in aiding injured workers with claim problems. They can give information on what benefits an injured worker is entitled to receive. Such problems as benefits not being paid on time, unpaid medical bills, questions in regard to proper settlement amounts, etc., should be brought to the attention of the **Ombudsman/Claims Advisory Section**. Our toll free telephone number: **1-800-332-0353**.

WHERE TO GET HELP WITH YOUR CLAIM:

Current claims are being administered by _____

The claims office is located at _____ telephone (____) _____

INFORMACIÓN SOBRE COMPENSACIÓN DE TRABAJADORES

La ley exige que cuando un trabajador llega a sufrir un accidente, una herida, o una enfermedad a causa de su empleo, el empleador debe proporcionarle al trabajador incapacitado tratamiento médico y otros beneficios sin ningún costo al trabajador. El trabajador incapacitado tiene derecho a recibir un sueldo reducido, mientras se restablece. La ley tambien protege los derechos del trabajador incapacitado en otras maneras, por ejemplo: se prohibe el desempleo de un trabajador solo por haber reclamado los beneficios de la compensación de trabajadores. Reporte cada accidente o lastimadura industrial inmediatamente al patrón, o al empleador.

<u>Su reclamo puede ser negado si usted no notifica (avisa) a su empleador (patrón) dentro de 10 días del accidente o lastimadura.</u> Por buena causa usted puede tener 75 días para avisarle a su empleador (patrón) de su accidente o lastimadura. De allí en adelante, usted debe entregar un aviso por escrito dentro de 200 días del accidente o último día que recibío tratamiento medico, o que recibío beneficios. Un reporte de accidente no constituta un aviso por escrito. Para mas información acerca de los beneficios o para recibir asistencia con un reclamo, llame al teléfono 1-800-332-0353 (gratis) o al 785-296-2996.

KANSAS
DEPARTMENT OF LABOR

Division of Workers Compensation
800 S.W. Jackson Street, Suite 600, Topeka, KS 66612-1227
Phone: 785-296-2996
Web site: www.dol.ks.gov • E-mail: wc@dol.ks.gov

K-WC 40 (Rev. 3-08)   Persons with impaired hearing or speech utilizing a telecommunications device may access the above number(s) by using the Kansas Relay Center at 1-800-766-3777.

FIGURE 8.9 ■ Individual states also require certain worker compensation posters. This one is from Kansas. *Source: U.S. Department of Labor.*

stand too long, or use awkward postures. Sometimes, equipment or furniture changes are the best solution to allow personnel to work comfortably. On other occasions, the equipment may be satisfactory but the task could be redesigned. For example, studies have shown that those working at computers have less discomfort with short, hourly breaks.

Situations in offices that can lead to injury or illness range from physical hazards (such as cords across walkways, leaving low drawers open, objects falling from above) to task-related (speed or repetition, duration, job control, etc.), environmental (chemical or biological sources), or design-related hazards (such as nonadjustable furniture or equipment). Job stress that results when the requirements of the job do not match the capabilities or resources of the individual also may result in illness. (Figure 8.10 offers a general safety checklist.)

General Safety Checklist

Work Environment
- [ ] Are all worksites clean, sanitary, and orderly?
- [ ] Are work surfaces kept dry, and are appropriate means taken to ensure the surfaces are slip resistant?
- [ ] Are all spilled hazardous materials or liquids, including blood and other potentially infectious materials, cleaned up immediately and according to proper procedures?
- [ ] Are combustible scrap, debris, and waste stored safely and removed from the worksite promptly?
- [ ] Are spilled materials cleaned up immediately?
- [ ] Are changes of direction or elevations readily identifiable?
- [ ] Are aisles or walkways that pass near moving or operating machinery, welding operations, or similar operations arranged so personnel will not be subjected to potential hazards?
- [ ] Is adequate headroom provided for the entire length of any aisle or walkway?
- [ ] Are standard guardrails provided wherever aisle or walkway surfaces are elevated more than 30 inches (76.20 centimeters) above any adjacent floor or the ground?
- [ ] Are bridges provided over conveyors and similar hazards?

Floor and Wall Openings
- [ ] Are floor openings guarded by a cover, a guardrail, or equivalent on all sides (except at stairways or ladder entrances)?
- [ ] Are toeboards installed around the edges of permanent floor openings where persons may pass below the opening?
- [ ] Are skylight screens able to withstand a load of at least 200 pounds (90.7 kilograms)?
- [ ] Is the glass in windows, doors, glass walls, and so on subject to possible human impact, and are they of sufficient thickness and type for the conditions of use?
- [ ] Are grates or similar types of covers over floor openings, such as floor drains, designed to allow unimpeded foot traffic and rolling equipment?
- [ ] Are unused portions of service pits and pits not in use either covered or protected by guardrails or the equivalent?
- [ ] Are manhole covers, trench covers, and similar covers and their supports designed to carry a truck rear axle load of at least 20,000 pounds (9,072 kilograms) when located in roadways and subject to vehicle traffic?
- [ ] Are floor or wall openings in fire-resistant construction provided with doors or covers compatible with the fire rating of the structure?

FIGURE 8.10 ■ Checklist for general safety. *Source: U.S. Department of Labor.*

- [ ] Is all regulated waste, as defined in OSHA Bloodborne Pathogens Standard 29 CFR 1910.1030 discarded according to federal, state, and local regulations?
- [ ] Are accumulations of combustible dust routinely removed from elevated surfaces, including the overhead structure of buildings?
- [ ] Is combustible dust cleaned up with a vacuum system to prevent suspension of dust particles in the environment?
- [ ] Is metallic or conductive dust prevented from entering or accumulating on or around electrical enclosures or equipment?
- [ ] Are covered metal waste cans used for oily or paint-soaked waste?
- [ ] Are all oil- and gas-fired devices equipped with flame failure controls to prevent flow of fuel if pilots or main burners are not working?
- [ ] Are paint spray booths and dip tanks cleaned regularly?
- [ ] Are the minimum number of toilets and washing facilities provided and maintained in a clean and sanitary fashion?
- [ ] Are all work areas adequately illuminated?
- [ ] Are pits and floor openings covered or otherwise guarded?
- [ ] Have all confined spaces been evaluated for compliance with 29 CFR 1910.146? (Permit required for confined spaces.)

Walkways
- [ ] Are aisles and passageways kept clear and marked as appropriate?
- [ ] Are wet surfaces covered with nonslip materials?
- [ ] Are holes in the floor, sidewalk, or other walking surface repaired properly, covered, or otherwise made safe?
- [ ] Is there safe clearance for walking in aisles where motorized or mechanical handling equipment is operating?
- [ ] Are materials or equipment stored in such a way that sharp projections will not interfere with the walkway? Is equipment provided with a self-closing feature when appropriate?

Stairs and Stairways
- [ ] Do standard stair rails or handrails on all stairways have at least four risers?
- [ ] Are all stairways at least 22 inches (55.88 centimeters) wide?
- [ ] Do stairs have landing platforms of not less than 30 inches (76.20 centimeters) in the direction of travel, and do they extend 22 inches (55.88 centimeters) in width every 12 feet (3.6576 meters) or less of vertical rise?
- [ ] Do stairs angle no more than 50 degrees and no less than 30 degrees?
- [ ] Are stairs of hollow-pan type treads and landings filled to the top edge of the pan with solid material?
- [ ] Are step risers on stairs uniform from top to bottom?
- [ ] Are steps slip resistant?
- [ ] Are stairway handrails located between 30 inches (76.20 centimeters) and 34 inches (86.36 centimeters) above the leading edge of stair treads?
- [ ] Do stairway handrails have at least 3 inches (7.62 centimeters) of clearance between the handrails and the wall or surface they are mounted on?
- [ ] Where doors or gates open directly on a stairway, is a platform provided so the swing of the door does not reduce the width of the platform to less than 21 inches (53.34 centimeters)?

FIGURE 8.10 ■ *(Continued)*

> [ ] Are stairway handrails capable of withstanding a load of 200 pounds (90.7 kilograms), applied within 2 inches (5.08 centimeters) of the top edge in any downward or outward direction?
> [ ] Where stairs or stairways exit directly into any area where vehicles may be operated, are adequate barriers and warnings provided to prevent personnel from stepping into the path of traffic?
> [ ] Do stairway landings have a dimension measured in the direction of travel at least equal to the width of the stairway?
> [ ] Is the vertical distance between stairway landings limited to 12 feet (3.6576 meters) or less?
>
> **Elevated Surfaces**
> [ ] Are signs posted, when appropriate, showing the elevated surface load capacity?
> [ ] Are surfaces that are elevated more than 30 inches (76.20 centimeters) provided with standard guardrails?
> [ ] Are all elevated surfaces beneath which people or machinery could be exposed to falling objects provided with standard 4-inch (10.16 centimeters) toeboards?
> [ ] Is a permanent means of access and egress provided to elevated storage and work surfaces?
> [ ] Is required headroom provided where necessary?
> [ ] Is material on elevated surfaces piled, stacked, or racked in a manner to prevent it from tipping, falling, collapsing, rolling, or spreading?
> [ ] Are dock boards or bridge plates used when transferring materials between docks and trucks?

FIGURE 8.10 ■ *(Continued)*

SAFETY AND HEALTH

Despite common belief that the office provides a safe environment to work in, many hazards cause thousands of injuries and health problems among office workers. In addition to the obvious hazards of slippery floors or open file drawers, the modern office may contain hazards such as poor lighting, noise, and poorly designed furniture and equipment (Figure 8.11).

Types of Disabling Accidents

It is estimated that office workers sustain approximately 76,000 fractures, dislocations, sprains, strains, and contusions annually. The leading types of disabling office accidents are falls and slips, strains and overexertion, being struck by or striking against objects, and being caught in or between objects.

There are a number of common office safety and health hazards. They include physical layout and housekeeping, **exits and egress**, **fire hazards**, handling and storage, **office furniture hazards**, **electrical equipment hazards**, **office machinery/tools hazards**, **computer terminal hazards**, **ventilation hazards**, **illumination hazards**, and **noise hazards**. These office hazards relate to essentially two areas: **physical layout** and **housekeeping hazards**. Poor design or poor housekeeping (Figure 8.11) can lead to crowding, lack of privacy, and slips, trips, and falls.

A number of important factors are related to office layout and orderliness. There should be a 3-foot distance between desks and at least 50 square feet of office space per person. Telephone and electric cords can create a hazard; they should be kept out of aisles and walkways. Cords create a tripping hazard, and if not properly secured, electrical cords create a fire hazard.

The placement of office machines should also be considered. They should be kept away from edges of desks and tables. This will help

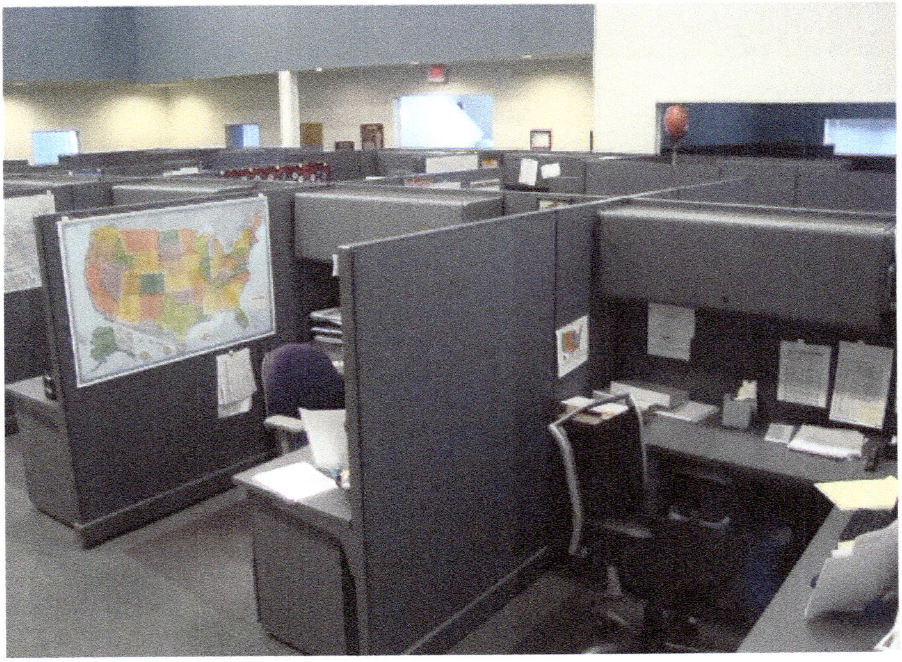

FIGURE 8.11 ■ In the sometimes limited space of a work environment, poor housekeeping can lead to crowding, lack of privacy, and slips, trips, and falls. *Courtesy of Jeffrey T. Lindsey, Ph.D.*

prevent them falling off the desk or table and injuring an individual. They also can cause other injuries, depending on the type of the machine and objects protruding from the machine.

You should regularly inspect, and repair or replace, faulty carpeting. Carpets that come in the form of individual squares are available. When replacing carpet in rooms, this type of carpet should be considered since it can be removed and replaced a lot easier than the traditional rolled carpet that is all one piece.

Some individuals tend to be pack rats. They love to store things in their office or cubicle. In many instances, storage or lack thereof, creates an environment in which individuals tend to keep more in their work area than they should. It is important to remove excess materials from the work area. Often these items need to be discarded or taken to a more suitable storage area.

When spills occur, they should be cleaned up promptly. Spills makes for poor traction and cause many slips and falls. After the spill is removed, and if the floor is wet from mopping the area, warning signs should be posted.

Exits and Egress Hazards

First, let's distinguish the difference between exits and egress. An exit is the place to leave a building. An egress is the path to exit the building. Blocked or improperly planned means of egress can lead to injuries as a result of slips, trips, and falls. If personnel becomes trapped during an emergency due to improper egress, more serious injuries or fatalities can result. There are many times when EMS personnel see blocked or poor means of egress at an emergency scene, yet in their own environments they tend to overlook such problems. Set the example in all that your EMS agency does.

Best Practice

Morgan Stanley, the famous investment bank, is a resilient company. Soon after the 1993 attack on the World Trade Center, the company recognized the grim reality of being in that building. Morgan Stanley's more than 2,700 employees occupied 32 floors (43–74) in the South Tower. In an effort to improve safety, the company hired Rick Rescorla (a highly decorated Vietnam veteran) and put him in charge of security. In addition, three alternative locations in which to conduct business were secured; if another such disaster were to happen again, Morgan Stanley would be able to conduct business again by the next day, which in fact did happen.

During the 9 years following the 1993 attack, Mr. Rescorla, with bullhorn in hand, conducted a monthly evacuation drill. He had a vision and a purpose: to save his friends and colleagues if an attack ever happened again. On September 11, 2001, after the first tower was hit, Mr. Rescorla got on the bullhorn and advised everyone to do what they had practiced over and over, month after month. He was doing this even when building managers were telling people to stay in their locations. People listened to Rick. As a result, Morgan Stanley lost only seven people; Rick Rescorla was among them.

A number of controls ensure proper and safe means of egress, including the following:

- Minimum access to exit should have a width of 28 inches.
- Generally, two exits should be provided.
- Exits and access to exits must be marked.

Means of egress, including stairways used for emergency exit, should be free of obstructions and adequately lit. Personnel must be aware of exits and trained in evacuation procedures. We take these for granted too often. (Figure 8.12 offers an exit and egress checklist.)

Fire Hazards

A serious problem associated with office design is the potential for fire hazards. Offices contain large amounts of combustible materials, such as paper, furniture, and carpeting, which can easily ignite and emit toxic fumes. The following are some ways to reduce office fire hazards:

- Place fire extinguishers and alarms in a conspicuous and accessible location.
- Store excess paper materials inside cabinets, files, or lockers.
- Use flame-retardant materials.

Just because EMS personnel are in the emergency services industry does not protect them from hazards. A fire can occur anywhere. There even have been fires in fire stations. Be sure to take the same precautions you would advise anyone else to take. (Figure 8.13 offers a fire safety checklist.)

Handling and Storage Hazards

The handling and storage of materials can cause a variety of hazards. Improper lifting of materials can cause musculoskeletal disorders such as sprains, strains, and inflamed joints. Office materials that are improperly stored can lead to hazards such as objects falling on personnel, poor visibility, and fires.

There are a number of ways to control those **handling and storage hazards**, including the following:

- An effective ergonomic control program incorporating personnel awareness and training and ergonomic design of work tasks

Exit/Egress Checklist
Exiting or Egress for Evacuation
[ ] Are all exits marked with an exit sign and illuminated by a reliable light source?
[ ] Are the directions to exits, when not immediately apparent, marked with visible signs?
[ ] Are doors, passageways, or stairways that are neither exits nor access to exits, but could be mistaken for exits, appropriately marked "NOT AN EXIT," "TO BASEMENT," "STOREROOM," and so on?
[ ] Are exit signs labeled with the word "EXIT" in lettering at least 5 inches (12.70 centimeters) high and the stroke of the lettering at least ½ inch (1.2700 centimeters) wide?
[ ] Are exit doors side-hinged?
[ ] Are all exits kept free of obstructions?
[ ] Are at least two means of egress provided from elevated platforms, pits, or rooms where the absence of a second exit would increase the risk of injury from hot, poisonous, corrosive, suffocating, flammable, or explosive substances?
[ ] Are there sufficient exits to permit prompt escape in case of emergency?
[ ] Are special precautions taken to protect members during construction and repair operations?
[ ] Is the number of exits from each floor of a building and the number of exits from the building itself appropriate for the building occupancy load?
[ ] Are exit stairways that are required to be separated from other parts of a building enclosed by at least 2-hour fire-resistive construction in buildings more than four stories in height, and not less than 1-hour fire-resistive construction elsewhere?
[ ] Where ramps are used as part of required exiting from a building, is the ramp slope limited to 1 foot (0.3048 meter) vertical and 12 feet (3.6576 meters) horizontal?
[ ] Where exiting will be through frameless glass doors, glass exit doors, or storm doors, are the doors fully tempered and meet the safety requirements for human impact?
[ ] Are exit plans or escape routes prominently displayed in every room?

Exit Doors
[ ] Are doors that are required to serve as exits designed and constructed so that the path of exit travel is obvious and direct?
[ ] Are windows that could be mistaken for exit doors made inaccessible by means of barriers or railings?
[ ] Can exit doors able be opened from the direction of exit travel without the use of a key or any special knowledge or effort when the building is occupied?
[ ] Is a revolving, sliding, or overhead door prohibited from serving as a required exit door?
[ ] Where panic hardware is installed on a required exit door, will it allow the door to open by applying a force of 15 pounds (6.80 kilograms) or less in the direction of the exit traffic?
[ ] Are doors on cold storage rooms provided with an inside release mechanism that will release the latch and open the door even if the door is padlocked or otherwise locked on the outside?
[ ] Where exit doors open directly onto any street, alley, or other area where vehicles may be operated, are adequate barriers and warnings provided to prevent personnel from stepping into the path of traffic?
[ ] Are doors that swing in both directions and are located between rooms where there is frequent traffic provided with viewing panels in each door?

FIGURE 8.12 ■ Checklist for exit and egress safety.

Fire Protection Checklist
[ ] Is your local fire department familiar with your facility, its location, and specific hazards?
[ ] If you have a fire alarm system, is it certified as required and tested annually?
[ ] If you have interior standpipes and valves, are they inspected regularly?
[ ] If you have outside private fire hydrants, are they flushed at least once a year and on a routine preventive maintenance schedule?
[ ] Are fire doors and shutters in good operating condition?
[ ] Are fire doors and shutters unobstructed and protected against obstructions, including their counterweights?
[ ] Are fire door and shutter fusible links in place?
[ ] Are automatic sprinkler system water-control valves, air, and water pressure checked periodically as required?
[ ] Is the maintenance of automatic sprinkler systems assigned to responsible persons or to a sprinkler contractor?
[ ] Are sprinkler heads protected by metal guards if exposed to potential physical damage?
[ ] Is proper clearance maintained below sprinkler heads?
[ ] Are portable fire extinguishers provided in adequate number and type and mounted in readily accessible locations?
[ ] Are fire extinguishers recharged regularly with this noted on the inspection tag?
[ ] Are personnel periodically instructed in the use of fire extinguishers and fire protection procedures?
[ ] Are fire extinguishers selected and provided for the types of materials in the areas where they are to be used?
[ ] Class A, Ordinary combustible material fires.
[ ] Class B, Flammable liquid, gas, or grease fires.
[ ] Class C, Energized-electrical equipment fires.
[ ] Are appropriate fire extinguishers mounted within 75 feet (22.86 meters) of outside areas containing flammable liquids and within 10 feet (3.048 meters) of any inside storage area for such materials?
[ ] Are extinguishers free from obstructions or blockage?
[ ] Are all extinguishers serviced, maintained, and tagged at intervals not to exceed 1 year?
[ ] Are all extinguishers fully charged and in their designated places?
[ ] Where sprinkler systems are permanently installed, are the nozzle heads so directed or arranged that water will not be sprayed into operating electrical switchboards and equipment?

FIGURE 8.13 Checklist for fire protection.

- No storage of materials on top of cabinets or in aisles or walkways
- Heavy objects stored on lower shelves and materials stacked neatly
- Flammable and combustible materials identified and properly stored

Another area that is important is training. Many EMS personnel are required to take hazmat training to respond to incidents. There is also a requirement for personnel to have hazard communication (hazcom) training. This training is separate from and in addition to hazmat training for field response. Its purpose is to explain and reinforce the information presented to personnel from labels and MSDSs, and to apply this information in the EMS environment.

Office Furniture Hazards
Many hazards are associated with office furniture. Whether it is the office or the station, serious injuries can result from defective

furniture, misuse of chairs, desks, or file cabinets, and improper use of ladders and stools. Particular attention must be paid to these issues in order to improve safety in the office environment.

Chairs. A properly fitting chair can make a significant difference to personnel. Every person is unique in structure, so it is important that individuals select a chair that fits the body well. Chairs also should be properly designed and regularly inspected for missing casters and loose parts. Safety should be enforced with the use of chairs. Never allow individuals to climb on a chair. Make sure ladders or stools are available in a location that is both convenient and readily accessible. Individuals should not be allowed to lean back in an office chair with feet up. Do not allow personnel to scoot across the floor while sitting in a chair, because the chair may catch on an object and flip, causing injuries to the individual.

File Cabinets. File cabinets can cause severe injury and even death if proper precautions are not taken. For example, individuals should open only one file drawer at a time. If more than one drawer is opened, the cabinet could fall forward and onto the person. The location of the file cabinet is important as well. Do not locate file cabinets close to doorways or in aisles where they can make it difficult to pass through or where they can block egress. File cabinets and shelving should also be anchored to the wall.

Desks. Desks can be another cause of injury. You should keep desks in good condition. They should be free from sharp edges, nails, or other sharp objects. Ensure that glass-top desks do not have sharp edges. Desk drawers should be kept closed when not in use. This will make the desk a lot safer for personnel who work at it and those passing by or approaching the desk.

Ambulances

In many EMS systems, personnel are deployed at the beginning of a shift and stationed at certain points in the district. In many instances personnel stay in the ambulance until they receive a call and only get out when they are on an incident. This has led to an increase in back pain for these providers. According to Morneau and Stothart (1999), 93% of paramedics said that they suffer from back pain or discomfort while simply sitting in an ambulance. (This was not pain or discomfort due to a lifting injury.) Interestingly, 88% of paramedics within their first 6 years of employment complained of suffering from this back pain/discomfort at least once a week or more often. Even more revealing was the fact that 90% of all respondents 30 years of age or younger complained of this pain/discomfort at least every other shift or more often.

Ladders

There are many different types of ladders. Ladders should be made available so personnel can access files or storage areas that are out of reach. As with any task, be sure that you provide the right ladder for the task at hand. Ensure that the ladder is in good condition and inspected regularly. Personnel should be warned not to use the top of a ladder as a step. A ladder of proper length should be used. Do not ever use a ladder that is too short and does not reach the intended point.

Personnel should be sure the ladder is fully open and the spreaders are locked. If not, the ladder could become unstable and collapse. The ladder also should be placed on a slip-free surface. The area around a ladder should be free of debris. Ladder safety should be stressed to all personnel. Falls from ladders are not uncommon (Figures 8.14 and 8.15).

In addition, there are weight limits to ladders. When purchasing a ladder, purchase the ladder that will do the job.

> **Volunteer Fire Fighter Dies After Nine-Foot-Fall from Ladder—Pennsylvania**
> On January 17, 2000, a 53-year-old male volunteer fire fighter (the victim) died after the extension ladder he was descending slipped out from under him while he was performing maintenance work on the previous day. The victim had been working on replacing a garage door opener in the middle bay of the fire station before the incident occurred. Access to the door opener was gained by placing a 14-foot fireground aluminum extension ladder against the side of a fire rescue truck, climbing the ladder to the roof of the fire rescue truck, and then accessing the garage door opener. The victim had removed the existing door opener and was in the process of assisting in getting the new door opener ready for installation. While descending the extension ladder, the ladder slipped out from under him and the victim fell headfirst to the concrete floor. Another firefighter, who was assisting the victim in the replacement of the door opener, saw the victim fall and immediately jumped down to the ground from the roof of the rescue truck to assist the victim. He summoned a civilian who was on the ground putting the new opener together. The firefighter who jumped from the roof of the rescue truck ran to a neighboring house to inform the victim's wife, while the civilian called 911. Within a few minutes, paramedics and a police officer arrived on scene. The victim was intubated and transported via a helicopter to the local hospital where he died of his injuries.
>
> NIOSH investigators concluded that, to minimize the risk of similar occurrences, fire departments should:
> * Ensure that ladders are used in accordance with existing safety standards.
> * Designate an individual as the fire station safety officer for all in-house maintenance to identify potential hazards and ensure that those hazards are eliminated.
> * Consider the use of mobile scaffolding, personnel lifts, scissor lifts, or boom lifts, instead of the top surface of a fire truck.

FIGURE 8.14 This NIOSH report (NIOSH, 2000) illustrates the importance of ladder safety.

Electrical Hazards

Electrical hazards should be considered in every safety program. Electrical accidents in offices, stations, and facilities usually occur as a result of faulty or defective equipment, unsafe installation, or misuse of equipment.

To prevent electrical hazards, equipment must be properly grounded to prevent shock injuries. A sufficient number of outlets will prevent overloading of circuits. This may not always be the case in older buildings. It is good practice to employ a licensed electrician to upgrade the electrical system and add receptacles as needed. Extension cords should be avoided. You should never allow the use of poorly maintained or nonapproved equipment. No type of electrical cord should be dragged over nails, hooks, or other sharp objects; this could cause the outer sheathing to wear away or damage the wires and cause a fire hazard or potential electrical shock to someone who comes in contact with the cord. You need to ensure that receptacles are installed and equipment maintained so that no live electrical parts are exposed.

Whether it is an office machine, a station machine, or a machine in the maintenance shop, all machines must be disconnected before cleaning or adjusting; this will help prevent electrical shock. Generally, machines and equipment must be locked or tagged out during maintenance. Shortcuts should never be allowed, and safety procedures should be followed at all times (Figure 8.16).

Ladder Safety Checklist
[ ] Are all ladders maintained in good condition, joints between steps and side rails tight, all hardware and fittings securely attached, and moveable parts operating freely without binding or undue play?
[ ] Are nonslip safety feet provided on each metal or rung ladder, and are ladder rungs and steps free of grease and oil?
[ ] Are personnel prohibited from placing a ladder in front of doors opening toward the ladder unless the door is blocked open, locked, or guarded?
[ ] Are personnel prohibited from placing ladders on boxes, barrels, or other unstable bases to obtain additional height?
[ ] Are personnel required to face the ladder when ascending or descending?
[ ] Are personnel prohibited from using ladders that are broken, have missing steps, rungs, or cleats, broken side rails, or other faulty equipment?
[ ] Are personnel instructed not to use the top step of ordinary stepladders as a step?
[ ] When portable rung ladders are used to gain access to elevated platforms, roofs, etc., does the ladder always extend at least 3 feet (0.9144 meters) above the elevated surface?
[ ] Are personnel required to secure the base of a portable rung or cleat-type ladder to prevent slipping, or otherwise lash or hold it in place?
[ ] Are portable metal ladders legibly marked with signs reading "CAUTION! Do Not Use Around Electrical Equipment" or equivalent wording?
[ ] Are personnel prohibited from using ladders as guys, braces, skids, gin poles, or for other than their intended purposes?
[ ] Are personnel instructed to only adjust extension ladders while standing at a base (not while standing on the ladder or from a position above the ladder)?
[ ] Are metal ladders inspected for damage?
[ ] Are the rungs of ladders uniformly spaced at 12 inches (30.48 centimeters) center to center?

FIGURE 8.15 ■ Checklist for ladder safety.

Office Machinery and Tool Hazards

Office machines have the potential to cause significant injury to the user. They can have hazardous moving parts, such as electric hole punches and paper shredders, which can cause lacerations, abrasions, and fractures. Misuse of office tools, such as pens, pencils, paper, letter openers, scissors, and staplers can cause cuts, punctures, and related infections.

Photocopying Machines. Photocopy machine hazards include excessive noise and intense light. During repair or troubleshooting, some parts of the copier may be hot. Proper precautions should be taken. Because it is quicker to lay the document on the glass and make the copy rather than open the lid, laying the document on the glass, closing the lid, making the copy, and opening the lid again to retrieve the document, you must encourage personnel to keep the document cover closed when making copies.

The location of the machine also is important. To reduce noise exposure, locate the machine in an isolated area or an area that will help reduce the amount of noise generated by the machine. Have the machines serviced routinely, and always follow the manufacturer's instructions for troubleshooting.

Electrical Safety Checklist
[ ] Do you require compliance with OSHA standards for all contract electrical work?
[ ] Are all personnel required to report any obvious hazard to life or property in connection with electrical equipment or lines as soon as possible?
[ ] Are personnel instructed to conduct preliminary inspections and/or appropriate tests to determine conditions before starting work on electrical equipment or lines?
[ ] When electrical equipment or lines are to be serviced, maintained, or adjusted, are necessary switches opened, locked out, or tagged whenever possible?
[ ] Are portable electrical tools and equipment grounded or of the double-insulated type?
[ ] Are electrical appliances, such as vacuum cleaners, polishers, vending machines, and so on, grounded?
[ ] Do extension cords have a grounding conductor?
[ ] Are multiple plug adaptors prohibited?
[ ] Are ground-fault circuit interrupters installed on each temporary 15 or 20 ampere, 120 volt alternating current (AC) circuit at locations where construction, demolition, modifications, alterations, or excavations are being performed?
[ ] Are all temporary circuits protected by suitable disconnecting switches or plug connectors at the junction with permanent wiring?
[ ] Do you have electrical installations in hazardous dust or vapor areas? If so, do they meet the National Electrical Code (NEC) for hazardous locations?
[ ] Are exposed wiring and cords with frayed or deteriorated insulation repaired or replaced promptly?
[ ] Are flexible cords and cables free of splices or taps?
[ ] Are clamps or other securing means provided on flexible cords or cables at plugs, receptacles, tools, equipment, and son, and is the cord jacket securely held in place?
[ ] Are all cord, cable, and raceway connections intact and secure?
[ ] In wet or damp locations, are electrical tools and equipment appropriate for the use or location or otherwise protected?
[ ] Is the location of electrical power lines and cables (overhead, underground, under floor, other side of walls, etc.) determined before digging, drilling, or beginning similar work?
[ ] Are metal measuring tapes, ropes, hand-lines, or similar devices with metallic thread woven into the fabric prohibited where they could come in contact with energized parts of equipment or circuit conductors?
[ ] Is the use of metal ladders prohibited where the ladder or the person using the ladder could come in contact with energized parts of equipment, fixtures, or circuit conductors?
[ ] Are all disconnecting switches and circuit breakers labeled to indicate their use or equipment served?
[ ] Are disconnecting means always opened before fuses are replaced?
[ ] Do all interior wiring systems include provisions for grounding metal parts of electrical raceways, equipment, and enclosures?
[ ] Are all electrical raceways and enclosures securely fastened in place?
[ ] Are all energized parts of electrical circuits and equipment guarded against accidental contact by approved cabinets or enclosures?
[ ] Are sufficient access and working space provided and maintained around all electrical equipment to permit ready and safe operations and maintenance?
[ ] Are all unused openings (including conduit knockouts) in electrical enclosures and fittings closed with appropriate covers, plugs, or plates?

FIGURE 8.16 ■ Checklist for electrical safety issues.

> [ ] Are electrical enclosures, such as switches, receptacles, junction boxes, and so on, provided with tight-fitting covers or plates?
> [ ] Are disconnecting switches for electrical motors in excess of 2 horsepower able to open the circuit when the motor is stalled without exploding? (Switches must be horsepower rated equal to or in excess of the motor rating.)
> [ ] Is low-voltage protection provided in the control device of motors of driving machines or equipment that could cause injury from inadvertent starting?
> [ ] Is each motor disconnecting switch or circuit breaker located within sight of the motor control device?
> [ ] Is each motor located within sight of its controller, or can the controller disconnecting means be locked open, or is a separate disconnecting means installed in the circuit within sight of the motor?
> [ ] Is the controller for each motor that exceeds 2 horsepower rated equal to or above the rating of the motor it serves?
> [ ] Are personnel who regularly work on or around energized electrical equipment or lines instructed in cardiopulmonary resuscitation (CPR)?
> [ ] Are personnel prohibited from working alone on energized lines or equipment over 600 volts?

FIGURE 8.16 ■ *(Continued)*

Paper Cutters. Paper cutters can cut more than paper. Safety precautions include keeping the blade down and locked when not in use. Also make sure a blade guard is provided and fingers kept clear of the blade. Caution should be used when operating a paper cutter.

Staplers. Automatic staplers can have the same effect as a nail gun, causing significant puncture wounds. Personnel always should use a stapler remover when removing staples from documents. Also, personnel should never test a jammed stapler with a thumb. Staplers can cause injury and should be treated accordingly.

Pencils, Pens, Scissors. Causing low-severity but frequent injuries such as puncture wounds and cuts, these implements should be stored in a drawer or with the point down if stored in a pencil holder. Do not allow them to lay cluttered on the desk or other areas. In addition, discourage individuals from putting these items behind their ears, and instead to store pens and pencils in their proper places when not in use.

Other Machines. In addition, a number of precautions and safety measures may be taken with various office machines to make the office, facilities, and stations safer places to work. For example, machines with nip points or rotating parts should be guarded so that office personnel cannot contact the moving parts. Machines that tend to move during operation should be secured. Personnel also should avoid wearing long or loose clothing or accessories around machinery with moving parts. All this will help to reduce the number of potential incidents within the office.

Computers

There are a number of health concerns that accompany computer usage. They include eye irritation; low back, neck, and shoulder pain; cumulative trauma disorders, such as carpal tunnel syndrome; and stress. However, all can be overcome by instituting proper ergonomic design tailored to prevent discomfort. There is a whole science in understanding the ergonomics of using a computer. You may need to have someone evaluate the individual who has issues when using the computer to determine the best remedy for the problem that is occurring.

Factors to consider when using a computer include relation of operator to screen, operator's posture, lighting and background, keyboard position, chair height, document holder, and screen design and color. All can make a difference in the comfort of the operator. If the operator is comfortable, the safety of the individual improves and so does the productivity.

The same considerations should be taken with mobile data computers (MDC), which are common in EMS units. (*Note:* The MDC should not be operated by a driver, especially when the vehicle is in motion. Therefore, place the MDC in the vehicle where it is not accessible to the driver.)

Ventilation

Ventilation has become a major concern within offices and stations. There are a number of sources of air pollution, including natural agents such as mold spores and synthetic chemicals such as cleaning fluids. When dealing with the station environment, be sure to consider sleeping quarters. In many instances, personnel live at the station for a 24-hour period, which gives them three times the exposure of a nine-to-five job. However, in either case, the air quality of the building must be considered and taken seriously.

An adequate ventilation system that delivers quality indoor air and provides comfortable humidity and temperature is a necessity. Ventilation system components should be checked and maintained on a regular basis by qualified technicians. In order for that to happen, you may need to hire or contract with a company that specializes in indoor air quality. In the same vein, you must be cautious when testing the indoor air quality so as not to spark a concern in personnel, especially when you receive the test results. Be sure you completely understand the results and what they mean before sharing them with personnel. Many organizations do not share the results; rather they notify the members that the air quality is being controlled. Consider these questions: Is there adequate circulation? Are intake and outflow vents and ducts cleaned regularly?

There are systems designed for the evacuation of exhaust from vehicle bays. Carbon monoxide should be monitored in all facilities that house vehicles, and proper exhaust evacuation systems should be installed.

Illumination

Lighting can be an issue within the office or station environment, including such related problems as glare, eyestrain, fatigue, and double vision. Keep in mind that poor lighting can be a contributing factor in accidents.

You can implement a few controls to assist in illumination issues. They include regular maintenance of the lighting system, light-colored matte finish on walls and ceilings to reduce glare, adjustable shades on windows, and indirect or task lighting.

Noise

EMS facilities can be very noisy. Printers and other office machines may be running. Telephones may be ringing, sirens and alarms sounding, and, of course, personnel are involved in all sorts of noise-producing job-related activities. Depending on the design of the facility, all those noises can become overwhelming. A high noise level can produce tension and stress, as well as damage hearing.

Noise in the environment can be controlled in various ways. Noisy machines should be placed in an enclosed space to help eliminate or reduce the sound in work areas. Carpeting, draperies, and acoustical ceiling tiles are great ways to help muffle noise. Telephone volume should be adjusted to its lowest level, which may be challenging to some individuals, especially if they have difficulty hearing already.

> **Noise Safety Checklist**
> [ ] Are there areas in the workplace where continuous noise levels exceed 85 decibels?
> [ ] Is there an ongoing preventive health program to educate personnel in safe levels of noise, exposures, effects of noise on their health, and the use of personal protection?
> [ ] Have work areas where noise levels make voice communication between personnel difficult been identified and posted?
> [ ] Are noise levels measured with a sound-level meter or an octave band analyzer, and are records being kept?
> [ ] Have engineering controls been used to reduce excessive noise levels? Where engineering controls are determined to be infeasible, are administrative controls (i.e., worker rotation) being used to minimize individual exposure to noise?
> [ ] Is approved hearing protective equipment (noise attenuating devices) available to every individual working in noisy areas?
> [ ] Have you tried isolating noisy machinery from the rest of your operation?
> [ ] If you use ear protectors, are personnel properly fitted and instructed in their use?
> [ ] Are personnel in high noise areas given periodic audiometric testing to ensure that you have an effective hearing protection system?

FIGURE 8.17 ■ Checklist for noise safety.

However, there are other means to alert individuals to incoming phone calls, such as with a flashing light. Traffic routes in the office should be arranged to reduce traffic within and between work areas. The location of the speakers for the siren should be mounted so that they do their job but have minimal effect on EMS personnel; typically, mounting them in the grill of the front of the vehicle has the best effect. (Figure 8.17 offers a noise safety checklist.)

■ VEHICLE MAINTENANCE AREAS—

Vehicle maintenance areas can be vulnerable to safety issues due to the type of work performed. It is essential that you ascertain that safety is integrated into this area. Personnel should be trained in safety measures, and periodic evaluations should be conducted to ensure that safety is part of the everyday work environment.

EYE PROTECTION AND PROTECTIVE CLOTHING

Eye injuries can be very common in the maintenance shop. They can also be easily prevented. Eye protection should be mandatory for all operations that produce sparks, chips, flying objects, or involve the use of corrosive chemicals. Face shields should be worn for all operations that involve use of a high-pressure steam system. Appropriate gloves and protective clothing also should be worn.

WORK CLOTHING

Emergency vehicle technicians and mechanics should not be allowed to wear loose clothing around rotating equipment. In addition, clothes saturated with oil, grease, or solvents should not be allowed to be worn. Personnel should have at least one change of clothes available to them in the workplace should their clothes become soiled. Thought EVTs tend to like to use compressed air to clean their clothing, this practice should be avoided as it may cause debris from the individual to cause injury to them or someone else.

HOUSEKEEPING

Maintenance areas can become dirty quickly. Shop floors need to be kept free of grease, oil, gasoline, and other slipping hazards. Personnel should not use defective electrical or mechanical shop equipment or hand tools. All automotive shop machinery must be grounded.

LIFTING DEVICES

Jacks, hoists, or other lifting devices should not be used beyond the safe load capacity recommended by the manufacturer. Personnel should not remain in vehicles being lifted by hydraulic lifts or jacks, even if it seems like a workable shortcut. These safety rules should be followed at all times and enforced by the leadership of the organization.

In addition, technicians should not work under vehicles that are not properly supported with approved stands. Makeshift stands made of wood, cement blocks, or boxes should never be used. Although doing so may save time and money, it is not worth the value of an EMS responder's life. Proper lifting of vehicles should be performed at all times.

FLAMMABLES

Flammable materials should be stored and used properly. Gasoline, acetone, kerosene, or similar solvents should never be used to clean hands, floors, walls, or other surfaces. Parts should be cleaned only in approved containers using appropriate solvents. Also, never use standard sanitary sewer drains for the disposal of gasoline, oil, or solvents. Contact your local environmental health and safety agency for disposal guidelines.

In addition, tanks or containers that are used for gasoline or other flammable solvents should never be mechanically opened or repaired by welding without purging and cleaning. Never take shortcuts to save time or money.

TOWING AND CHANGING TIRES

EMS personnel tend to improvise at times. However, if a vehicle must be towed or removed from a roadway, personnel should attempt to do so only if they are properly trained and have the proper equipment.

Changing tires is another common necessity. However, EMS personnel generally should avoid changing tires for safety reasons. If tires must be changed and the tires are not on split-rim wheels, EMS personnel may be allowed to do so, but not on the road unless wheel chocks and warning devices are used. Flares should be set out to warn others whenever a vehicle tire is changed while on a heavily used road. In many instances, it is better to call a professional or a technician to change the tire.

Changing of tires on split-rim wheels should only be performed by individuals with proper training and using only appropriate equipment.

A few areas should be considered when reviewing tire-changing procedures. Personnel should not begin tire inflation before the rim is properly seated, and they should not attempt to adjust the tire with a hammer as it is being inflated. Personnel should not place hands or arms between mounted dual tires during inflation. They should always use a long air chuck for inflation. These rules should be emphasized for all personnel if individuals are allowed to inflate tires on ambulances and other vehicles with dual wheels.

COMPRESSED GASES

Compressed gases, including oxygen, are found in virtually every vehicle and EMS station. EMS is neither isolated nor exempt from the safe and proper storage of compressed gases. For a safety checklist, see Figure 8.18.

Compressed Gas Safety Checklist
[ ] Are cylinders with a water weight capacity over 30 pounds (13.6 kilograms) equipped with a means to connect a valve protector device, or with a collar or recess to protect the valve?
[ ] Are cylinders legibly marked to clearly identify the type of gas?
[ ] Are compressed gas cylinders stored in areas protected from external heat sources such as flame impingement, intense radiant heat, electric arcs, or high-temperature lines?
[ ] Are cylinders located or stored in areas where they will not be damaged by passing or falling objects or subject to tampering by unauthorized persons?
[ ] Are cylinders stored or transported in a manner to prevent them from creating a hazard by tipping, falling, or rolling?
[ ] Are cylinders containing liquefied fuel gas stored or transported in a position so that the safety relief device is always in direct contact with the vapor space in the cylinder?
[ ] Are valve protectors always placed on cylinders when the cylinders are not in use or connected for use?
[ ] Are all valves closed off before a cylinder is moved, when the cylinder is empty, and at the completion of each job?
[ ] Are low-pressure fuel gas cylinders checked periodically for corrosion, general distortion, cracks, or any other defect that might indicate a weakness or render them unfit for service?
[ ] Does the periodic check of low-pressure fuel gas cylinders include a close inspection of the cylinders' bottoms?

Flammable and Combustible Materials
[ ] Are combustible scrap, debris, and waste materials (oily rags, etc.) stored in covered metal receptacles and promptly removed from the worksite?
[ ] Is proper storage practiced to minimize the risk of fire, including spontaneous combustion?
[ ] Are approved containers and tanks used to store and handle flammable and combustible liquids?
[ ] Are all connections on drums and combustible liquid piping, vapor, and liquid tight?
[ ] Are all flammable liquids kept in closed containers when not in use (e.g., parts cleaning tanks, pans, etc.)?
[ ] Are bulk drums of flammable liquids grounded and bonded to containers during dispensing?
[ ] Do storage rooms for flammable and combustible liquids have explosion-proof lights and mechanical or gravity ventilation?
[ ] Is liquefied petroleum gas stored, handled, and used in accordance with safe practices and standards?
[ ] Are "NO SMOKING" signs posted on liquefied petroleum gas tanks and in areas where flammable or combustible materials are used or stored?
[ ] Are liquefied petroleum storage tanks guarded to prevent damage from vehicles?
[ ] Are all solvent wastes and flammable liquids kept in fire-resistant, covered containers until they are removed from the worksite?
[ ] Is vacuuming used whenever possible rather than blowing or sweeping combustible dust?
[ ] Are firm separators placed between containers of combustibles or flammables that are stacked one upon another to ensure their support and stability?
[ ] Are fuel gas cylinders and oxygen cylinders separated by distance and fire-resistant barriers while in storage?
[ ] Are safety cans used for dispensing flammable or combustible liquids at the point of use?
[ ] Are all spills of flammable or combustible liquids cleaned up promptly?
[ ] Are storage tanks adequately vented to prevent the development of excessive vacuum or pressure as a result of filling, emptying, or atmosphere temperature changes?
[ ] Are storage tanks equipped with emergency venting that will relieve excessive internal pressure caused by fire exposure?
[ ] Are rules enforced in areas involving storage and use of hazardous materials?

FIGURE 8.18 ■ Checklist for compressed gas safety.

CHAPTER REVIEW

Summary

EMS tends to focus on incident safety and sometimes forgets about safety for the office staff, stations, and other facilities. But it must be focused on. The first thing is to conduct a self-inspection. This will help to identify any areas of concern. Once you identify those areas, determine a solution that will improve safety in that area.

A bottom-line question each organization must ask is this: Even if many of the facility issues mentioned in this chapter are in place, is there a process in management to emphasize and prioritize the importance each and every day? *Remember:* Without management's commitment, the success of the whole safety program is in jeopardy.

WHAT WOULD YOU DO? Reflection

You are now more prepared to deal with office and facility safety issues. The first thing you need to do is a self-inspection. This will give you a basis or foundation for where some of the issues may lie. You know you want to look at the physical layout of the work area to make sure it is the proper size and that there are no housekeeping issues. You will want to evaluate the machines and make sure they have the proper safety features and are located in the most effective and efficient area of the building. You will want to pay particular attention to the work process and the staff. This includes checking out the furniture and activities such as filing and storing. You know that there are many areas that you can improve on in order to make it safer in the environment. You also know that you will need to do a self-inspection of each of the stations and the maintenance facility to look for any areas that could be improved to make the environment a safer environment.

Review Questions

1. What should be included in a self-inspection? List the items.
2. What are the leading types of disability accidents in an office environment?
3. What controls ensure proper and safe means of egress?
4. Construct a checklist for a self-inspection of your EMS station.
5. You have an employee who complains of lower back, neck, and shoulder pain. She works in the EMS office. Describe what you would do with this complaint.
6. Describe at least two safety issues pertaining to vehicle maintenance areas.

References

Morneau, P. M., and J. P. Stothart. (1999). "System Status Management and Ambulance Design: Negative Effects on Paramedics (My Aching Back)." *Journal of Emergency Medical Services 24*(8), 36–50, 78–81.

National Institute for Occupational Safety and Health. (2000, July 11). "Death in the Line of Duty: Volunteer Fire Fighter Dies After Nine-Foot Fall from Ladder, Pennsylvania." Report F2000-07. Washington, DC: Author. (See the organization website.)

Occupational Safety and Health Administration. (2005). "OSHA Handbook for Small Businesses." OSHA #2209. Washington, DC: Author. (See the organization website.)

U.S. Department of Labor. (n.d.). "Summary of the Major Laws of the Department of Labor." Washington, DC: Author. (See the organization website.)

Washington State Department of Labor and Industries. (2010, May). "Office of Safety and Health." [PowerPoint slides]. Olympia, WA: Author. (See the organization website.)

Key Terms

computer terminal hazards Dangers or safety risks associated with the use of computers in buildings and in vehicles.

egress The pathway out of a building.

electrical equipment hazards Dangers or safety risks associated with office equipment, electrical components of a building, and electricity in general.

exit The place to leave a building.

fire hazards Dangers or safety risks of any kind that can result in a fire if left uncorrected.

handling and storage hazards Dangers or safety risks associated with the handling and storage of various materials, including medical supplies, cleaning supplies, and office supplies.

housekeeping The task of keeping an area clean and free of clutter and debris, especially as it relates to dangers or safety risks.

housekeeping hazards Dangers of safety risks associated with crowding, lack of privacy, and slips, trips, and falls.

illumination hazards Dangers or safety risks associated with lighting in a building or environment in which personnel work.

noise hazards Dangers or safety risks associated with noise in the work environment, such as the ambulance siren or machines in vehicle maintenance bays.

office furniture hazards Dangers or safety risks associated with various types of office furniture, including desks, chairs, and filing cabinets, such as using a chair instead of a ladder to reach.

office machinery/tools hazards Dangers or safety risks associated with various office machinery and tools, which include photocopiers, paper cutters, staplers.

physical layout The actual arrangement of an office or room of a building and its contents.

self-inspection An essential activity if you are to know where probable hazards exist and whether they are under control.

vehicle maintenance areas Areas of a facility where vehicle maintenance is conducted.

ventilation hazards Dangers or safety risks associated with air quality and air flow, including the exhaust from vehicles parked inside of stations.

Accident Investigation

CHAPTER 9

Objectives

After reading this chapter, the student should be able to:

9.1 Identify and analyze the major causes involved in line-of-duty deaths related to health, wellness, fitness, and vehicle operations.
9.2 Identify the components of an accident investigation.
9.3 Conduct an accident investigation.
9.4 Compare and contrast the accident causation theories.
9.5 Discuss how to create recommendations, based on accident investigations, to improve safety.

Overview

This title on EMS safety and risk management has been written to assist EMS providers in the reduction of line-of-duty injuries, illnesses, and fatalities. It provides a framework for developing programs that will create an appropriate margin of health and safety for providers during the performance of EMS duties.

Key Terms

action
actor
analysis
hazardous conditions
material evidence
system weaknesses
unsafe behaviors

WHAT WOULD YOU DO?

It is after lunch when you arrive back in your office. The first week as safety officer has been pretty uneventful, yet overwhelming with things to do. But things are about to change. Your pager goes off for a motor vehicle crash involving Medic 102. Injuries reported. You immediately go to your vehicle and respond to the scene. En route you begin to play your priorities through your head. There is a whole lot to remember!

Questions

1. What is the first thing you should do when you arrive on the scene?
2. What if there are injuries to your personnel?
3. Who do you need to call?
4. What needs to be done after the incident?
5. Who should you interview?

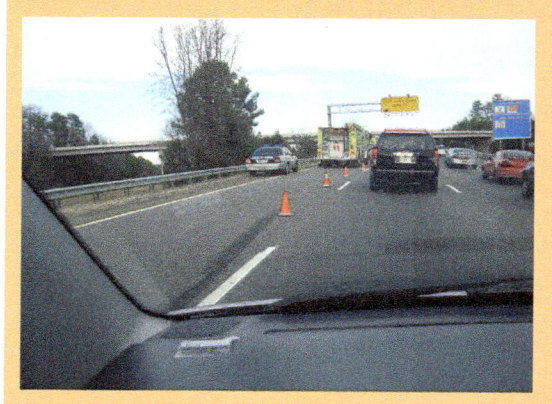

As the safety officer, you may be called on at any time to respond to investigate an incident.
Courtesy of Jeffrey T. Lindsey, Ph.D.

INTRODUCTION

How many times have you said or heard the phrase "Accidents happen"? But it is technically not true that accidents always happen unexpectedly or unplanned. Often accidents result from **hazardous conditions** and **unsafe behaviors** that have been ignored or tolerated for weeks, months, or even years. In such cases, it is not a question of "if" the accident is going to happen; it is only a matter of "when." Yet the decision is made to take the risk.

It is always less expensive to prevent accidents or crashes from occurring than to investigate the reasons for one after the fact. However, if your hazard identification and control program fails to eliminate a workplace hazard, it is important to conduct a thorough and effective analysis of the incident. The only way to receive full benefit from the investigation is to make sure as many root causes as possible are uncovered and permanently corrected.

The intent of an accident investigation is for future prevention and mitigation. The process should be promoted as a positive process and a means to improve the safety culture of the organization. An accident investigation should never be used to blame. Blame is counterproductive and will cause lack of cooperation in future investigations. There are times and places for investigations that find fault, such as in criminal cases or as a matter of discipline, but in safety's realm the intent of an accident investigation is to find ways to prevent and mitigate.

Accident review can be an integral part of the role of the safety committee. It is more valuable to have a committee review the accident than to have one person do it.

So what needs to be investigated? As a general rule, you should investigate the following:

- All injuries, even the minor ones
- All accidents with potential for injury
- Property damage, patient care errors, and near-miss situations in order to identify the root causes
- Every injury or illness entered on the OSHA Injury and Illness Log

The term *accident* is defined as an event that results in injury or illness to an individual and possibly property damage. An event occurs when one **actor** (one person/thing) performs an **action** (does something). In this definition, a person or thing will do something that results in a change of state (an injury). An accident may be the result of many factors (simultaneous, interconnected, cross-linked events) that have interacted in some dynamic way. The term *accident* is used in this chapter to encompass all incidents including motor vehicle crashes, medical errors, personnel injuries, and other events as described previously.

THE ACCIDENT/INCIDENT INVESTIGATION

Every accident, whether a near miss or an actual injury-related event, should be investigated. Near-miss reporting and investigation allow you to identify and control hazards before they cause a more serious incident. An accident investigation is a tool for uncovering hazards and risks that either were missed earlier or have managed to slip out of the controls planned for them. Such an investigation is useful only when done with the aim of discovering every contributing factor to the accident to improve the condition and/or activity and prevent future occurrences. In other words, your primary objective is to identify root causes to correct, not to set blame.

NEAR MISSES

Near misses describe incidents in which no property was damaged and no personal injury was sustained, but given a slight shift in time

Best Practice

EMSCloseCalls.com was an idea born from www.FirefighterCloseCalls.com. Like FirefighterCloseCalls.com, it also has roots within "The Secret List," an independent email newsletter produced since 1998 in an effort to bring forward the issues involving injury and death to firefighters and now also a focus on EMS personnel and issues that are ignored, quickly forgotten, or just not talked about. Originally started as an email group among some close friends in the fire/EMS service, "The Secret List" is currently received by thousands of fire and EMS members.

The newsletter supports the attitude that in order for EMS personnel to survive the dangers of the job, EMS personnel must learn how other fire and EMS members have had "close calls" and even been injured or killed. The intent is not to Monday-morning quarterback or to purposely embarrass anyone, but to provide information that is as factual as possible, is provided by commentary from visitors, and allows the reader to *think* and decide if, or what, they want to do to prevent the bad stuff from occurring again. The editors always welcome corrections or updated information.

Just like FirefighterCloseCalls.com helps set the tone, EMSCloseCalls.com exhibits that same attitude by providing its site as well as *solutions* to help make the job safer.

EMSCloseCalls.com is owned by FirefighterCloseCalls.com but, due to the need for "EMS expertise," International Association of Fire Chiefs EMS Section members play an active role in the day-to-day operations of EMSCloseCalls.com to ensure that the site is *for* EMS Personnel *by* EMS personnel.

Source: EMS Close Calls, www.emsclosecalls.com.

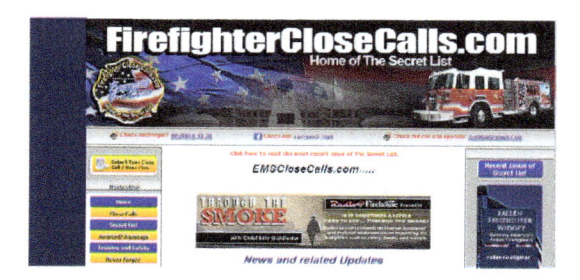

FIGURE 9.1 ■ EMSCloseCalls.com has become a portal through which EMS personnel can input close calls of accidents and incidents. *Courtesy of www.FirefighterCloseCalls.com, Home of "The Secret List."*

or position damage and/or injury easily could have resulted. A website is devoted to near-miss incidents (Figure 9.1). The site is dedicated to EMS providers recording near-miss incidents. Near misses are an important of the safety element for EMS personnel.

THE INVESTIGATOR

The accident investigator for incidents can any of a variety of individuals depending on the organization, the incident, and the organization's accident investigation policy. This could be you as the EMS safety officer. Who does the investigation will depend on the organization and its policy. For purposes of this text, assume that you will assume the role of the investigator. Keep in mind that your role may change depending on your organization's policy.

ACCIDENT INVESTIGATIONS

Accident investigations represent a good way to involve personnel in safety. Personnel involvement will not only give you additional expertise and insight, but it also will lend credibility to the results. Personnel involvement also benefits personnel by educating them on potential hazards, and the experience usually makes them believers in the importance of safety, thus strengthening the safety culture of the organization.

The EMS safety officer should participate in the investigation or review the investigative findings and recommendations regardless of whether or not he is the designated investigator. Many organizations use a team or a subcommittee or the joint personnel-management committee to investigate incidents involving serious injury or extensive property damage.

Training

No one should investigate accidents without appropriate accident investigation training (Figure 9.2). Many safety consultants and professional organizations provide this type of training. You should check with your insurance carrier because some insurers provide an accident investigation program for their clients.

Investigative Techniques

During an accident investigation, six key questions should be answered: Who? What? When? Where? Why? How? Fact should be distinguished from opinion, and both should be presented carefully and clearly. The report should include thorough interviews with everyone who has any knowledge of the incident.

A good investigation is likely to reveal several contributing factors, and it probably will reveal several preventive actions as well.

Avoid the trap of laying blame solely on injured personnel. Even if injured personnel openly blame themselves for making the mistake of not following prescribed procedures, the accident investigator must not be satisfied that all contributing causes have been identified. In fact, the error made by the injured individual may not be the most important contributing cause.

The individual who has not followed prescribed standard operating procedures and/or guidelines may have been encouraged directly or indirectly by a supervisor. The prescribed procedures may not be practical, or even safe, in the eyes of personnel. Sometimes where elaborate and difficult procedures are required, engineering

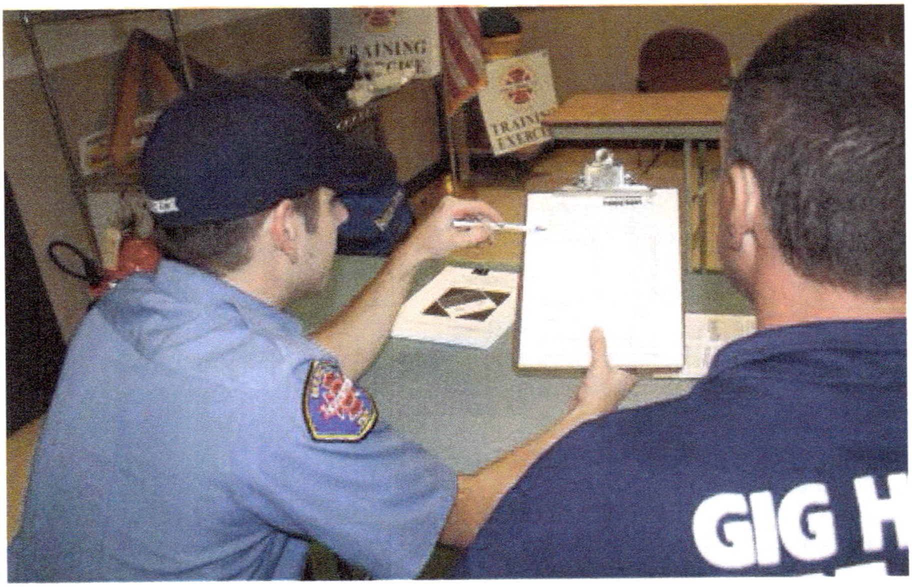

FIGURE 9.2 ■ Anyone who is assigned to conduct an accident investigation must have had the proper training. *Courtesy of 24-7 EMS®, a member of the HSI family of brands.*

redesign might be a better answer. In such cases, management error, not personnel error, may be the most important contributing cause.

The investigator should be held accountable for describing causes objectively. When reviewing accident investigation reports, the safety committee or safety officer should be on the lookout for catch phrases, such as "Individual did not plan job properly." Although such a statement may suggest an underlying problem with the injured individual, it is not conducive to identifying all possible causes, preventions, and controls. Certainly, it is too late to plan a job when personnel are about to perform that job. Further, it is unlikely that safe work will always result when personnel are expected to plan procedures alone.

PURPOSE OF AN INVESTIGATION

The purpose of an investigation is the key to the success of the entire program. To determine the purpose of a process or procedure, it is important to look at the output of that process. The fatality investigation report is the output of the investigation process.

"Analyze to fix the system" should be the organization's mandate. Unfortunately, some organizations believe that the investigation process ends once blame has been established. The problem is that once the purpose of the **analysis** process has been achieved, analysis stops. When organizations investigate to place blame, no further analysis is conducted to fix the underlying safety management **system weaknesses** failures that contributed to the accident.

Even when an individual has disobeyed a required practice, it is critical to ask "Why?" An analysis will generally reveal a number of deeper factors that permitted or even encouraged an individual's action. Such factors may include a supervisor's allowing or pressuring the individual to take shortcuts in the interest of inadequate equipment, or a work practice that is difficult for the individual to carry out safely. An effective analysis will identify actions to address each of the causal factors in an accident or near-miss incident.

The bottom line is that the output of the organization's accident investigation process should not end with merely identifying violations of organization safety rules, procedures, protocols, and guidelines. The final report should focus on identifying safety management system weaknesses, which will result in long-term returns that are substantially greater than the investment in the process.

A trained, competent person can examine workplace conditions, behaviors, attitudes, and underlying systems to predict closely what kind of accidents will occur in the EMS workplace. The most effective accident investigation addresses liability only after an evaluation is completed by a qualified person. In addition, it concludes that all relevant elements of the safety management system are effectively designed and implemented.

Granted, EMS is a business that is sometimes unpredictable and dangerous, but it is unacceptable to have or to promote a concept of helplessness. Organizations with a healthful attitude about accidents consider them to be inexcusable and demand that hazards be corrected before they cause an injury.

Implications

Implications from the root causes of the accident need to be analyzed for their impact on all other operations and procedures. Recommended preventive actions should make it very difficult, if not impossible, for the incident to recur. The investigative report should list all the ways to improve the safety of the condition or activity. Considerations of cost or engineering should not enter at this stage. The primary purpose of accident investigation is to prevent future occurrences. Beyond this immediate purpose, the information obtained through the investigation should be used to update and revise the inventory of hazards and/or the program for hazard prevention and control. For example, the job safety analysis should be revised and personnel retrained to the extent that the analysis fully reflects the recommendations made by an incident report.

EFFECTIVE INVESTIGATION PLANNING

An effective plan for an accident investigation and analysis program includes the following characteristics: It is guided by a written plan (SOP, SOG, protocol) that identifies specific procedures and responsibilities, each clearly stated and easy to follow in a step-by-step fashion. It assigns responsibility for conducting accident investigations, usually a supervisor, management/labor team, EMS safety officer, or safety committee member. Whoever conducts the investigation must understand his role. Usually, two heads work better than one, especially when gathering and analyzing material facts about the accident. Therefore, a team approach is recommended.

An effective plan requires accident investigators to be formally trained in accident investigation techniques and procedures. Investigators should attend accident investigation training presented by educational institutions or other training conducted by a qualified person and provides a course completion of a recognized training program. It is separate from any potential disciplinary procedures resulting from the accident. The purpose of the accident investigation is to get the facts, not find fault. The accident investigator must be able to state with complete sincerity that he is conducting the investigation only for the purpose of determining cause, not blame. It addresses in writing both the surface causes and the root causes. Most accident reports are ineffective precisely because they neglect to uncover the contributing underlying reasons or factors. Only by digging deep, can the investigator eliminate the hazardous conditions and work practices that, on the surface, caused the accident.

An effective plan makes recommendations to correct hazardous conditions, work practices, and those underlying system weaknesses that caused them. In many instances, the surface causes for the accidents are corrected on the spot and will be reported as such. However, the investigator must make recommendations for long-term corrections in the safety system to ensure that those surface causes do not reappear. It includes follow-up procedures to ensure short- and long-term corrective actions are completed.

An effective plan and analysis also require an annual review of accident reports. Safety committee members should evaluate accident reports for consistency and quality. They also should make sure root causes are being addressed and corrected and that information about the types of accidents, locations, trends, and so on are gathered and evaluated.

INITIATING THE PROCESS

First things first: Lay the groundwork. When a serious accident occurs, everyone will be too busy dealing with the emergency at hand to worry about putting together an investigation plan. So before any accident occurs, develop an effective written accident analysis plan that will determine who should be notified of the accident. Establish who is authorized to notify outside agencies (fire, police, and so on). Determine who is assigned to conduct investigations. Identify required training for accident investigators. Determine who receives and acts on investigation reports. Establish timetables for conducting the investigation and follow-up actions such as hazard correction.

The first step in an effective accident investigation procedure is to secure the accident scene as soon as possible so that initial data can be collected. Sometimes, the investigator may actually be able to begin the investigation, while the victim(s) is being assisted by other emergency responders. In this case, the investigator needs to make sure he does not interfere in any way with the emergency responders. The first responsibility is to make sure the victim receives care. At this early point, the investigator is primarily making initial observations, taking photographs, making notes, and doing audio recordings for later analysis.

Most of the time, the investigation will not begin until emergency response is completed. In this situation, **material evidence** most likely will not be in its original location. Of course, this will make it more difficult for the investigator to determine the original location of evidence, but effective interviews will help to reconstruct the scene. In either situation, the investigator is not yet interested in what "caused" the accident, just gathering as much pertinent information as possible for later analysis.

It is important to start the investigation as soon as possible in order to accurately determine the surface and root causes for the accident. The longer an investigator waits to investigate, the more unlikely it will be to fulfill this very important purpose.

Two things disappear after an accident occurs. The first is material evidence. Somehow, tools, equipment, and sometimes people just seem to move or disappear from the scene. Understandably, the organization is eager to "clean up" the accident scene (remember accident scenes include falls and other traumatic events, not just vehicle crashes) so people can get back to work or so that roadways can be reopened. It is important that an effective procedure be developed to protect material evidence so that it does not get moved or disappear.

The second thing to disappear is memory. Accidents are traumatic events. There are varying degrees of psychological trauma depending on how "close" an individual is to the accident or victim. There may be physical trauma to the victim and others whenever a serious accident occurs in the workplace. Everyone is affected somehow. As time passes, conversations with others and individual emotions distort what people believe they saw and heard. After a while, the memory of everyone affected by the accident will be altered in some way. This type of distortion can have nothing but negative effects on your success as an accident investigator.

Secure the Accident Scene

The first step in the accident investigation process is to physically secure (close off) the accident scene to prevent material evidence from being removed or relocated in any way. This is especially true if the accident is a reportable (serious or fatal) injury that might trigger an OSHA accident investigation. Depending on the scene, law enforcement may handle this need.

Securing the accident scene is not difficult, but it is critically important to do it quickly. You may use tape, cones, even personnel to secure the accident scene. It is important in preventing the loss or misplacement of material evidence.

Document the Accident Scene

There are many ways to document a scene, so it may become quite difficult for one person to effectively complete all actions. The most effective strategy is to document as much as possible, even if you question relevancy. It is easy to discard clues or leads if they appear to be unrelated to or not useful to the investigation. It is not at all easy to find material evidence later. All items found at the accident scene should be considered important and potentially relevant. Consequently, a team approach is probably the most efficient strategy for conducting accident investigations when very serious injuries or fatalities are involved. This includes working with agencies such as law enforcement and fire, and others that are also conducting an investigation or documenting the incident.

ACCIDENT INVESTIGATOR'S KIT

A ready-and-waiting accident investigator's kit is important to any investigation (Figure 9.3). The investigator will not be able to fulfill the purpose of the job unless prepared to do so.

METHODS TO DOCUMENT THE ACCIDENT

To document the scene of an accident, the investigator should first make personal observations. With clipboard in hand, the investigator should take notes on those observations. Document what the scene looks like. Be sure to identify any materials, vehicles, buildings, equipment, and any other item that has an impact or potential impact on the accident. The environment includes gouges, scratches, dents, and smears. If vehicles are involved, check for tracks and skid marks. Look for irregularities on surfaces. Are there any fluid spills, stains, contaminated materials, or debris? Include the weather conditions. Record the time of day, location, lighting conditions, and so on. Note whether the terrain is flat or rough, for example. Document the activity that was occurring around the accident scene. Identify the individuals who were witnesses to the accident. It is important to obtain initial statements and interviews from those people. Measure distances and positions of anything and everything that could have an impact on the investigation.

Initial Statements

Hopefully, one or more eyewitnesses will have seen the accident. You should ask each eyewitness for an initial statement. The intent is to have them describe what they saw. Also, try to obtain other information from the witness,

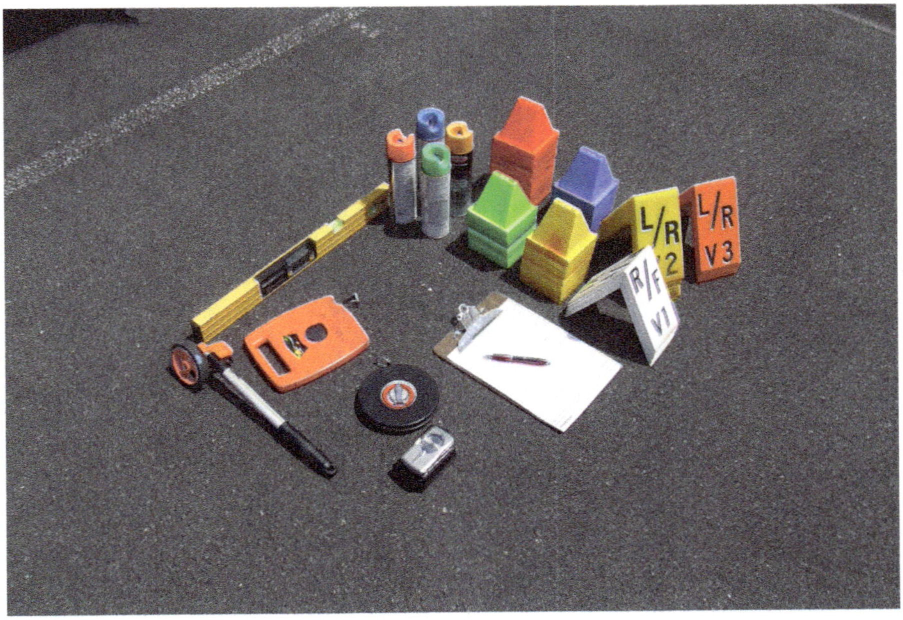

FIGURE 9.3 ■ An accident investigator's kit should include a camera (35mm, Polaroid, panoramic); tape recorder; tape measures (25 and 50 foot lengths); clipboard, paper, pencils, or electronic device on which notes may be written; plastic bags with ties; a square and a French curve template; personal protective equipment including respirators, eye and ear protection, gloves and other protective clothing; string and scene tape; and stakes. *Courtesy of Bruce Evans.*

including the names of other possible witnesses for subsequent interviews; the names of responding rescuers and emergency response services; and the materials, equipment, and articles that were moved or disturbed during the emergency.

Photos

Take photos of the workplace accident scene. It is recommended that you start with distance shots, then move in closer with each photo. Also, include notes about the photos in the report. Remember to consider patient confidentiality when taking photos of the injured, even if they are personnel from your organization.

Some important points to remember about taking photos include the following (Oregon OSHA, n.d.-b): Take photos at different angles—for example, shoot 360 degrees of the scene as well as from above and to the left, right, and rear of the scene to show the relationship of objects and details such as defective equipment, medications, wet areas, containers, other vehicles. Take panoramic photos to help present the entire scene, from top to bottom and side to side. Make notes about each photo. For example, a note to describe the direction of the photo or an object that was photographed may need additional detail so it makes sense when reviewing the report. These notes will be included in the appendix of the report along with the photos. Identify the type of photo, date, time, location, subject, weather conditions, measurements, and so on. Place an item of known dimensions in the photo if hard-to-measure subjects are being photographed. Document who took the photo. Correlate the photos to your sketches.

Videotape

Videotape the scene. The earlier you can begin videotaping the scene, the better. Once your EMS organization or other emergency responders are attending to the victim, you should begin videotaping the scene for documentation purposes. The video recorder will pick up details and conversations that can add much valuable information to the investigation. Just remember not to get in the way when you are doing the investigation. Also, maintaining patient confidentiality is imperative when videotaping the scene even if the patient is part of your organization.

Some important points to remember when videotaping include (Oregon OSHA, n.d.-a). Have witness(es) describe what happened. If possible, have them reenact the event. Use a tripod when taping. To get the "lay of the land," stand back at a distance and zoom into the scene. Scan slowly 360 degrees left and right to establish location. Narrate what is being taped while describing objects, size, direction, location, and so on. If a vehicle was involved, tape the direction of travel going and coming. Before you tape, make sure your video camera is operating properly, the battery is charged, and the lens cap is off.

Other videotape may be available for your use as part of the investigation in motor vehicle collisions. It is also common for video recording devices to capture video in public areas and even in occupancies. It may be difficult to obtain any video footage from cameras in a private occupancy, but you should always try to review any materials available. A number of organizations have dash-mount cameras in their units. These devices capture the event as it occurs. The vehicle also may be equipped with a recording device similar to what the aviation industry calls a black box. This device records a number of different factors including seat belt use, speed, and braking of the unit. Be sure to look at all available technology that may provide assistance in your investigation.

Sketch

Sketch the accident scene. According to Oregon OSHA (n.d.-b), sketches are very important because they compliment the information in photos and are good at indicating distances among the various elements of the accident scene that establishes "position evidence." It is important to be as precise as possible when making sketches. The basic components of the sketch are documentation of date, time, and location; identity of objects, victims, and so on; spatial relationships and measurements; and location from which photos were taken.

Sketches are valuable because they reconstruct the accident in model form and are best able to indicate movement through time. They also help establish testimony if it becomes necessary to defend against a damage or injury claim. The sketch also may help establish a claim against a supplier or manufacturer. You do not have to be a professional illustrator to make a decent sketch, but you must be accurate in your measurements.

The following are some sketching pointers to take into consideration (Oregon OSHA, n.d.-b). Make sketches large, preferably 8 inches × 10 inches.

Make sketches clear. Include information pertinent to the investigation. Include measurements. Establish precise, fixed, identifiable reference points. Print legibly. All printing should be on the same plane. Indicate directions by using the cardinal points north, south, east, and west. Always tie measurements to a permanent point, such as a telephone pole or building. Mark where people were standing. Use sketches to help illustrate what you are speaking about when interviewing people. Show where photos were taken.

Review Documents

Review documents. Some records you might want to review during the investigation include the following (Oregon OSHA, n.d.-b):

- *Maintenance records* to determine the maintenance history of the tools, medication, PPE, equipment, or vehicles involved in the accident
- *Training records* to determine the quantity and quality of the training received by the victim of your organization
- *Standard operating procedures* to identify the formally established steps in the procedures
- *Safety policies, plans, and rules* to determine their presence and adequacy
- *Shift schedules* to determine if the victim might have been fatigued or otherwise overworked
- *Disciplinary records*, if discipline is considered justified, to determine if disciplinary actions have occurred previously
- *Medical records*, if permission is granted or otherwise allowed, to determine potential physical or mental contributing factors
- *EMS patient care reports* to determine quality of response procedures
- *Safety committee minutes* to determine the history of any discussion of related hazardous conditions, unsafe behaviors, or program elements
- *Medical examiner/coroner's report* to determine direct cause of injury that lead to the fatality
- *Police report* to determine facts when criminal negligence is in question

Note: When criminal negligence is suspected, stop the investigation and coordinate all activities with legal advisors such as your organization's attorney.

Documenting the scene is important for so many reasons. *Remember*: The team approach works best because accuracy in reconstructing the accident is the final criteria.

Conduct Interviews

Once you have completed the initial documentation of the accident scene, it becomes important to research the details through the interview process. Conducting interviews is perhaps the most difficult part of an investigation (Figure 9.4). The purpose of the accident investigation interview is to obtain an accurate and comprehensive picture of what happened by obtaining all pertinent facts, interpretations, and opinions. Your job, as the investigator, is to construct a composite story using the various accounts of the accident and other evidence. The effective investigator will have a firm understanding of the techniques for interviewing and the skills acquired through experience and training to apply those techniques.

Prepare for the Interview. The first task is to determine who needs to be interviewed. Questions must be designed for the interviewee. Consequently, each interview will be a unique experience. Interviews should occur as soon as possible. The interviews may include the following (Oregon OSHA, n.d.-b):

- *The victim* to determine specific events leading up to and including the accident
- *Co-workers* to establish what actual versus appropriate procedures had been used
- *Direct supervisor* to get background information on the victim (He can provide procedural information about the task that was being performed.)
- *Supervisor/division chief* to get the main information on related systems or procedures
- *Training department* to get specific content and assessment of the learner on the quantity and quality of training the victim and others have received
- *Human resources department* to get information on the victim's and others' work histories, discipline, and performance appraisals
- *Maintenance personnel* to determine background on equipment and machinery maintenance
- *Emergency responders* to learn what they saw when they arrived and during the response

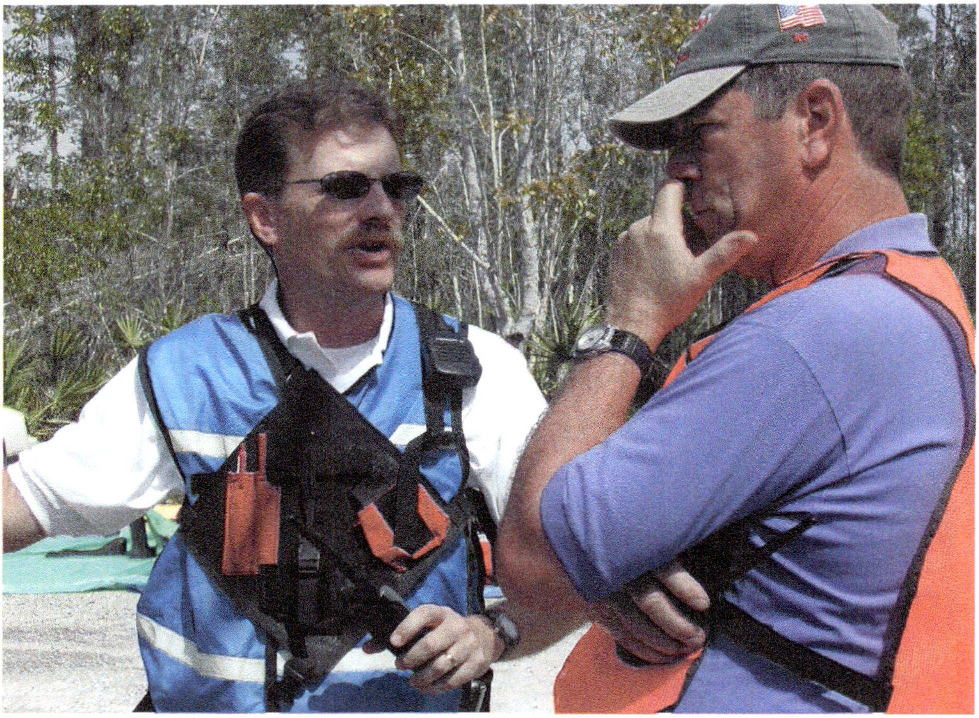

FIGURE 9.4 ■ Conducting interviews can be one of the more difficult jobs of an accident investigator. *Courtesy of Estero Fire Rescue.*

- *Medical personnel* to get medical information (as allowed by law)
- *Coroner/medical examiner* to get the determination on type/extent of fatal injuries
- *Police*, if they filed a report
- *The victim's spouse and family* to get any insight into the victim's state of mind or other work issues.
- *Other interested persons*, if there is anyone else you believe would provide valuable information

Cooperation, not intimidation, is the key to a successful accident investigation interview. The purpose of the accident interview is to uncover additional information about the hazardous conditions, unsafe work practices, and related system weaknesses that contributed to the accident. Consequently, it is very important that effective techniques to establish a cooperative atmosphere be used by the investigator during the process.

Effective Interviewing Techniques. As you conduct interviews, gaining experience along the way, you will further develop the art of interviewing by improving your ability to apply effective techniques.

Some effective techniques that will ensure you get to the facts, not find fault, are as follows (Oregon OSHA, n.d.-b):

- *Keep the purpose of the investigation in mind.* To determine the cause of the accident so that similar accidents will not recur. Make sure the interviewee understands this.
- *Approach the investigation with an open mind.* It will be obvious if you have preconceptions about the individuals or the facts.

- *Go to the scene.* Even if you are familiar with the location or the victim's job, do not assume that things have remained the same. If you cannot conduct a private interview at the location, find an office or meeting room that the interviewee considers a "neutral" location.
- *Interview the people involved* (victim, witnesses, people involved with the process such as the driver of the striking vehicle, or mechanic that repaired or provided maintenance on the vehicle).
- *Put the person at ease.* Explain the purpose and your role. Sincerely express concern regarding the accident and desire to prevent a similar occurrence.
- *Listen with interest.* Express to the individual that the information he or she offers is important. Be friendly, understanding, and open minded. Be calm and unhurried.
- *Let the individual talk.* Ask for background information, name, job, and so on first. Ask the witness to tell you what happened, but do not ask leading questions. Do not interrupt, and do not respond by way of facial or verbal expressions of approval or disapproval.
- *Avoid asking "Why?"* because it tends to make people respond defensively. Instead of asking "Why did you drive the ambulance with underinflated tires?" ask "What are ambulance inspection procedures? What are ambulance safety hazard reporting procedures?"
- *Ask open-ended questions.* Avoid questions that can be answered with a "Yes" or "No." For example, you should say, "Tell me what happened." Don't make a request, such as "Could you tell me what happened?" If you do, the witness may respond with a simple "No," and that's that.
- *Check your understanding.* Repeat the facts and sequence of events back to the person to avoid any misunderstandings.
- *Document what you are told.* Your notes should be taken very carefully and as casually as possible. Let the individual read them if desired. Give the interviewee a copy of the notes you take.
- *Use a tape recorder*, but do not do so unless you get permission first. Tell the interviewee that the purpose of the recorder is to ensure accuracy. Offer to give the interviewee a copy of the tape.
- *Ask for lessons learned.* Ask for the witness's suggestions as to how the accident/incident could have been avoided.
- *Thank the witness.* Conclude the interview with a statement of appreciation for the witness's contribution. Ask the witness to contact you if he thinks of anything else. If possible, advise witnesses personally of the outcome of the investigation before it becomes public knowledge.

Understanding and applying these techniques during the interview process will help ensure the establishment of a cooperative relationship that will reveal the facts. Intimidation and blaming always results in an ineffective interview process.

ANALYZE THE ACCIDENT PROCESS

Over the past century, safety professionals have tried to effectively explain how and why accidents occur. As you will read in the following section of this chapter, their explanations were at first rather simplistic. Theorists gradually realized that it was not sufficient to explain workplace accidents as simple cause-and-effect events. Therefore, they developed new theories that better explained the complicated interaction among conditions, behaviors, and systems that result in an accident.

ACCIDENT CAUSATION THEORIES

There are a number of different theories on the causes of accidents. The following subsections will discuss some of the better-known theories and those that are typically used: the domino, energy-transfer, single-event, pure-chance, accident-proneness, and multiple-causation theories.

The Domino Theory

In 1931 W. H. Heinrich developed the domino theory, which argues that 88% of all accidents are caused by the unsafe acts of people, 10% by unsafe actions, and 2% by "acts of God." (Mitterer and Patrick, n.d.; Oregon OSHA, n.d.-a). He believed a five-step accident sequence occurred in which each factor would actuate the next step, much like we see in a row of falling dominoes. Heinrich's sequence of accident factors were these:

1. Ancestry and social environment
2. Worker fault
3. Unsafe act together with mechanical and physical hazard
4. Accident
5. Damage or injury

Heinrich believed that by removing a single domino in the row, the sequence would be interrupted, thus preventing the accident. The key domino to be removed from the sequence, according to him, was domino number 3. It is surprising how firmly this theory took hold in the safety profession, given that he provided no data for his theory.

The domino theory ignores important underlying system weaknesses and root causes for accidents. However, it is a valuable tool for use in identifying losses so that effective countermeasures, or actions designed to counter the effect of the loss, can be developed and implemented. Look at the dominos in Table 9.1.

Dominos 4 and 5 are concerned with the consequences/result and the transfer of energy that caused the loss or damage. The major focus should be on Dominos 1 to 3. In this way we can proactively identify actual or potential hazards that can be reduced or eliminated to prevent the mishap from ever occurring.

Domino 5 refers to the major loss. This is what you are left with after an accident: injury to personnel, bystanders, stockholders, and others; and damage to your equipment and that of others.

Domino 4 refers to the transfer of energy beyond the threshold limits of what causes damage and injury. Common forms of energy transfer include mechanical, radiant, chemical, thermal, and electrical.

Domino 3 refers to the immediate causes or symptoms. These are usually obvious and generally attributable to individuals and the actions they take or the conditions within which they operate. Domino 3 comprises many of the classic human errors. These include substandard practices or substandardized conditions. Significant Domino 3 human errors include failed to follow instructions; blundered ahead without knowing how to do the job; bypassed or ignored a rule, regulation, or procedure to save time; failed to use protective equipment; did not think ahead to possible consequences; used the wrong equipment to do the job; used equipment that needed repair or replacement; did not look; did not listen; did not recognize

TABLE 9.1 ■ The Domino Theory

Domino 1	*Domino 2*	*Domino 3*	*Domino 4*	*Domino 5*
Management Dysfunction	Basic Cause	Immediate Cause	Energy Transfer	Accident Result
Planning	System	Individual	Chemical	Injury
Organizing			Mechanical	Damage
Directing			Thermal	
Controlling			Radiation	
Staffing			Electrical	

physical limitations; failed to use safeguards or other protective devices; did not pay attention.

Domino 2 refers to the basic causes of incidents. Sometimes these causes are referred to as root causes or indirect causes. Basic causes are frequently classified into two categories: personal factors and job factors. The basic causes referred to as personal factors explain why people engage in substandard practices. Similarly, the basic causes referred to as job factors explain why substandard conditions are created or exist. These hazards usually affect many people in the organization. They may include, for example, incomplete training for personnel in proper patient transfers; management pressure to make a profit as quickly as possible; and absence of formal training.

Domino 1 refers to lack of control or leadership dysfunction. In this context, control refers to one of the following classical functions of management:

> *Planning.* Defining organizational goals, strategies for achieving those goals, developing a hierarchy to integrate and coordinate activities
>
> *Organizing.* Determining the structure, outlining the tasks, who will do them, how they are grouped, who reports to whom, where decisions are made
>
> *Directing.* Motivating subordinates, directing activities, selecting modes of communication, conflict resolution, directing change
>
> *Controlling.* Ensuring things are going as they should, comparing actual performance with previously set goals and objectives; if deviations exist, taking action to correct them; also includes routine evaluations, such as audits

Though Dominos 4 and 5 are concerned with the consequences/results and the transfer of energy that caused the loss or damage, it is Dominos 1, 2, and 3 that allow you to proactively identify actual or potential hazards and reduce or eliminate them to prevent the mishap from ever occurring. Domino 5 refers to major loss, which is what you are left with after an accident.

The domino theory provides a structured process for understanding the cause of accidents. In addition, it furnishes a framework for implementation of measures developed to counter the actual or potential effects of hazards associated with EMS operations. It is a process that should be used by management personnel to assist in identification and analysis. It explains not only the cause of losses; more important, it provides a means of correcting those things that are likely to cause a loss.

Haddon's Energy Transfer Theory

Haddon's energy transfer theory claims that an individual incurs injury from exposure to a harmful change of energy (Mitterer and Patrick, n.d.). For every change of energy, there is a source, a path, and a receiver. This theory is useful for evaluating work for energy hazards and engineering control methods.

Instead of concentrating on human behavior, Haddon treats accidents as a physical engineering problem. That is, he says that accidents result when energy that is out of control puts more stress on a structure (property or person) than that structure can tolerate. Situations in which energy could be "out of control" include fire losses, industrial injuries, and virtually any other situation in which injury or damage can result.

Haddon suggested strategies to suppress conditions that produce accidents or to enhance conditions that retard accidents. They include these:

- Prevent the creation of the hazard or limit the amount of energy that is created.
- When the hazard cannot be prevented or limited, separate in time or space the hazard and that which is to be protected.
- Make what is to be protected more resistant to damage from the hazard.
- When damage has occurred, act to repair the damage caused by the hazard. (Mitterer and Patrick, n.d.)

Single-Event Theory

In the single-event theory, an accident is thought to be the result of a single, one-time, easily identifiable, unusual, unexpected occurrence that results in injury or illness (Mitterer and Patrick, n.d.). Some still believe this explanation to be adequate, and they find it convenient to blame the victim when an accident occurs. For instance, if an individual cuts her hand on a sharp edge of a work surface in the ambulance, her lack of attentiveness may be explained as the cause of the accident. With this theory, all responsibility for the accident is placed squarely on the shoulders of the individual.

Pure-Chance Theory

According to the pure-chance theory, every individual has an equal chance of being involved in an accident (Mitterer and Patrick, n.d.; Oregon OSHA, n.d.-a). Therefore, no single discernible pattern of events leads to an accident. All accidents correspond to acts of God, and no interventions exist to prevent them. This theory contributes nothing at all toward developing preventive actions for avoiding accidents.

Accident-Proneness Theory

The accident-proneness theory says that there exists within a workplace a subset of individuals who are more liable to be involved in accidents (Mitterer and Patrick, n.d.; Oregon OSHA, n.d.-a). Contradictory research and professional consensus do not generally support this theory and, if accident proneness is supported by any empirical evidence at all, it probably accounts for only a very low proportion of accidents.

Multiple-Cause Theory

This explanation takes us beyond the simplistic assumptions of the single-event and domino theories. Once again, accidents are not assumed to be simple events (Mitterer and Patrick, n.d.; Oregon OSHA, n.d.-b). Rather, they are the result of a series of random related or unrelated acts/events that somehow interact to cause the accident. Unlike the domino theory, this theory causes the investigator to realize that eliminating one of the events does not ensure prevention of future accidents. Removing or padding the sharp edge of a work surface does not guarantee a similar injury will be prevented. Many other factors may have contributed to an injury. An accident investigation will not only recommend corrective actions to remove or pad the sharp surface, it also will address the underlying system weaknesses that caused it.

DETERMINING THE SEQUENCE OF EVENTS

As the investigator, you have documented your observations and gathered all relevant reports, interviewed witnesses and other interested parties, and determined the theory to pursue in the investigation. Now you must accurately determine the sequence of events so that you can effectively analyze the accident process (Figure 9.5). Once the steps in the process are determined, you can then

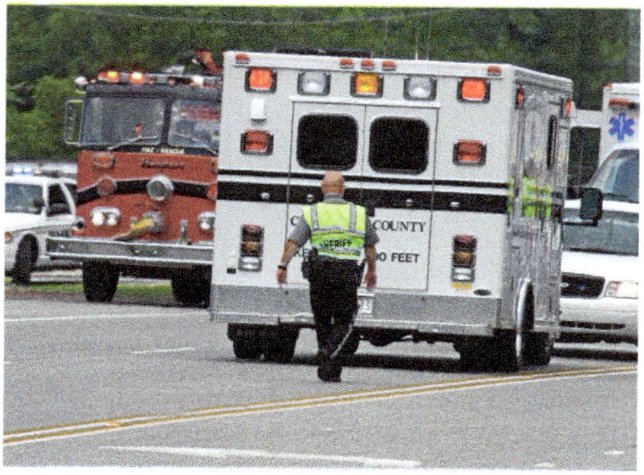

Figure 9.5 ■ Conducting an investigation can be challenging, especially when determining the sequence of events in the accident process.
Source: Fotolia/© Sir_Eagle.

study each event to identify related details (Oregon OSHA, n.d.-b):

Hazardous conditions. Things and states that directly caused the accident.

Unsafe behaviors. Actions taken/not taken that contributed to the accident.

System weaknesses. Underlying inadequate or missing programs, plans, policies, processes, and procedures that contributed to the accident.

When you understand that the accident is actually the final event in an unplanned process, you will naturally want to know what the initial event was. When the initial event occurs, it affects the actions of others, setting in motion a potentially very complicated process eventually ending in an injury or illness. The trick is to take the information gathered and arrange it so that you can accurately determine what initial condition and/or action transformed the planned work process into an unplanned accident.

Remember: In the multiple-cause approach to accident investigation, many events may occur, each contributing to the final event. For instance, if a supervisor ignores an unsafe behavior because doing so is not thought to be his responsibility, the failure to enforce behavior represents an event in the production process that may contribute to or increase the probability of an accident.

Each event in the unplanned accident process describes a unique facet (Oregon OSHA, n.d.-b):

Actor. An individual or object that directly influenced the flow of the sequence of events. An actor may participate in the process or merely observe the process. An actor initiates a change by performing or failing to perform an action.

Action. Something that is done by an actor. Actions may or may not be observable. An action may describe something that is done or not done. Failure to act should be thought of as an act in itself.

It is important when describing events to first indicate the actor, and then tell what the actor does. Remember, the actor is the doer, not the person or object being acted on or otherwise having something done to them. For instance, take a look at the following statement:

John unbuckled the seatbelt in the captain's seat in the back of the ambulance.

In this example, "John" is the actor and "unbuckling" is the action. First, describe the actor, John. Then describe the action, unbuckling. The seat belt and the captain seat are objects, not actors; they are not performing an action. Rather, something is being done to them. Also note that the statement is written in active tense.

Paint a word picture. It is important that the sequence of events clearly describes what occurred so that others unfamiliar with the accident are able to visualize it happening as they read. If an event is difficult to understand, it may be that the description is too vague or general. The solution to this problem is to increase the detail by determining if anything else was said/done before or after the event you are currently assessing. You need to separate actors. Remember, an actor may be a person or a thing accomplishing a given action. If an event includes actions by more than one actor, separate the event into two events.

Once you have determined the sequence of events, you can begin the analysis by examining each event for potential causes of the accident.

DETERMINING SURFACE AND ROOT CAUSES

To effectively fulfill the responsibilities of an accident investigator, you must not close the investigation until the root causes have been identified.

MANAGEMENT PERCEPTIONS

It is a common struggle to try to overcome long-held perceptions about safety and how accidents occur. In that struggle, it is important to understand that management perceptions and subsequent actions reflect both traditional thinking and progressive thinking.

Traditional thinking about the causes of accidents assumes that the individual makes a choice to work in an unsafe manner. It implies that there are no outside forces acting upon the individual and influencing his actions and that there are simple reasons for the accident. Traditional thinking also considers accidents solely as the result of personnel error (such as a lack of common sense) and the locus of the problem. To prevent accidents, the individual must work more safely. This thinking results in blaming and short-term fixes, which is inefficient, ineffective, and in the long run more expensive to implement and maintain.

In contrast, the progressive or systems approach takes into account the dynamics of systems that interact within the overall safety program. It concludes the idea that accidents are considered defects in the system. People are only one part of a complex system composed of many complicated processes (more than most realize). Accidents are the result of multiple causes or defects in the system. It becomes the investigator's job to uncover the root causes (defects) in the system. Fixing the system and not the individual is the heart of the investigation. To prevent accidents, the system must work more safely. This thinking results in long-term fixes, which are less expensive to implement and maintain.

ANALYZE FOR CAUSE

You have gathered information and used it to develop an accurate sequence of events. You have a good mental picture of what happened. Conduct an analysis of each event to determine causes. The next subsections present injury analysis, event analysis, systems analysis, direct causes of injury, surface causes of accidents, and root causes of accidents (Oregon OSHA, n.d.-b).

As mentioned earlier, accidents are processes that culminate in an injury or illness. An accident may be the result of many factors (simultaneous, interconnected, cross-linked events) that have interacted in some dynamic way. In an effective accident investigation, the investigator will conduct three levels of cause analysis.

Injury Analysis

At this level of the accident investigation, do not attempt to determine what caused the accident, but rather focus on trying to determine how harmful energy transfer caused the injury. Remember, the outcome of the accident process is an injury.

Event Analysis

The next step is to examine each event to determine the hazardous conditions and unsafe or inappropriate behaviors that represent the *surface* causes for the incident or accident. All hazardous conditions and unsafe behaviors are clues pointing to possible system weaknesses. This level of investigation is called a special-cause analysis because the analyst can point to a specific thing or behavior.

You usually can trace surface causes to inadequate safety policies, programs, plans, processes, or procedures. Each level of questioning will get you closer to the root cause(s) that allowed the hazardous condition or unsafe behavior.

Systems Analysis

At this level, you need to analyze the *root* causes contributing to the accident. Once you start identifying the surface causes—inadequate policies, programs, plans, processes, and procedures—you also are beginning to get to the real root causes. The root causes for accidents are the underlying safety system weaknesses that have somehow contributed to the existence of hazardous conditions and unsafe behaviors that represent surface causes of accidents. These weaknesses can take two forms: design and implementation (Oregon OSHA, n.d.-b).

Design Root causes lie in the inadequate planning and design of the system. The development of formal (written) safety management system policies, plans, processes, and procedures is very important to make sure appropriate conditions, activities, behaviors, and practices occur.

Implementation Root causes lie in inadequate implementation of the designed system. Failure to effectively carry out the safety management system is critical to the success of the system. You can develop a wonderfully designed system, yet if it is not implemented correctly, it will not work.

It is important to understand that root causes always exist prior to surface causes. Indeed, inadequately designed and implemented system components have the potential to feed and nurture hazardous conditions and unsafe behaviors. If root causes are left unchecked, surface causes will flourish. Examples of safety management system functions are as follows:

- *Safety systems* are developed to promote commitment/leadership, increase member involvement, establish accountability, identify and control hazards, investigate incidents/accidents, educate and train, and evaluate the safety program.
- *System components* include policies, programs, plans, processes, procedures, budgets, reports, and rules.

TABLE 9.2 ■ Hazardous Conditions

- Are basically things or objects that cause injury or illness
- May also be thought to be defects in a process—for example, medication packaging that looks the same
- May exist at any level of the organization

The biggest challenge to effectively conduct an accident investigation is to transition from event analysis to systems analysis.

The Surface Causes of the Accident

The surface causes of accidents are those specific hazardous conditions and unsafe personnel/supervisor behaviors that have directly caused or contributed in some way to the accident. See Tables 9.2 and 9.3.

It is important to know that most hazardous conditions in the EMS environment are the result of specific unsafe behaviors that produced them. See Table 9.4.

TABLE 9.3 ■ Categories of Hazardous Conditions

- Materials
- Machinery
- Equipment
- Tools
- Chemicals
- Environment
- Workstations
- Facilities
- People
- Workload
- Body fluids

TABLE 9.4 ■ Unsafe Behaviors

- Actions you take or do not take that increase risk of injury or illness
- May also be considered errors in a process or procedure
- May occur at any level of the organization

Examples of Unsafe Personnel/Supervisor Behaviors

- Failing to comply with rules
- Using unsafe methods
- Taking shortcuts
- Horseplay
- Failing to report injuries
- Failing to report hazards
- Allowing unsafe behaviors
- Failing to train
- Failing to supervise
- Failing to correct
- Scheduling too much work
- Ignoring worker stress

Role of Safety Engineers

Safety engineers are an integral part of equipment and vehicle design. In most instances, the recognition of a safety engineer is not considered at the organization level. A safety engineer closely analyzes all the surface-cause categories and attempts to eliminate, reduce, or reduce exposure to the harmful source.

They do this by designing safety features directly into tools, machinery, equipment, facilities, and so on. Most safety engineers in EMS are found with the equipment and vehicle manufacturers, working together to eliminate or reduce exposure to hazards through effectively improving safety system components. The EMS safety officer can assist in the design of equipment and vehicles by getting involved with the manufacturer and working with the safety engineer in the design of the equipment or vehicle.

DEVELOPING RECOMMENDATIONS

An accident investigation is generally thought to be a reactive safety process because it is initiated only after an accident has occurred. However, if you propose recommendations that include effective control strategies and system improvements, you transform the investigation into a valuable proactive process that ensures similar accidents do not recur.

Some organizations may assign the responsibility for making recommendations to safety officers. However, you, as the accident investigator, may be required to take on this very important responsibility. Consequently, it is a good idea to know where to start, and how to write strong proposals. One tip up front: If you find the responsibility is yours, be sure to get the help of experts if you are unsure how to proceed. Consultants with your workers' compensation insurer or vehicle-and-liability insurer can be a great source for help.

EFFECTIVE RECOMMENDATIONS

To make sure recommendations are effective, you must address effective control strategies that will eliminate or reduce the specific surface causes of the accident. You also must propose system improvements to missing or inadequate safety system components that contributed to the accident.

HIERARCHY OF CONTROLS

The Hierarchy of Controls, or hazard-control strategies, when used separately or in combination may be quite effective in eliminating or greatly reducing the probability of a similar accident recurring. However, to make sure long-term risk reduction is achieved throughout the entire company, system improvements must be made.

Engineering Controls

Sometimes the cause of an accident is corrected most effectively by removing or reducing the hazard itself. This may be done in a number of ways, including redesigning the hazard out, replacing the unsafe item with a safe item, enclosing the hazard, and substituting an unsafe item with a different item.

Engineering out the hazard is the top priority. Engineering controls remove the hazard itself. You are somehow changing a thing/condition in the EMS environment. It has the potential to completely remove a hazard and, as you know, you cannot be exposed to a hazard if it does not exist: No hazard, no exposure, no accident.

Management Controls

EMS safety officers employ management control strategies to eliminate or reduce the frequency and duration of exposure to hazards. This is accomplished through either *managing EMS work practices* (effectively designing and implementing safe EMS work procedures and practices) or *managing work schedules* (including job rotation, breaks, shift work, and so on).

These control strategies are less effective in the long term than engineering controls because they do not remove the hazards themselves. Rather, they attempt to reduce exposure to hazards by controlling human behavior or by attempting to change "things you do or don't do."

As long as personnel behave or comply with the changed procedures or schedules, management controls work. Sometimes safe work procedures are not perceived as most efficient, so you may not use them. Supervisors must diligently oversee and maintain management control strategies or those controls may become ineffective.

Personal Protective Equipment

The personal protective equipment (PPE) control strategy is used in conjunction with the other control strategies. It should not be used to replace them. When engineering and/or administrative controls do not adequately eliminate or reduce the hazard(s) of a task, PPE may be needed in addition to those strategies. PPE places a barrier between workers and the hazard (Figure 9.6). Remember, PPE does not eliminate or reduce the hazard itself; it merely sets up a barrier between the personnel and the hazard. In all cases, to be successful it is highly dependent on safe behaviors.

RECOMMEND SYSTEM IMPROVEMENTS

Root causes for accidents are usually a result of missing or inadequate safety system components in EMS. Surface causes represent symptoms of system weaknesses. Therefore,

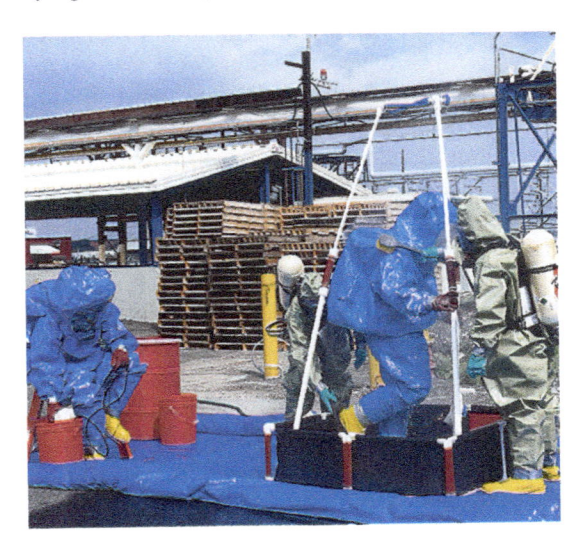

FIGURE 9.6 ■ Not every hazard can be eliminated. However, the use of proper PPE can place a barrier between personnel and the hazard.

every effort should be made to improve system components to ensure long-term safety in the EMS work environment.

The most successful accident investigator is actually a systems analyst. Making system improvements might include some of the following:

- Incorporate "safety" into your organization's mission statement.
- Improve safety SOPs/SOGs so that it clearly establishes responsibility and accountability.
- The daily checklists that personnel complete should incorporate safety into them.
- Revise the purchasing policy to include safety considerations as well as cost.

Behavior-Based Safety

Behavior-based safety, a type of formal observation process, is successful when the data-gathering process is clearly understood by observer and observed, and the data collected is analyzed only to fix the system, not to fix blame. Any changes in expectations must be clearly communicated to everyone through effective education and training to ensure behavioral changes are understood. Behavior-based safety is not usually successful if the process is, in any way, tied to discipline. The only consequences that work in behavior-based safety are positive consequences for making observations and being observed demonstrating safety leadership.

It is important to understand that once improvements have been designed and implemented, they then should be tied to accountability. Only effective consequences will ensure the changed behaviors are sustained long term. When carefully designed, bottom-line, behavior-based safety is another useful analysis tool that can be quite successful in helping the organization improve the safety management system. When supervisors do not respond to a recommendation, it may be that they do not have enough useful information. What is commonly applied to data entry and computer programming (garbage in, garbage out) applies equally well to the process of making effective recommendations: Useful information must be presented to managers so they are able to make correct decisions.

Proactive Recommendations

To speed up the process and to improve the approval rate, you must learn to anticipate the concerns and questions that supervisors have when deciding what actions to take. The more pertinent the information included in the recommendation, the greater the likelihood for approval. To make sure you do provide good information, ask some important proactive questions.

The following six points can help you develop and justify recommendations.

Pinpoint the Problem. Identify the problem and the specific hazardous conditions. Note any unsafe work practices that caused the problem. Define the system components: the inadequate or missing policies, processes, procedures, and SOPs/SOGs that allowed the conditions and practices to exist.

Know the History of the Problem. Have similar accidents occurred previously? If so, probability for similar accidents occurring runs the gamut from highly likely to certain. What are previous direct and indirect costs for similar accidents? How have similar accidents affected production and morale?

Pinpoint the Specific Solution. What are the solutions that would correct the problem? What are the specific engineering, administrative, and PPE controls that, when applied, will eliminate or at least reduce exposure to the hazardous conditions? What are the specific system improvements needed to ensure a long-term fix?

Identify the Decision Maker. Who is the person who can approve, authorize, and act on corrective measures? What are the possible objections that he might have? What are the arguments that will be most effective in overcoming objections?

Know Why the Decision Maker Is Doing Safety. It is important to know what is motivating the supervisor. The following may be some of the motivations:

- Fulfill the legal obligation? You may need to emphasize possible penalties if corrections are not made.
- Fulfill the fiscal obligation? You may want to emphasize the costs/benefits.
- Fulfill the moral obligation? You may want to emphasize improved morale, public relations.

Estimate the Cost/Benefits of Approving and of Not Approving the Recommendation. What are the estimated costs and benefits of taking corrective action, as contrasted with the possible costs and harm that might occur if the hazardous conditions and unsafe work practices remain? What are the organization's obligations under administrative law? What is the message sent to the personnel as a result of action or inaction? The maintenance supervisor may be able to help you determine these estimates. Also, detail the costs associated with any training that might be required.

Simple Cost-Benefit Analysis

A simple cost-benefit analysis assumes that there is a reasonable expectation that a disabling injury is likely in the foreseeable future (5 years) when personnel are exposed (place themselves within a danger zone) to a hazard in the EMS environment. The objective is to contrast the relatively high cost-low benefit if the hazard is not eliminated, with the low cost-high benefit if the hazard is eliminated.

The analysis answers the following questions:

- What are the potential costs to the organization if the hazard is not eliminated?
- What are the potential costs to the organization if the hazard is eliminated?
- How soon will the corrective action pay for itself?
- What is our return on investment (ROI) if corrective actions are taken?

Consider the following as an example:

You watch your personnel lift and move patients every day. You notice that the amount of claims for your organization on back injuries seem higher than normal. You know there must be a way to reduce these claims.

To construct a cost-benefit analysis for this situation you would answer the four questions listed above as follows:

To be effective, recommendations should be supported by a bottom-line cost-benefit analysis that contrasts the relatively high costs of accidents against the much lower costs associated with corrective actions. Doing a cost-benefit analysis is even more important when recommending corrective actions before an accident occurs.

Next to headaches, medical experts note that back problems are the most common medical complaint (National Safety Council, 2012). Back pains also are found to be second only to the common cold as the greatest cause of lost workdays. Back injuries alone cost U.S. industry $10 billion to $14 billion in workers' compensation costs and about 100 million lost workdays annually. The National Safety Council tracks and reviews the costs of injuries in general, and not necessarily in specific industries. Because obtaining information on the number and severity of nonfatal injuries for home, public non–motor vehicle, and work is difficult, the best approach is to estimate total costs on the per death basis using the

TABLE 9.5 ■ Average Economic Cost of Fatal and Nonfatal Injuries by Class of Injury, 2010

Home injuries (fatal and nonfatal) per death	$ 3,300,000
Public non–motor vehicle injuries (fatal and nonfatal) per death	$ 4,400,000
Work injuries (fatal and nonfatal) per death	
• without employers' uninsured costs	$ 44,100,000
• with employers' uninsured costs	$ 46,800,000

Source: National Safety Council (2012).

averages listed in Table 9.5; the averages are based on their respective injury:death ratio. Table 9.6 shows the per-case average cost of wage and productivity losses, medical expenses, and administrative expenses.

Indirect costs can be as much as 2 to 50 times the direct costs, or more. *Remember:* When estimating, the lower the direct cost, the higher the ratio between the direct and indirect costs. For instance, if someone suffers only minor injury requiring a few hundred dollars to close the claim, the indirect:direct costs ratio may be much higher than the national average. Capital-intensive operations, where large sums have been invested in facilities, realize higher than average indirect:direct cost ratios. For example, if someone is seriously or fatally injured in an ambulance crash resulting in operations shutting down for a day or so,

the organization may be out of business or significantly impacted for days to months. In high-end capital-intensive work processes, the expected ratio between direct and indirect costs may be 5:50. Labor-intensive operations, where more investment is made in personnel than in capital assets, realize lower indirect:direct cost ratios. In labor-intensive operations, someone may suffer a serious injury, but operations are not as likely to be significantly impacted, so in labor-intensive operations the expected ratio between direct and indirect costs may be 2:10.

You can use the following figures to demonstrate the benefits of taking corrective action. For example, *what are the estimated costs to an organization if the hazard is eliminated?* Costs: $15,000 needed to purchase new stretcher. *How soon will the corrective action*

TABLE 9.6 ■ Average Economic by Class and Severity, 2010

Average Economic Cost by Class and Severity, 2010

Death	Disabling	Injury
Home injuries	$1,070,000	$7,900
Public injuries	$1,070,000	$8,800
Work injuries		
without employer costs	$1,330,000	$48,000
with employer costs	$1,350,000	$53,000

Source: National Safety Council (2012).

pay for itself? If a disabling injury occurs within the next 5 years, using the National Safety Council (2012) figures, you can estimate a direct:indirect cost to the company of approximately $53,000. Given the cost to purchase the stretcher at $15,000, the corrective action will pay for itself in just 18 months: $15,000/($53,000/60 months).

It is important to provide alternatives to make it more likely that corrective actions will be taken, as in this example. *First option: If you had all the money you needed, what could you do?* Eliminate the hazard with primarily engineering controls and additional administrative controls if required. *Second option: If you have limited funds, what would you do?* Eliminate the hazard using work practice and/or administrative controls, plus engineering controls if required. *Third option: If you don't have any money, what can you do?* Reduce exposure to the hazard with work practice/administrative controls and/or PPE.

It is important to remember that your organization should first try to engineer out the hazard if feasible before using administrative controls or PPE. Of course, some tasks require the use of PPE.

WRITING THE REPORT

Now that you have accurately assessed and analyzed the facts related to the accident, you must report your finding(s) to those who have authority and accountability and can take action. This individual is called the "A Person" (Figure 9.7).

Never forget that your primary objective as an accident investigator is to uncover the causal factors that contributed to the accident. It is not your job to place blame. Your responsibility is to be as objective and accurate as possible. Your findings, and how you present them, will shape perceptions and subsequent

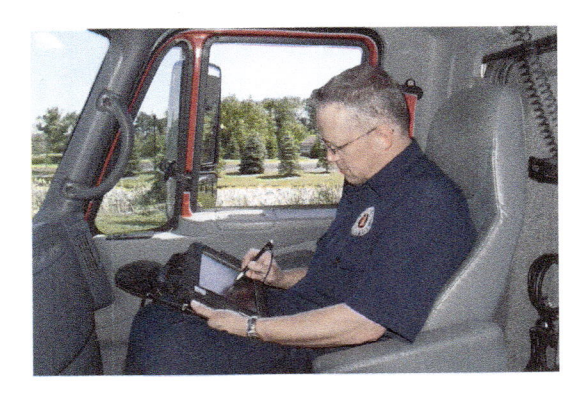

FIGURE 9.7 ■ Once you have accurately assessed and analyzed the facts, you need to make a written report.

corrective actions. If your report arrives at conclusions such as "Sue should have used common sense" or "Suzie forgot to use PPE," how effective will that be? Of course, it will not be effective at all. If your report concludes with such statements, it will be virtually impossible to take corrective actions that permanently eliminate the causes. It is likely that similar accidents will repeatedly occur. *Bottom line:* If the accident investigation does not fix the system, it most likely has been a waste of time and effort.

So the challenge is to report your findings in a well-thought-out manner so that management will be more likely to adopt your recommendations for improving its safety processes, thus solving problems long term.

THE ACCIDENT REPORT FORM

The primary reason accident investigations fail to help eliminate similar accidents is that report forms are poorly designed (Oregon OSHA, n.d.-b). In many cases the form design actually makes it possible to identify and correct only surface causes; root causes are often ignored. An example of a format designed to give emphasis to root causes is illustrated in Figures 9.8 and 9.9.

242 CHAPTER 9 Accident Investigation

VFIS
A Division of Glatfelter Insurance Group

Vehicle Accident/Loss Investigation Report
(This is not a claim form)

Fire Department _____ Date _____

Address _____

Name of Driver _____ Vehicle ID/Unit Number _____

Type of Vehicle _____

Date Driver Last Certified On Above Vehicle _____

Date of Accident _____ Time _____ Date Reported _____

Location of Accident _____

Roadway
- ☐ Straight _____
- ☐ Curve _____
- ☐ On Grade _____
- ☐ Level _____
- ☐ Hillcrest _____
- ☐ Dry _____
- ☐ Wet _____
- ☐ Muddy _____
- ☐ Snowy _____
- ☐ Icy _____
- ☐ Oily _____

- ☐ 2-lane
- ☐ 3-lane
- ☐ 4-lane
- ☐ Divided
- ☐ Rural
- ☐ Other _____
- ☐ Lanes marked
- ☐ Lanes unmarked
- ☐ No road detects
- ☐ Holes, ruts, etc.
- ☐ Loose material
- ☐ Other

Accident Occurred:
- ☐ At station
- ☐ Responding to emergency
- ☐ At emergency scene
- ☐ Returning from emergency
- ☐ Training
- ☐ Convention or parade
- ☐ Other _____
- ☐ Sleet

Type of Loss
- ☐ Personal injury
- ☐ Property damage
- ☐ Vehicle damage

Weather
- ☐ Clear
- ☐ Rain
- ☐ Snow
- ☐ Fog
- ☐ Other _____

Description Of Accident _____
_____
_____
_____
_____
_____

Motor Vehicle Diagram

Complete the following diagram showing direction and positions of automobiles involved, designating clearly point of contact.

Indicate North ↑

Instructions:
1. Show vehicles and direction of travel
2. Use solid line to show path of each vehicle before accident ▭▭▶ dotted line after accident...

Give Street Names and Directions
Your Vehicle ▭▶   Other Vehicle ◁1 ◁2

-over-

FIGURE 9.8 Example Vehicle Accident/Loss Investigation Form. *Reprinted with permission of VFIS.*

VFIS.
A Division of Glatfelter Insurance Group

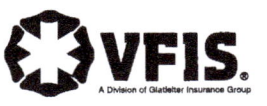

Please Note: This report is intended to be used by Emergency Service Organizations for internal use only. It is not an acceptable VFIS Claims form and therefore should not be submitted to VFIS.

Personal Injury/Illness Investigation Report

Emergency Service Organization _____ Date _____
Address _____
Name of Injured _____ Date of Birth _____
Address of Injured _____
Phone( ) _____ Age _____ Sex _____ Height _____ Weight _____ Occupation _____
Job Title _____ Social Security Number _____ Years with Dept. _____
Date of Injury _____ Time of Injury _____
Date Reported _____ Time Reported _____
Accident Reported To _____

Nature of Injury

- ☐ Fractures
- ☐ Inflammation
- ☐ Infectious Disease
- ☐ Frostbite, Cold Exposure
- ☐ Pinched Nerve, Ruptured Disk
- ☐ Electric Shock
- ☐ Chemical Injury

- ☐ Multiple Injury
- ☐ Recurrence
- ☐ Strain, Sprain, Torn Ligament
- ☐ Cuts, Lacerations, Punctures
- ☐ Inhalation, Fumes
- ☐ Inhalation, Smoke

- ☐ Heat Exhaustion, Fatigue
- ☐ Abrasions, Contusions, Bruises
- ☐ Heart Malfunction
- ☐ Eye Injury
- ☐ Burns
- ☐ Other _____

Parts of Body Affected

- ☐ Multiple Parts
- ☐ Head
- ☐ Eye(s)
- ☐ Ear(s)
- ☐ Neck
- ☐ Shoulder
- ☐ Chest
- ☐ Lung

- ☐ Abdomen
- ☐ Back
- ☐ Heart
- ☐ Groin
- ☐ Arm
- ☐ Hand
- ☐ Finger
- ☐ Leg(s)

- ☐ Knee(s)
- ☐ Ankle(s)
- ☐ Foot/Feet
- ☐ Ribs
- ☐ Hip
- ☐ Other _____

Where Injury Occurred

- ☐ Station Maintenance
- ☐ Apparatus Maintenance
- ☐ Emergency Scene
- ☐ Private Auto to Emergency
- ☐ Private Auto Non-Emergency

- ☐ Fundraising
- ☐ Convention
- ☐ Emergency Vehicle to Emergency
- ☐ Emergency Vehicle Non-Emergency
- ☐ Parades, Picnics, Contests

- ☐ Standing By Station for Call
- ☐ Training
- ☐ Auxiliary Services
- ☐ Responding/Returning to Emergency (Non-Vehicle)
- ☐ Other _____

FIGURE 9.9 ■ Example Personal Injury/Illness Investigation Form. *Reprinted with permission of VFIS.*

Cause of Injury

- ☐ Fall
- ☐ Weather
- ☐ Making Safety Devices Inoperative
- ☐ Using Defective Equipment
- ☐ Using Equipment Improperly
- ☐ Failure to Use Personal Protection Equipment
- ☐ Struck By Object
- ☐ Improper Lifting
- ☐ Horseplay
- ☐ Structural Collapse
- ☐ Inadequate Guards or Protection
- ☐ Back Draft
- ☐ Improper Placement
- ☐ Civil Disturbance
- ☐ Inadequate Illumination
- ☐ Inadequate Ventilation
- ☐ Lack of Knowledge or Skill
- ☐ Irrational Civilian
- ☐ Communication
- ☐ Abuse or Misuse
- ☐ Other _____

Injury Occurred - Performing What Task?

- ☐ Forcible Entry
- ☐ Using Ladders
- ☐ Advancing/Directing Hose Line
- ☐ Ventilating
- ☐ Overhauling
- ☐ Salvage
- ☐ Servicing/Repairing Equipment
- ☐ Extrication
- ☐ Rescue Operation
- ☐ Administering Medical Aid
- ☐ Physical Fitness
- ☐ Other _____

Witness(es) to Injury: _____

Injured Person's Signature _____ Date _____

Investigation Report

Thoroughly describe accident: (What, How, Where, Equipment, Activity, etc.) _____

_____
_____
_____
_____
_____

Hospitalized or Treated, Where? (Include Address) _____

Name and Address of Physician: (Include Referral) _____

Did the injury require individual to perform limited duties, or to be assigned to other duties or positions? YES or NO

If yes, what duties or position? _____

And, what period of time? _____

Investigated by _____ Title _____ Date _____

Safety Officer's Report

What Acts, Failures to Act and/or Conditions Contributed Most Directly to This Accident? (Immediate Cause)

_____
_____
_____

FIGURE 9.9 ■ *(Continued)*

> What Are the Basic or Fundamental Reasons for the Existence of These Acts and/or Conditions? (Fundamental Cause)
> _____
> _____
> _____
>
> What Action Has or Will Be Taken to Prevent Recurrence? Place "X" By Items Completed.
> _____
> _____
> _____
> _____
> _____
> _____
> _____
>
> Reviewed by Safety Officer _____ Title _____ Date _____

FIGURE 9.9 ■ (*Continued*)

Demographic Information
Most forms are very straightforward. Fill in all the requested pertinent information, including checkbox data.

Description of the Accident
The "Description of the Accident" on the form requires a narrative description of the events leading up to, including, and immediately after the accident. It is important that the narrative paint a vivid word picture so that someone unfamiliar with the accident can clearly see what happened. The format you choose is important. You can use a format similar to that which you see in most prehospital care reports.

Findings
The findings section of an accident report form should be used to describe the hazardous conditions, unsafe behaviors, and system weaknesses your investigation has uncovered. Each description of surface and root cause also will include justification for the finding. The justification will explain how you came to your conclusion. Some report forms used today force the investigator to list only surface causes for accidents. Consequently, the investigator believes the job is done without ferreting out the root causes. Other types of forms offer very little space to write findings. As a result, the form does not report the root causes associated with each surface cause. It is not the object of this section to find fault or place blame.

Just state the facts: the hazardous conditions, unsafe procedures, inadequate or missing policies, training, accountability, and so on. Be sure to write complete descriptive sentences, not short cryptic phrases.

Primary Surface. The findings describe the hazardous conditions and unsafe behaviors that directly caused injury. They exist or occur immediately prior to the injury event. *Example:* hazardous condition (there was heavy traffic at the intersection); unsafe behaviors (the responder was not wearing a seat belt).

Secondary Surface. These findings describe conditions and behaviors produced by individuals at some point prior to the injury event. The conditions, activities, practices, and behaviors can exist at any time, in any place, and be produced by any person in the organization. *Example:* hazardous condition (the vehicle was responding to an emergency at a physician's office for a stable patient); unsafe behaviors (the vehicle did not come to a complete stop at the red light).

Implementation Root Cause. These findings describe management failures to implement programs, processes, plans, and procedures within the safety management system. The failures result in secondary surface causes, or those conditions and behaviors common to groups or the entire organization. *Example:* inadequate process (personnel are not being properly trained in safe-driving procedures while responding emergency to calls; supervisors are unfamiliar with rules and have not received training in this subject); inappropriate behaviors (supervisors generally allow unsafe work practices associated with emergency vehicle operations).

Design Root Cause. These findings describe one or more inadequate safety management system policies, programs, and processes in any of the seven element areas: commitment, accountability, involvement, identification/control, incident/accident analysis, education/training, and evaluation. These deep root causes result in inadequate implementation of the safety management system. *Example:* conditions (emergency vehicle response policy statement does not exist; safety training plan does not include policies and practices for responding to incidents; safety training plan does not include supervisor-level training on this subject).

RECOMMENDATIONS

If root causes are not addressed properly in the accident report form, it is doubtful recommendations will include improving system inadequacies. Effective recommendations will describe ways to eliminate or reduce both surface and root causes. They also will detail estimated investments involved with implementing corrective actions and system improvements.

Primary Surface Causes

These recommendations describe how to correct those unique hazardous condition(s) and unsafe behaviors that directly resulted in injury. The recommendations will impact only the unique condition or behavior:

- To correct a condition (e.g., for a lifting injury, correct it by purchasing a stretcher with battery-powered lifting)
  Benefit: This hazardous condition is eliminated. Estimated investment: $12,000.
- To correct a behavior (e.g., educate and train personnel on proper lifting techniques)
  Benefit: The injured responder will understand and gain the skills necessary to prevent a similar accident. Estimated investment: $300.00.

Secondary Surface Causes

These recommendations describe how to correct common hazardous conditions and unsafe or inappropriate behaviors that eventually "set up" or produce the unique conditions and behaviors of the injury event. Correcting secondary surface causes is accomplished by improving the implementation of the safety management system. These recommendations will have a generally positive impact throughout the organization.

- Implement an effective education and training process covering proper lifting and moving techniques for all personnel
  Example benefit: Affected personnel will understand and be skilled in proper lifting and moving techniques. Estimated investment: $2,500.00.

- Implement improved personnel orientation that includes education and training on lifting and moving techniques
  Example benefit: New personnel will understand and gain skills in appropriate lifting and moving procedures. Estimated investment: $300.
- Conduct supervisor training on new policies, SOPs, SOGs, and protocols
  Example benefit: Management will better understand and gain skills in their responsibilities in lifting and moving techniques. Estimated investment: $800.

Sample Recommendations that Correct Implementation-and-Design Root Causes

Solving implementation weaknesses is accomplished by improving system design. Recommendations may include improvements in more than one of the seven safety management system element areas discussed earlier. In most instances, safety committees and/or safety officers will be involved in this process. Policies, plans, procedures, and protocols are drafted, developed, and forwarded to upper management for approval.

- *Review and improve* (e.g., review and improve the training plan to ensure it includes lifting and moving procedures)
  Benefit: Ensures the safety training plan addresses affected responder responsibilities regarding lifting and moving. Estimated investment: $1,500.00.
- *Develop organization safety policy and safe work plan* (e.g., by addressing lifting and moving of patients)
  Example Benefit: Ensures safe work policies and procedures regarding lifting and moving of patients are detailed and properly implemented. Estimated investment: $1,000.
- *Include supervisor education and training in accountability principles and application*
  Example benefit: Ensures management is effectively educated and trained in accountabilities to the organization and personnel, and how to administer corrective actions. Estimated investment: $800.
- *Include supervisor education and training in recognition principles and application*
  Example benefit: Ensures management is effectively educated and trained in methods to motivate hazard reporting and discretionary behaviors such as suggesting and involvement. Estimated investment: $800.

ACCIDENT SUMMARY

The accident summary contains a brief review of the causes of the accident and recommendations for corrective actions. In your review, it is important to include language that contrasts the costs of the accident with the benefits derived from investing in corrective actions. Including bottom-line information will ensure that your recommendation will be understood and appreciated by management and the leadership of the organization.

REVIEW AND FOLLOW-UP ACTIONS

The review and follow-up actions parts of the report should describe the actions taken to repair equipment/vehicles, conduct training, revise policies, and so on. It also should describe the persons responsible for carrying out corrective actions and system improvements.

ATTACHMENT

The attachment should describe all of the photos, sketches, interview notes, and other items pertinent to the investigation. Of course, the more comprehensive the investigation, the more supporting documentation will be included.

CHAPTER REVIEW

Summary

Accident scenes can challenge the best investigator. Utilize the resources available and follow the guidelines established to conduct an accident investigation. Good documentation is critical for later recall. Accident investigations can take on many forms. Unless you have the credentials to conduct an accident investigation for who is at fault, the intent of the accident investigation should be solely for the purpose of making corrective actions to improve safety.

WHAT WOULD YOU DO? Reflection

What is the first thing you should do when you arrive on the scene? You know to begin the investigation process as soon as you hear the call. This is very similar to responding to a vehicle crash when you were a care provider on the street. You begin by thinking of the area where the incident occurred. You know that when you get on scene you want to get as much information as possible without getting in the way of the other responders.

What if there are injuries of your personnel? If there are injuries, you know that you will need to gather as much information as possible on the scene and then head to the hospital emergency room to find out the extent of injuries and the status of personnel and civilians. You also will want to get as much information as possible, and you will try to interview the crew members at the hospital if they are able to be interviewed.

Whom do you need to call? You need to make sure upper management is notified, especially your direct supervisor. Management is typically aware of such situations, but you want to make sure they are aware. In addition, you need to make sure your insurance carrier is notified as soon as possible.

What needs to be done after the incident? You know that there will be lots of time spent writing reports, conducting additional interviews. In addition, the safety committee will need to review the incident.

Who should you interview? You need to interview as many people as possible on the scene, at the hospital, and after the event. The more information you can obtain the easier it is to put things together.

Review Questions

1. Explain the difference between a near miss and an accident.
2. What are the six key questions you should ask in the investigative report?
3. What are the characteristics of an effective incident/accident analysis program?
4. List at least five documents you would review during your accident/incident evaluation.
5. Describe at least five techniques that will ensure you get the facts when you interview someone as part of an accident/incident investigation.
6. Describe at least three theories cause-and-effect of an accident.
7. What are the four ways to utilize engineering controls?

References

Mitterer, D., and R. Patrick. (n.d.). *Risk Management for EMS and the Ambulance Transport Industry*. York, PA: VFIS

National Safety Council. (2012). "Estimating the Costs of Unintentional Injuries." (See the organization website.)

Occupational Safety and Health Administration. (n.d.) Safety and Health Management Systems eTool: "Accident/Incident Investigation." Washington, DC: Author. (See the organization website.)

Occupational Safety and Health Administration. (n.d.) Safety and Health Management Systems eTool: "Accident/Incident Investigation Tips and Tools." Washington, DC: Author. (See the organization website.)

Oregon OSHA. (n.d.-a). "Oregon OSHA Online Course 100: Incident/Accident Analysis." Salem, OR: Author. (See the organization website.)

Oregon OSHA. (n.d.-b). Oregon OSHA Online Course 102: "Conducting an Accident Investigation." Salem, OR: Author. (See the organization website.)

Key Terms

action Something that is done by an actor. Actions may or may not be observable. An action may describe something that is done or not done. Failure to act should be thought of as an act in itself.

actor Person who conducts an act. An individual or object that directly influenced the flow of the sequence of events. An actor may participate in the process or merely observe the process. An actor initiates a change by performing or failing to perform an action.

analysis Separation of an intellectual or substantial whole into its parts for individual study.

hazardous conditions Things and states that directly cause an accident.

material evidence Items valuable to an accident investigation, such as tools, equipment, and people.

system weaknesses Underlying inadequate or missing programs, plans, policies, processes, and procedures that contributed to an accident.

unsafe behaviors Actions taken/not taken that contributed to the accident.

Recordkeeping

10 CHAPTER

Objectives

After reading this chapter, the student should be able to:

10.1 Discuss the various types of recordkeeping needed.
10.2 Explain how to maintain the various records.
10.3 Identify the requirements of recordkeeping.

Overview

This title on EMS safety and risk management has been written to assist EMS providers in the reduction of line-of-duty injuries, illnesses, and fatalities. It provides a framework for developing programs that will create an appropriate margin of health and safety for providers during the performance of EMS duties.

Key Terms

job transfer
OSHA 300 log
recordkeeping
restricted work

WHAT WOULD YOU DO?

The training chief comes to you and says she heard you were very knowledgeable about recordkeeping. You wish this was the case. You have no clue about the different types of recordkeeping but will hear her out. She tells you that she was just audited by the state and must establish a recordkeeping program for the training she has been conducting. She would like to know what components should be part of the document. This doesn't sound like it is something that would be too hard to figure out. You tell her that you will confirm the requirements and get back to her. You must start looking for a good model to cover the bases you must provide for her.

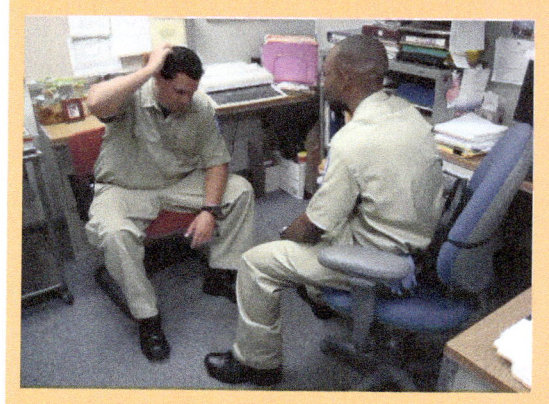

You may be asked to share your knowledge on recordkeeping. You must prepare yourself to be able to assist others as requested. *Courtesy of Jeffrey T. Lindsey, Ph.D.*

Questions

1. What information can you find from OSHA?
2. What other resources could you use as part of your presentation?
3. What five specific elements would you address in your training document?

INTRODUCTION

Recordkeeping is an important element for the EMS organization. It is your job to make sure the appropriate safety records are kept according to federal, state, and local requirements. This chapter will look at various recordkeeping issues, including how to make sure that the appropriate postings are displayed in your organization.

RECORDKEEPING

Recordkeeping is a critical component of the safety program. Regardless of who is deemed responsible for the task, it must be done. The following is a list of questions to answer to attest to your organization's compliance with various recordkeeping requirements:

* Are occupational injuries or illnesses, except minor injuries requiring only first aid, recorded as required on the OSHA 300 log?
* Are personnel medical records and records of personnel exposure to hazardous substances or harmful physical agents up to date and in compliance with current OSHA standards?
* Are personnel's training records kept and accessible for review by personnel, as required by OSHA standards?
* Have arrangements been made to retain records for the time period required for each specific type of record? (Some records must be maintained for at least 40 years.)

- Are operating permits and records up to date for items such as elevators, air pressure tanks, liquefied petroleum gas tanks, and so on?
- Are your personnel medical records kept in a separate place from all other records, and are they accessible only by those individuals whose job requires the information?

DOCUMENTING YOUR ACTIVITIES

It is essential that you document your activities, such as policy statements, training sessions, safety meetings, safety information distributed to personnel, and medical documentation related to safety factors such as injury reports (Figure 10.1). The essential records to maintain include those legally required under workers' compensation requirements, requested by insurance audits, and any government inspections requirements, or if there is a need or a requirement by law. You must be very familiar with your state recordkeeping laws and requirements. Maintaining essential records also will demonstrate sound management practice as supporting proof for showing "good faith" in reducing any proposed penalties from OSHA inspections, being prepared for insurance and other audits, aiding efficient review of your current safety and health activities for better control of your operations, and planning improvements.

SAFETY AND HEALTH RECORDKEEPING

EMS personnel are very familiar with documenting patient assessment and treatment on a patient care report. There is also an understanding of the importance of patient care records. Records of accidents, related injuries, illnesses, and property losses can serve the same purpose, if they are used in the same way. The primary purpose of OSHA-required recordkeeping is to retain information about accidents that have happened to help determine the causes and develop procedures to prevent a recurrence. Successful organizations strive to maintain appropriate records.

INJURY/ILLNESS RECORDS

OSHA rules for recording and reporting occupational injuries and illnesses affect 1.4 million businesses (OSHA, 2005). Small organizations with 10 or fewer employees throughout the year are exempt from most of the requirements of the OSHA recordkeeping rules (OSHA). Keep in mind that OSHA uses the term *employee* generically, which means it does not matter if people are paid or volunteer; they are still considered employees of the organization. Success can be measured by a reduction or elimination of personnel injuries and illnesses during a calendar year.

Periodically, review the records to look for any patterns or repeat situations. The records can help you identify high-risk areas that require your immediate attention.

Basic OSHA recordkeeping requirements address only injuries and illnesses, so you might consider expanding your own records to include all incidents, including those where no injury or illness resulted. This information may assist you in pinpointing unsafe conditions and/or procedures. Safety councils, insurance carriers, and

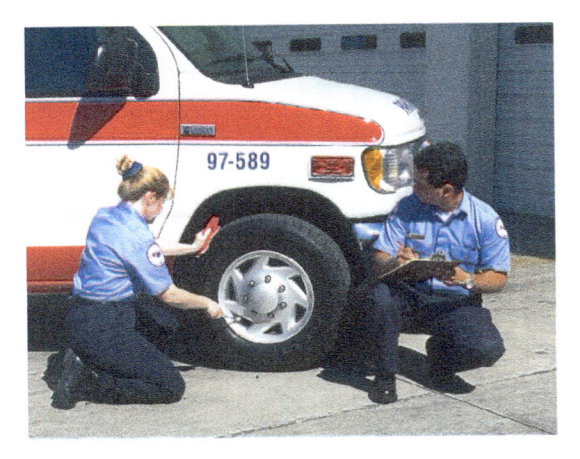

FIGURE 10.1 Document virtually everything you do. The records then must be filed appropriately.

others can assist you in instituting such a system. You are required to report to OSHA, within 8 hours of the accident, all work-related fatalities or multiple hospitalizations that involve three or more personnel. Even if your organization is exempt from routine recordkeeping requirements, you may be selected by the Federal Bureau of Labor Statistics (BLS) or a related state agency for inclusion in an annual sample survey. You will receive a letter directly from the agency with instructions, if you are selected. This is not common among EMS agencies. EMS is diverse and not every agency will fall under the same guidelines. It will depend on the type of agency and the laws for your state.

INJURY REPORTS

Injury reports fall under OSHA (2005) Section 1904.29 Subpart C—Recordkeeping Forms and Recording Criteria (66 FR 6123, Jan. 19, 2001). This subpart describes the work-related injuries and illnesses that an organization must enter into the OSHA records and explains the OSHA forms that organizations must use to record work-related fatalities, injuries, and illnesses.

You must use OSHA 300, 300-A, and 301 forms, or equivalent for recordable injuries and illnesses. The formal name for the **OSHA 300 log** is the Log of Work-Related Injuries and Illnesses; the 300-A is the Summary of Work-Related Injuries and Illnesses; and the OSHA 301 form is the Injury and Illness Incident Report.

You must enter information about your organization at the top of the OSHA 300 log, enter a one- or two-line description for each recordable injury or illness, and summarize this information on the OSHA 300-A at the end of the year. You must complete an OSHA 301 Incident Report form, or an equivalent, for each recordable injury or illness entered on the OSHA 300 log. You must enter each recordable injury or illness on the OSHA 300 log and 301 Incident Report within 7 calendar days of receiving information that a recordable injury or illness has occurred.

You can use an equivalent form that contains the same information and is as readable and understandable as the original, and is completed using the same instructions as the OSHA form it replaces. Many organizations use an insurance form instead of the OSHA 301 Incident Report, or supplement an insurance form by adding any additional information required by OSHA.

You can use computer records (Figure 10.2) of injuries and illnesses if the computer can produce equivalent forms when they are needed, as described under OSHA Sections 1904.35 and 1904.40. You may keep your records using the computer system.

If you have a case with privacy concerns, you may not enter the person's name on the OSHA 300 log. Instead, enter "Privacy Case" in the space normally used for the individual's name. This will protect the privacy of the injured or ill individual when another individual, former personnel, or an authorized individual representative is provided access to the OSHA 300 log under Section 1904.35(b)(2). You must keep a separate, confidential list of the case numbers and personnel names for your privacy-concern cases so you can update the cases and provide the information to OSHA if asked to do so.

The following injuries or illnesses are considered to be privacy-concern cases:

- An injury or illness to an intimate body part or the reproductive system
- An injury or illness resulting from a sexual assault
- Mental illnesses
- HIV infection, hepatitis, or tuberculosis
- Needlestick injuries and cuts from sharp objects that are contaminated with another person's blood or other potentially infectious material
- Other illnesses, if the individual independently and voluntarily requests that his or her name not be entered on the log

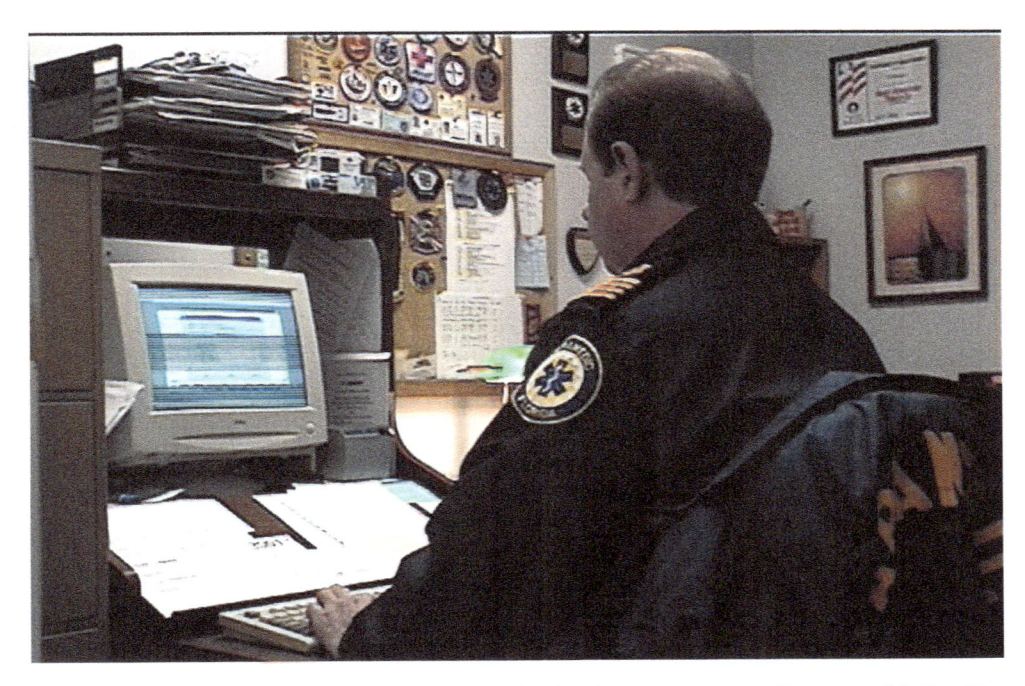

FIGURE 10.2 ■ Injury and illness records may be maintained on a computer. *Courtesy of Jeffrey T. Lindsey, Ph.D.*

Paragraph 1904.29(b)(3) establishes the requirement for how quickly each recordable injury or illness must be recorded into the records. It states that the organization is to enter each case on the OSHA 300 log and OSHA 301 Form within 7 calendar days of receiving information that a recordable injury or illness has occurred.

Defining Lost Workdays

The 300 log has four check boxes to be used to classify the illness or injury incident: death, day(s) away from work, day(s) of **restricted work** or duty transfer, and cases meeting other recording criteria. The person completing the form must check the single box that reflects the most severe outcome associated with a given injury or illness. Thus, for an injury or illness during which the injured individual first stayed home to recuperate and then was assigned to restricted duty for several days, the organization is required only to check the box for days away from the person's duties (Column I). For a case with only duty transfer or restriction, the person completing the log must check the box for days of restricted duty or duty transfer (Column H). However, the log still allows organizations to calculate the incidence rate formerly referred to as a "lost workday injury and illness rate" despite the fact that it separates the data formerly captured under this heading into two separate categories. Because the OSHA Form 300 has separate check boxes for days away from work cases and cases where the individual remained on duty but was temporarily transferred to another duty or assigned to restricted duty, it is easy to combine the totals from these two columns to obtain a single total to use in calculating an injury and illness incidence rate for total days away from duty and restricted duty cases.

Restricted Work or Job Transfer

Although the OSHA recordkeeping rule does not use the term *lost workday*, which formerly applied both to days away from duty and days of restricted or transferred duty, it continues OSHA's longstanding practice of requiring organizations to keep track of the number of days on which an individual is placed on restricted duty or is on duty transfer because of an injury or illness.

In the rule, OSHA has decided to require employers to record the number of days of restriction or transfer on the OSHA 300 log. From the comments received, and based on OSHA's own experience, the agency finds that counts of restricted days are a useful and needed measure of injury and illness severity. OSHA's decision to require the recording of restricted and transferred work cases on the log also was influenced by the trend toward restricted work rather than days away from work.

Exposure Records and Others

In addition to injury/illness records, certain OSHA standards require records on the exposure of personnel to toxic substances and hazardous exposures, physical examination reports, and service or employment records. As you identify hazards, you will be able to determine whether these requirements apply to your organization. Your records should be used in conjunction with your control procedures and with your self-inspection activity. They should not be considered merely as bookkeeping. OSHA is not the only agency that requires and governs recordkeeping. You must make sure you know and understand the state statutes that govern your organization for your state.

INFECTIOUS DISEASES

Recordkeeping in regard to exposures to infectious diseases can be found in Section 1904.8 of the OSHA regulation on infectious diseases. There is quite an extensive amount of information about specific diseases and recordkeeping for exposure to the disease.

Recording needlesticks and injuries from sharps is covered under this section. You must record all work-related needlestick injuries and cuts from sharp objects that are contaminated with another person's blood or other potentially infectious material as defined by 29 CFR 1910.1030. You must enter the case on the OSHA 300 log as an injury. To protect the member's privacy, you may not enter the member's name on the OSHA 300 log (see the requirements for privacy cases in paragraphs 1904.29[b][6] through 1904.29[b][9]).

If you record an injury and the individual is later diagnosed with an infectious blood-borne disease, you are to update the OSHA 300 log if the case results in death, days away from work, restricted work, or **job transfer**. You are also to update the description to identify the infectious disease and change the classification of the case from an injury to an illness.

The OSHA rule requires the recording of all workplace cut and puncture injuries resulting from an event involving contaminated sharps; however, it does not require the recording of all cuts and punctures. For example, a cut made by a knife or other sharp instrument that was not contaminated by blood or other potentially infectious materials would not generally be recordable, and a laceration made by a dirty aluminum can or greasy tool would also generally not be recordable, providing that the injury did not result from a contaminated sharp and did not meet one of the general recording criteria of medical treatment, restricted work.

OSHA requires only that lacerations and puncture wounds that involve contact with another person's blood or other potentially infectious materials be recorded on the log. Exposure incidents involving exposure of the eyes, mouth, other mucous membranes or non-intact skin to another person's blood or other potentially infectious material (OPIM) need not be recorded unless they meet one or more of the general recording criteria, result in a positive blood test (seroconversion), or result in the diagnosis of a significant illness by a health care professional. Otherwise, these exposure incidents are considered only to involve exposure and not to constitute an injury or illness. In contrast, a needlestick laceration or puncture wound is clearly an injury and, if it involves exposure to human blood or other potentially infectious materials, it rises to the level of seriousness that requires recording. For splashes and other exposure incidents, the case does not rise to this level any more than a chemical exposure does. If an individual who has been exposed via a splash in the eye from the blood or OPIM of a person with a blood-borne disease actually contracts an illness, or seroconverts, the case would be recorded (provided that it meets one or more of the general recording criteria).

Medical Records

In addition to Section 1904.8 of the OSHA regulation on infectious diseases, Section 1910.1030 has requirements for infectious disease exposure recordkeeping. The EMS organization must establish and maintain an accurate record for each individual with occupational exposure, in accordance with 29 CFR 1910.1020. This record must include the following:

- The name and Social Security number of the individual
- A copy of the individual's hepatitis B vaccination status, including the dates of all the hepatitis B vaccinations, and any medical records relative to the individual's ability to receive vaccination
- A copy of all results of examinations, medical testing, and follow-up procedures as required by paragraph (f)(3)*1910.1030*(h)(1)(ii)(D)
- The individual's copy of the health care professional's written opinion
- A copy of the information provided to the health care professional

Confidentiality

The EMS organization must ensure that personnel medical records required by the OSHA standard are kept confidential and not disclosed or reported without the individual's express written consent to any person inside or outside the organization except as required by the standard or as may be required by law. The organization must maintain the records in accordance for at least the duration the individual is with the organization plus 30 years.

It is important to remember that these records also fall under the Health Insurance Portability and Accountability (HIPAA) Act of 1996. You should refer to your organization's privacy act to determine the policy for your organization as required by law under those governance standards.

Training Records

Blood-borne pathogen training records must include the following information:

- Dates of the training sessions
- Contents or a summary of the training sessions, including a lesson plan
- Names and qualifications of persons conducting the training, including the person's résumé or curriculum vitae (CV)
- Names and job titles of all persons attending the training sessions

Training records must be maintained for 3 years from the date on which the training occurred.

Transfer of Records

The organization must comply with the requirements involving transfer of records. If your organization no longer provides services and no longer exists, then you must contact the director of OSHA of the situation. The director of OSHA will make a determination of what to do with the records. This must be completed within a 3-month period from the time the organization no longer exists.

Sharps Injury Log

The organization must establish and maintain a sharps injury log for the recording of percutaneous injuries from contaminated sharps. The information in the sharps injury log must be recorded and maintained in such manner as to protect the confidentiality of the injured member. The sharps injury log shall contain, at a minimum, the following:

- Type and brand of device involved in the incident
- Department or work area where the exposure incident occurred
- Explanation of how the incident occurred

PRIVACY ISSUES

The recordkeeping rule addresses this issue by prohibiting the entry of the individual's name on the OSHA 300 log for injury and illness cases involving blood and OPIM. Further, by requiring organizations to record all needlestick and sharps incidents—regardless of the seroconversion status of the individual—co-workers, and organization representatives who have access to the log will not be able to ascertain the disease status of the injured person.

OSHA believes that hepatitis C cases should, like other illness cases, be tested for recordability using the geographic presumption that provides the principal rationale for determining work-relatedness throughout this OSHA Standard 1910.1030.

According to Section 1910.1030(h)(5), the organization is to establish and maintain a sharps injury log for the recording of percutaneous injuries from contaminated sharps. The information in the sharps injury log must be recorded and maintained in such manner as to protect the confidentiality of the injured individual. The sharps injury log must contain, at a minimum, the type and brand of device involved in the incident, the department or work area where the exposure incident occurred, and an explanation of how the incident occurred.

The requirement to establish and maintain a sharps injury log applies to any organization that is required to maintain a log of occupational injuries and illnesses under 29 CFR 1904. You can use the OSHA 300 log to meet the requirements of the sharps injury log. To do this you must enter the type and brand of the device causing the sharps injury on the log, and you must maintain your records in a way that segregates sharps injuries from other types of work-related injuries and illnesses, or allows sharps injuries to be easily separated.

TUBERCULOSIS CASES

Section 1904.11 covers the recording criteria for work-related tuberculosis (TB) cases. If any of your personnel has been occupationally exposed to anyone with a known case of active TB, and that individual subsequently develops a tuberculosis infection, as evidenced by a positive skin test or diagnosis by a physician or other licensed health care professional, you are to record the case on the OSHA 300 log by checking the "Respiratory Condition" column.

A positive tuberculin skin test indicates that the individual has been exposed to *Mycobacterium tuberculosis* and has been infected with the bacterium. Although the individual may or may not have active tuberculosis disease, the individual has become infected. Otherwise, his or her body would not have formed antibodies against these pathogens. OSHA notes that, in rare situations, a positive skin test result may indicate a prior inoculation against TB rather than an infection.

OSHA believes that TB infection is a significant change in the health status of an individual and, if occupational in origin, is precisely the type of illness Congress envisioned including in the OSHA injury and illness statistics. Contracting a TB infection from a patient, or other person in the EMS environment would cause serious concern, in OSHA's view, in any reasonable person. Once an individual has contracted the TB infection, he or she will harbor the infection for life. At some time in the future, the infection can progress to become active disease, with pulmonary infiltration, cavitation, and fibrosis, and may lead to permanent lung damage and death. A member harboring TB infection is particularly likely to develop the full-blown disease if he or she must undergo chemotherapy, contracts another disease, or experiences poor health.

When an individual is exposed to an infectious agent in the workplace, such as TB, chicken pox, and so on, either by a co-worker, client, patient, or any other person, and the individual becomes ill, workplace conditions have either caused or contributed to the illness, thereby making it work related. TB infection is clearly a serious condition; it is not minor and must be recorded.

OSHA agrees that a case of TB should be recorded only when an individual has been exposed to TB in the workplace (i.e., that the positional theory of causation applies to these cases just as it does to all others). OSHA has added an additional recording criterion in this case: For a TB case occurring in an individual to be recordable, that member must have been exposed at work to someone with a known case of active tuberculosis.

The rule's criteria for recording TB cases include three provisions designed to help organizations rule out cases where occupational exposure is not the cause of the infection in the individual (i.e., where the infection was caused by exposure outside the work environment). An organization is not required to record a case involving a member who has a positive skin test and who is exposed at work if (1) the individual is living in a household with a person who has been diagnosed with active TB, (2) the public health department has identified the individual as a contact of a case of active TB unrelated to the workplace, or (3) a medical investigation shows that the individual's infection was caused by exposure to TB away from work or proves that the case was not related to the workplace TB exposure.

RESPIRATOR FIT TESTING

The respiratory protection program specifies a number of areas that should be documented with recordkeeping in place. The following basic elements regarding these areas should be maintained in writing and as records applicable to your personnel's duties and issuance of respirators (OSHA, n.d.-a):

- Procedures for selecting respirators for use in the workplace
- Medical evaluations of personnel required to use respirators
- Fit testing procedures for tight-fitting respirators
- Use of respirators in routine and reasonably foreseeable emergency situations
- Procedures and schedules for cleaning, disinfecting, storing, inspecting, repairing, and otherwise maintaining respirators
- Procedures to ensure adequate air quality, quantity and flow of breathing air for atmosphere-supplying respirators
- Training of personnel in the respiratory hazards to which they are potentially exposed
- Training of personnel in the proper use of respirators, including putting on and removing them, any limitations on their use, and maintenance procedures
- Procedures for regularly evaluating the effectiveness of the program

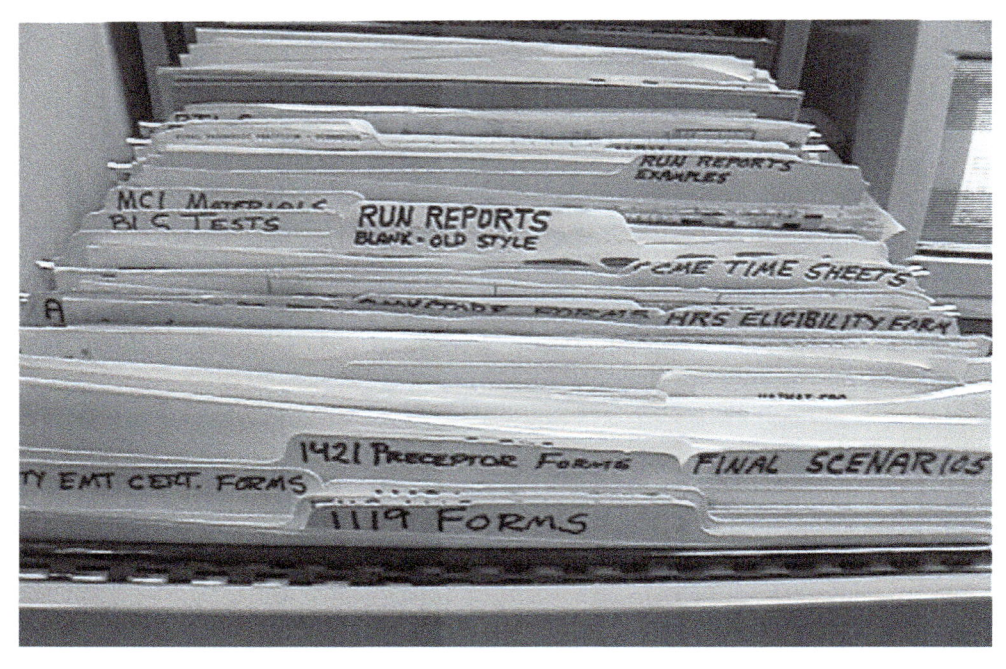

FIGURE 10.3 ■ Recordkeeping is an essential part of a safety program. Every EMS organization must maintain training records for a minimum of 3 years. *Courtesy of Jeffrey T. Lindsey, Ph.D.*

TRAINING

It is important to document any training sessions that you have (Figure 10.3). In EMS we are very familiar with providing documentation for continuing education in order to maintain our EMT or paramedic certification. It also is important to document any other type of training conducted. In addition, individuals who are not EMS certified should not be left out. These individuals require various types of training, and the training must be documented.

OSHA dictates that training records must be maintained for 3 years from the date of training. The following information should be documented in order to meet OSHA's requirements:

- Dates of the training sessions
- Outline describing the material presented and lesson plans
- Names and qualifications of persons conducting the training, including the person's CV or résumé illustrating competency as an instructor
- Names, job titles, and evaluations of all persons attending the training sessions

The true measurement of training performance is the training record. The basic objective in keeping training records is to record training in the simplest manner possible. Training records should regularly be examined as part of the quality improvement process. A variety of individuals may inspect these training records. If any type of legal action is waged against the department, the training records may be subpoenaed to determine whether existing training requirements are adequate to prevent further injuries or damage.

Another resource to look at in regard to training records is the National Fire Protection Association (NFPA) 1401 standard (NFPA,

2006). It is not necessarily exclusive to the fire service. It provides the elements of training documents. Five specific elements of information that must be included in a training document—who, what, when, where, and why:

- *Who.* Who was the instructor? Who participated? Who was in attendance? Who is affected by the documents?
- *What.* What was the subject covered? What equipment was utilized? What operation was evaluated or affected? What was the stated objective and was it met?
- *When.* When did the event take place?
- *Where.* Where did the event take place?
- *Why.* Why was the event necessary?

SAFETY AUDITS

Safety audits should be conducted to ensure that your organization is carrying out its mission in the safest manner possible. As a result of your audit, you should generate a safety audit document. There is no specific period within which you are required to maintain the safety audit records. However, it is always good practice to maintain the records to show that you do safety audits. Your insurance carrier may also be interested in these documents. How long you maintain the files can be based on the length of time you keep your training files, which is a period of 3 years.

ACCIDENT REPORTS

A number of documents are produced in response to accident investigations. You must remember there may be two separate tracks for accident investigations. There is the internal investigation that may be conducted for safety improvement reasons. Then there is the formal investigation that will include everything about the accident, including police reports, insurance claims, repair bills, and other documents required or completed. In many instances, agencies require that personnel complete an accident report for the agency. The accident record file should include all these documents.

For recordkeeping purposes, an accident involving a motor vehicle is defined as a collision that results in any of the following:

- Fatality at the scene or within 30 days
- Bodily injury to a person who, as a result of the injury, immediately receives medical treatment away from the scene of the accident
- One or more vehicles incur "disabling damage," requiring the vehicle(s) to be transported away from the scene by a tow truck or other vehicle

A record of the event including all documentation should be kept for each accident for at least 1 year. In many instances, it is good practice to maintain the files for at least 7 years. As with any recordkeeping, you should check with your state for other requirements imposed on you for recordkeeping. The information on the register should include the following:

- Date of the accident
- City or town nearest the accident site
- State in which the accident occurred
- Driver's name
- Number of persons injured
- Number of fatalities
- Whether hazardous materials were released (other than fuel spilled from the fuel tanks of vehicles involved in the accident)

BENEFITS OF RECORDKEEPING

Accident recordkeeping has benefits. First, it identifies high-risk or problem routes and types of equipment that can pose a safety problem. This can result in using different response routes during different times of day or different locations in a given area. It may identify a problem with a piece of equipment that needs the manufacturer to make changes in order to resolve the problem.

Another benefit is that it gives you and the safety committee the ability to evaluate the impact of the safety program on reducing the frequency and severity of accidents. If a program is not showing an effect, the program may need to be revised. You can also compare the time period of accidents to identify any correlation of accident experiences. Efforts may be needed to change shift schedules or practices as a result.

There are benefits in being able to formulate solutions to safety problems. By gathering the data and taking it into account, the information may enable you and the safety committee to implement new procedures or processes to reduce the number of accidents. In addition, it can identify individuals who are prone to accidents. This will help focus attention on correcting these issues, including changing the duties of personnel in order to reduce the number of incidents caused by them.

Recordkeeping provides a starting point for accident investigations and analysis. Reviewing various records can give clues to the potential cause of an incident. Further, it creates an interest in safety and accident prevention among supervisors and drivers. It also helps in complying with state and federal regulations.

Another benefit of recordkeeping is that it can illustrate the strengths and weaknesses in the management system. This can be helpful; however, it is also important to have management buy-in for this to be beneficial. This information should be shared only with management for purposes of improvement.

Finally, recordkeeping assists your insurance company in the expeditious handling of claims. The insurance company's access to your records will help them process the claim.

SAFETY MEETINGS

A record of these safety meetings must be maintained (Figure 10.4). The records will serve in the future as a record of any items discussed. They also will serve as proof to any regulatory agency or your insurance carrier should you be audited and a copy of the meeting notes be requested. The record of the safety meeting should include the names of the attendees. A sign-in sheet typically suffices for this portion. The records should also include the date, topic(s) discussed, and person leading the meeting.

It is also a good idea to follow up on items discussed at safety meetings and to note any outcomes as a result of the work completed or in effect. You can note any training that has been implemented, and if there has been a decrease in lost work days, this can be noted in the meeting minutes. Regardless, documentation of the progress of the safety committee and the meetings is important to maintain on file (Figure 10.5). You must check with any regulatory agency that requires you to maintain records of your safety meetings to determine the length of time to keep the meeting records. If there are no requirements, it is always a good practice to maintain files for at least 3 years.

VEHICLE AND EQUIPMENT MAINTENANCE

Inspections and preventive maintenance efforts (including repairs and malfunctions) should be documented, and a record should be kept during the life of the vehicle or piece of equipment. The records should include a vehicle/equipment log, a maintenance file, and all work order request forms.

VEHICLES

If an emergency vehicle is involved in a crash, and it is possible that a mechanical malfunction was the cause, the courts will be very interested in reviewing the maintenance records of the emergency vehicle. If

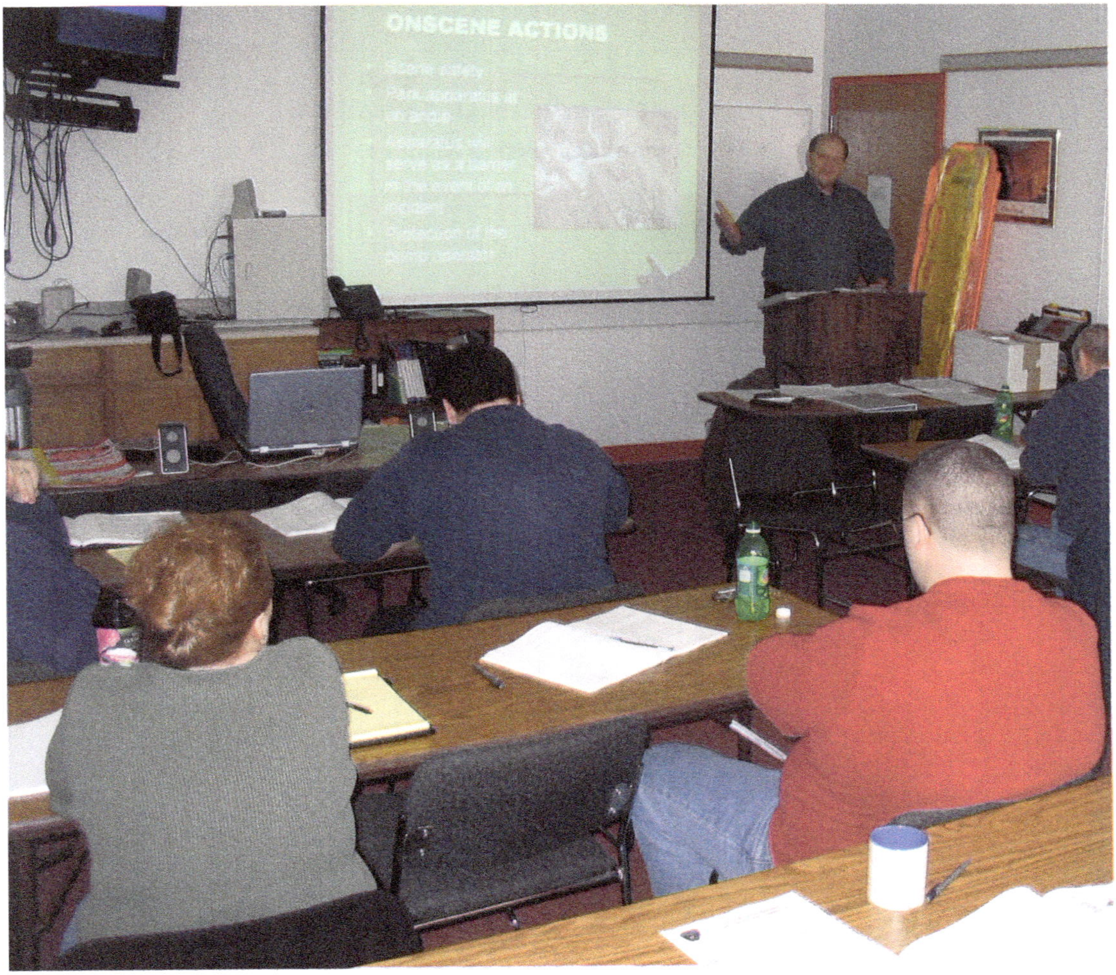

FIGURE 10.4 ■ Safety meetings must be documented for future reference. *Courtesy of Lawrence T. Bennett.*

the operating organization knew in advance of the malfunction and continued to operate the vehicle, it may be found negligent and held liable for all damages resulting from the crash.

Maintenance departments must be able to document in writing the servicing, maintenance, and repair of all vehicles and equipment. A good general guideline for documenting inspections and maintenance actions is "If it is not in writing, it did not happen."

Work Requests

A work request tells maintenance department what work is needed on a vehicle. When the maintenance department finishes the work, the work performed, tests run, and the results should be recorded on the

ABC Emergency Services Organization
Safety Committee Meeting Minutes

Meeting Date:
_____

Members Present:
_____
_____
_____
_____
_____

Review of Old Business:
_____
_____
_____
_____
_____
_____
_____
_____
_____
_____

New Business: (Review of accidents; review of feedback from emergency services organizations on safety related issues.)
_____
_____
_____
_____
_____
_____

FIGURE 10.5 Sample format for safety committee meeting minutes.

Best Practice

Sunstar EMS is a public utility model based in Pinellas County, which is on the west coast of Florida. Pinellas County is part of the Tampa Bay metropolitan area and is home to St. Petersburg and Clearwater. Sunstar EMS performs all vehicle maintenance and repair work for critical failures in-house, except major body repair and vehicle towing. This practice allows the organization to control the quality of work on its units and related costs. Direct control of maintenance guarantees that the units are safe, reliable, and available in numbers sufficient to meet normal as well as extraordinary demands. Sunstar's maintenance personnel are all certified to work on the vehicles and equipment.

The preventive maintenance program pursues the goal of zero critical failures by constantly monitoring component life and mechanic performance. A critical failure is any incident in which a specific ambulance dispatched to or needed for a call cannot respond to the patient or complete a call, due to mechanical problems with the vehicle itself.

Every Sunstar EMS ambulance receives scheduled services at intervals of 4,000 miles or 300 engine hours, whichever comes first. Certain vehicles require customized service intervals, depending on the year of manufacture, type of transmission, chassis, and brake system. The preventive maintenance program is also adjusted for administrative and support vehicles, since they are subject to less strenuous use than ambulances.

Sunstar EMS scientifically studies wear and tear on parts to ensure they do not exceed their safe useful life. For example, to determine the best interval for oil changes, it contracted with a vehicle performance research company to run ambulances on a track for extended periods. The results determined that a 5,000-mile interval was appropriate. To exceed these requirements, Sunstar EMS performs the service every 4,000 miles.

Through extensive recordkeeping and monitoring, Sunstar is able to provide a model preventive maintenance program for its units.

Source: Based on Sunstar Paramedics. (2011). "Fleet Maintenance." (See the organization website.)

---

work request form. This document covers those problems that the driver finds during an inspection as well as routine preventive maintenance. An organization may or may not use a work request to track maintenance and repairs.

Vehicle Maintenance Logs

Information from the inspection checklists and work requests are written into a vehicle maintenance log. The vehicle maintenance log is a vehicle's central record for listing all maintenance needed and done, including routine maintenance and problems identified by inspections, and for supporting the preventive maintenance program. To document that the vehicle has been properly maintained, vehicle maintenance log pages are usually organized into binders and saved in an inspection file for use by a maintenance supervisor or manager.

EQUIPMENT

If a piece of equipment fails (Figure 10.6), and a mechanical malfunction may have been the cause, the courts would be very interested in reviewing the maintenance records of the piece of equipment. If the operating organization knew in advance of

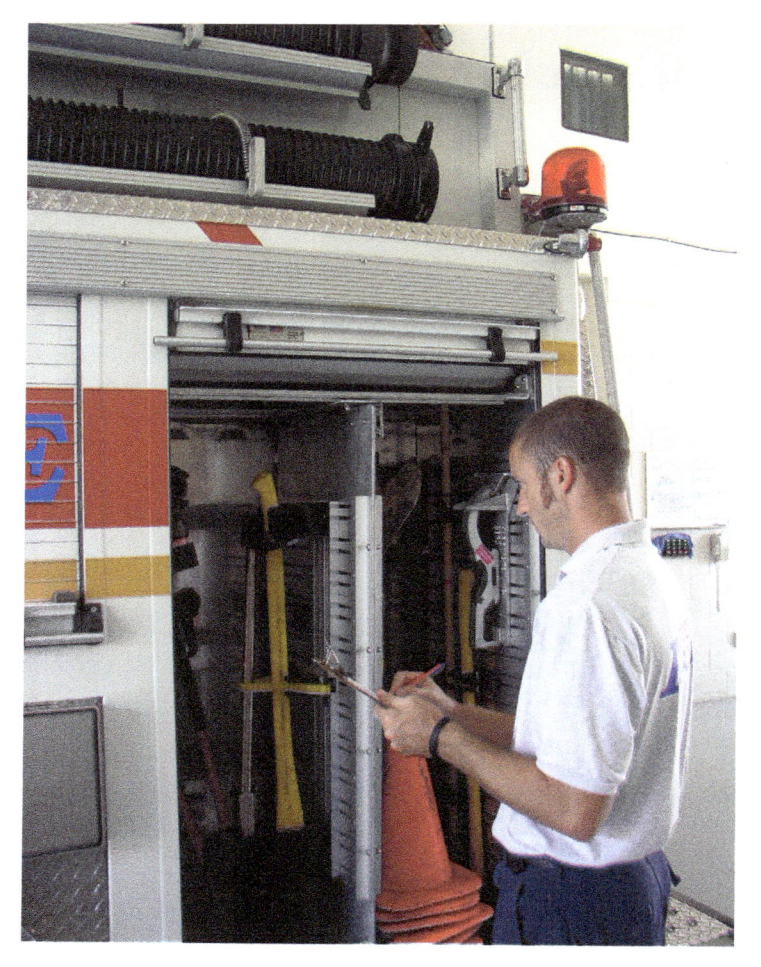

FIGURE 10.6 ■ It is essential to document any equipment failure. *Courtesy of Jeffrey T. Lindsey, Ph.D.*

the malfunction and continued to use the piece of equipment, it may be found negligent and held liable for all damages resulting from the incident.

Organizations must be able to document in writing the servicing, maintenance, and repair of the equipment. A good general guideline for documenting inspections and maintenance actions is, as it is for vehicles, "If it is not in writing, it did not happen."

It is also critical that any maintenance or repairs on equipment are conducted by an individual certified to work on the equipment. If an individual makes adjustments to a medical device and is not certified or licensed to work on that particular equipment, the organization could face significant fines, lawsuits, and the person making the alteration could face prison time while the administrator and/or person directing the alteration could be liable, too.

Work Requests

A work request is used to tell the individuals performing maintenance on the equipment what work is needed. When the maintenance department finishes the work, the work performed, tests conducted, and results should be recorded on the work request form. This document covers those problems that the individual finds during an inspection, as well as routine preventive maintenance. Virtually all equipment repair vendors will provide to the organization a document of repair or maintenance, which should be kept in the file for that piece of equipment. Certain pieces of equipment, such as stretchers and cardiac monitors, require scheduled maintenance. You should refer to the manufacturer's recommendations to plan those scheduled events.

Equipment Maintenance Logs

Information from the inspection checklists and work requests are written into an equipment maintenance log. The equipment maintenance log is a piece of equipment's central record used to list all maintenance needed and completed, including routine maintenance and problems identified by inspections, as well as to support the preventive maintenance program. To document that the equipment has been properly maintained, the equipment maintenance log pages are usually organized into binders and saved in an inspection file for use by a maintenance supervisor or manager.

■ RECORDKEEPING CHECKLIST

The following checklist should assist you in making sure you are in compliance with recordkeeping. Remember that each state may have its own recordkeeping requirements, and you will need to ascertain that your recordkeeping is in compliance within your state. Depending on the type of organization you are associated with also dictates what records you are required to maintain. You can ask the following questions:

- Are occupational injuries or illnesses, except minor injuries requiring only first aid, recorded as required on the OSHA 300 log?
- Are individuals' medical records and records of exposure to hazardous substances or harmful physical agents up to date and in compliance with current OSHA standards?
- Are individual training records maintained and accessible for review by individuals, as required by OSHA standards?
- Have arrangements been made to retain records for the time period required for each specific type of record?
- Are operating permits and records up to date for items such as elevators, air pressure tanks, liquefied petroleum gas tanks, and so on?

CHAPTER REVIEW

Summary

Recordkeeping is an important component of a risk and safety program. Appropriate documentation and recordkeeping are important in a variety of areas. It is crucial that you check with your state statutes in regard to recordkeeping to be sure your recordkeeping meets your state's requirements. OSHA also has a number of requirements for recordkeeping. Maintaining a good recordkeeping system can make all the difference when you are in need of demonstrating proficiency in a certain area of concern.

WHAT WOULD YOU DO? Reflection

You did your research and think you have some good information to present to your training chief so she can establish a solid recordkeeping program for her training program. The first example would be what OSHA provides for information that should be documented:

- Dates of the training sessions
- Outline describing the material presented
- Names and qualifications of persons conducting the training
- Names and job titles of all persons attending the training sessions

Another resource to look at in regard to training records is the National Fire Protection Association (NFPA) 1401 standard (NFPA, 2006). It provides the elements of training documents, which are not necessarily exclusive to the fire service. You include five specific elements of information in your training document: who, what, when, where, and why.

The training chief thanks you for the assistance and now has a great basis to establish a recordkeeping program for her training program.

Review Questions

1. What are some of the essential records that document your EMS organization's activities?
2. List the five steps of the OSHA recordkeeping system.
3. What privacy concerns are related to injury or illness recordkeeping?
4. You have a member who had a significant exposure to an infectious disease. How long must you maintain his medical records for this event?
5. What are the components that must be recorded and maintained in the medical record of a member who has an occupational exposure to infectious diseases?
6. Develop a training record with the required information. Include an outline of the specific elements.
7. For recordkeeping purposes, what are the three items that define a collision? Include the information you should maintain as a result of a recordable collision.
8. What are the elements that should be included on an equipment maintenance log?

References

Hanover Insurance Company. (2006). "Accident Record Keeping. Reducing Your Risk of Loss Series." Howell, MI: Author. (See the organization website.)

Lindsey, J. (2006). *Fire Service Instructor.* Upper Saddle River, NJ: Brady Publishing.

Lindsey, J., and R. Patrick. (2007). *Emergency Vehicle Operations.* Upper Saddle River, NJ: Prentice Hall.

National Fire Protection Association (NFPA). (2006). "NFPA 1401: Recommended Practice for Fire Service Training Reports and Records." (See the organization website.)

Occupational Safety and Health Administration. (2001). "OSHA Fact Sheet: Highlights of OSHA's Recordkeeping Rule." Washington, DC: OSHA, U.S. Department of Labor. (See the organization website.)

Occupational Safety and Health Administration. (n.d.-a). "OSHA Technical Manual (OTM) Section VIII: Chapter 2—Respiratory Infection." Washington, DC: Author. (See the organization website.)

Occupational Safety and Health Administration. (2005). "OSHA Recordkeeping Handbook." Washington, DC: OSHA, U.S. Department of Labor. (See the organization website.)

Occupational Safety and Health Administration. (n.d.-b). "Recording and Reporting Occupational Injuries and Illness: Recordkeeping Forms and Recording Criteria 1904.4." *Regulations Standards—29 CFR: 29 Code of Federal Regulations (CFR) 1904*. Washington, DC: Author. (See the organization website.)

Occupational Safety and Health Administration. (n.d.-c). "Recording and Reporting Occupational Injuries and Illness: Recordkeeping Forms and Recording Criteria 1904.8." From *Regulations Standards—29 CFR: 29 Code of Federal Regulations (CFR) 1904*. Washington, DC: Author. (See the organization website.)

Key Terms

job transfer When a member is placed into another position because of an illness or injury that prevents him from performing his normal functions. In many organizations this is referred to "light duty."

OSHA 300 log A record of injury and illnesses from an on-the-job occurrence.

recordkeeping The process of documenting and maintaining documents.

restricted work Occurs when a member can still function in his role, but has restrictions.

CHAPTER 11
EMS Provider Health and Wellness

Objectives

After reading this chapter, the student should be able to:

11.1 Identify and analyze the major causes involved in line-of-duty deaths related to health, wellness, fitness, and vehicle operations.
11.2 Identify and assess safety needs for both emergency and nonemergency situations.
11.3 Describe the benefits of risk management and safety programs.
11.4 Identify the role of EMS personnel in risk management and safety.

Overview

This title on EMS safety and risk management has been written to assist EMS providers in the reduction of line-of-duty injuries, illnesses, and fatalities. It provides a framework for developing programs that will create an appropriate margin of health and safety for providers during the performance of EMS duties.

Key Terms

carcinogens
content validity
criterion validity
critical incident stress management
construct validity
early return-to-work (ERTW) program
employee assistance programs (EAPs)
exercise program
fitness assessment
fitness standards
heat stress index
medical screening
nutrition
peer fitness trainer

CHAPTER 11 *EMS Provider Health and Wellness* **271**

permissible exposure limit
physical ability testing (PAT)
physical fitness programs
post-exposure exams
stress
transitional employment
windchill index

WHAT WOULD YOU DO?

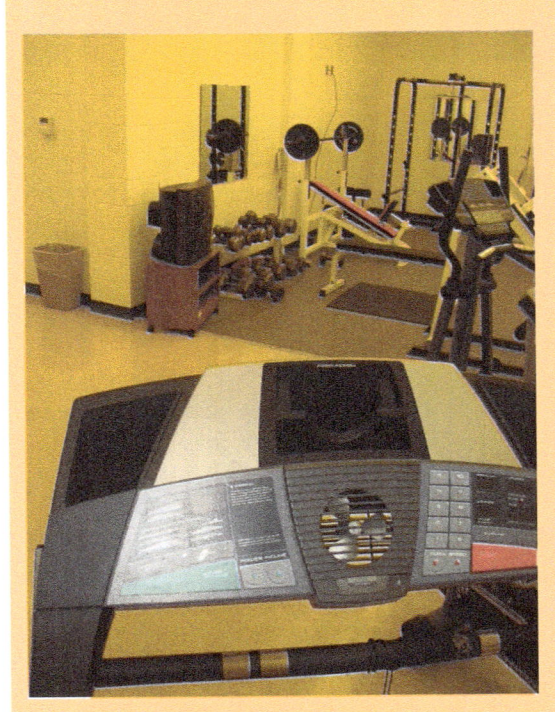

Your organization is in the process of establishing a physical fitness program. The majority of the organization's personnel have bought into the idea and want to implement a program so they can be more physically fit to do the job. You are asked to develop a program with recommendations on how to implement it. There is concern that the program will fail if it is not done properly.

Questions

1. What components would you consider?
2. Who are some resources you could consult with in order to develop your program?
3. Who would you get involved in your organization?

A physical fitness program is a valuable benefit for both personnel and the organization.
Courtesy of Lawrence T. Bennett.

INTRODUCTION

Although some aspects of EMS workforce occupational illness and injury have been relatively well studied (e.g., ambulance crashes), a review of the literature demonstrates that studies are limited in other areas. Further, as one would expect, with the exception of a handful of pioneering efforts the existing literature has been built around information from systems developed for purposes other than studying EMS workforce illness and injury. Some areas, such as cardiovascular fitness of EMS workers, are almost wholly unexplored.

HIGH RISK FACTORS

A number of factors can create a high risk for EMS personnel. As the EMS safety officer, you will need to consider various programs to assist in reducing these high-risk factors for your personnel.

LACK OF PHYSICAL FITNESS

Overweight EMS personnel are at increased risk for injury. Excess weight can increase the chances of back injuries as well as sprains and strains. It also is well-known that being overweight increases ones odds for cardiovascular (CV) diseases and diabetes, among other chronic diseases.

EMS personnel do not always have the ability to exercise while on duty as a result of high call volumes, not being stationed at a fixed location, and working long hours on varied shifts. Regardless, there is no excuse for lack of physical fitness. It is critical for the EMS safety officer to encourage, assist, and create programs to enhance the physical fitness program for providers.

LACK OF PRE-EMPLOYMENT PHYSICAL ABILITY TESTING

The fire service created an initial testing process to assess applicants on their physical ability. **Physical ability testing (PAT)** for applicants can identify whether or not the applicant can actually do the physical activity of the job. It should not matter whether individuals are paid or volunteer; they are doing the same job and should be physically able to do so.

HISTORY OF ILLNESS

> **Side Bar**
>
> **Alcohol Abuse**
>
> EMS personnel who abuse alcohol have more chronic problems than do personnel who do not. Nearly all of the body's tissues and organs are affected by alcohol abuse.

Many illnesses may affect EMS personnel, including communicable and noncommunicable diseases. EMS personnel face the same risk of heart attacks and strokes as the general population. In addition, they are prone to many traumatic injuries, which may create chronic conditions and influence other illnesses.

Like most individuals, EMS personnel typically are not aware of any CV disease problem. Nonetheless, they should monitor their blood pressure, and if they have a family history of CV disease should get regular physical exams until they begin to develop problems or have acute signs and symptoms.

Best Practices

Austin-Travis County EMS Physical Ability Course

Austin-Travis County EMS is a forerunner in developing a physical ability test for EMS applicants. The test includes a 1.5-mile walk/run warmup. A pre-employment physical ability assessment includes an obstacle course and mannequin drag, an equipment carry, stair climb, lifting and moving a scoop stretcher and hydraulic ambulance stretcher, a fine motor skills assessment, and a hydraulic stretcher course. The critical failures are identified for each component of the test. The most recent information on the test can be found at http://atcems.org/home/and searching for "physical ability" or you can contact Austin-Travis EMS for further information.

The use of caffeine and nicotine should be avoided because they increase the risk of CV conditions. Prevention is the key.

EMS personnel who were injured on the job should be monitored. If they return to work before completely recovering, they may actually cause additional injuries or increase their stress, which can cause other conditions, including a heart attack or stroke.

EMS personnel must take their health seriously, and it is wise to encourage your personnel to do so. Health fairs and annual exams are great benefits and can help reduce costs for the organization in the long run.

MEDICATIONS

Certain medications can have an adverse effect on EMS personnel (Figure 11.1). Such effects can be long term. Some of the over-the-counter medications that can cause an adverse effect on the EMS provider are these:

- *Antihistamines.* Antihistamines, such as Benadryl and Actifed, are typically taken for sinus problems and the common cold. These can cause drowsiness.
- *Stimulants.* Stimulations, such as caffeine, decongestants, and diet pills, can be found in various drinks, over-the-counter medications, and supplements. These can cause hyperactivity and nervousness.

A policy should be in place to address personnel taking any type of medication while functioning as EMS providers. The policy must be specific about what personnel can and cannot do while taking medications. Every medication has different side effects and can affect each person differently.

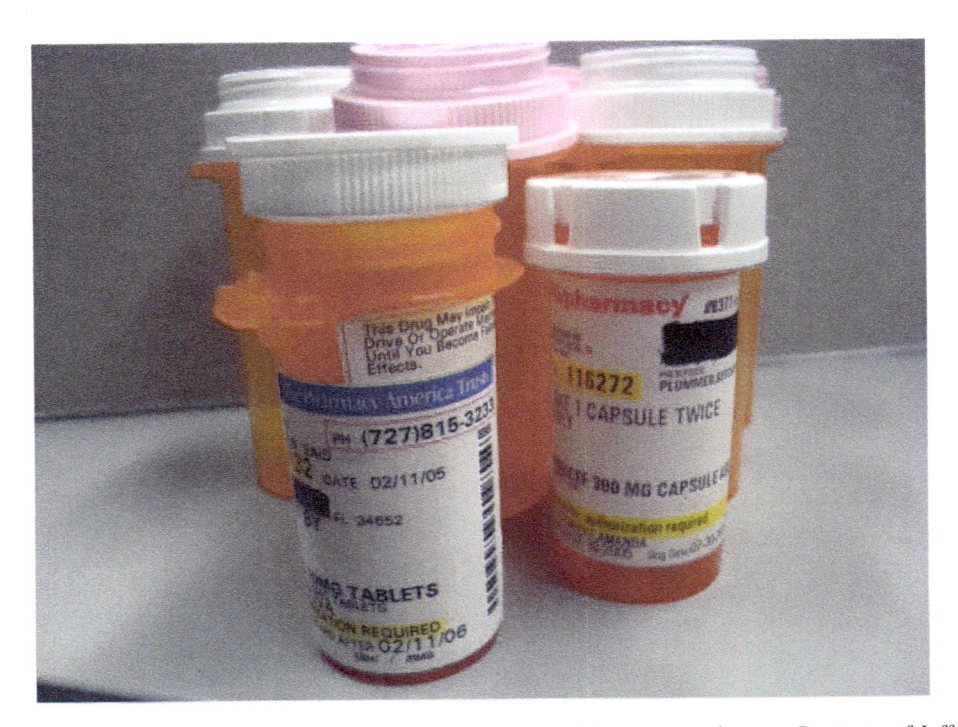

FIGURE 11.1 ■ Medications can have various effects on providers, some adverse. *Courtesy of Jeffrey T. Lindsey, Ph.D.*

Drug/ETOH (alcohol) testing is a controversial topic, and you must determine your organization's limits regarding how to implement such tests. The Fourth Amendment of the United States Constitution is used by personnel to prevent employers or organizations from conducting drug testing on personnel. EMS personnel have access to controlled drugs and proper procedures must be implemented to monitor and control these medications in addition and prevent drug use and abuse. In fact, legal advice from a labor attorney should be obtained to determine the organization's ability to conduct any type of drug testing.

USE OF TOBACCO

Smoking causes heart problems, respiratory problems, cancer, and other medical conditions. Chewing tobacco has been known to cause cancer. Thus, the use of tobacco products should be discouraged. A number of EMS organizations have adopted a tobacco-free environment. This means there is no tobacco use on vehicles, at incident scenes, at any of the organization's facilities, or at organization-sponsored events. This goes not only for personnel but also for those visiting the facility.

Consider having your board or council pass a resolution to create a tobacco-free environment policy. If your EMS personnel are also firefighters, tobacco use could jeopardize their public safety officer benefits should they develop a heart or lung disease. In many states, firefighters are prohibited from using tobacco products or risk losing their public safety benefits entirely. EMS personnel should be no different. You are in the medical field and know the ramifications of using such substances. You should be setting the example.

HEARING LOSS

Hearing loss is caused by the destruction of cells in the inner ear as a result of exposure to continual noise. Currently, ambulances are constructed to protect personnel from the sounds of the siren on the units. Emphasis is needed on proper construction of all emergency vehicles to help reduce the amount of noise generated from the sirens and other audible devices.

Personnel also should be provided with personal hearing protection. When operating on the scene of various incidents, personnel are exposed to loud noises from equipment. OSHA noise requirements set a maximum **permissible exposure limit (PEL)** of 90dB for an 8-hour period. Hearing loss is recognized as a significant exposure for EMS personnel and should always be a consideration.

Personnel should be given a baseline audiometry test when starting with your organization and then annually to measure any changes. A hearing-loss program should be established and adhered to by your organization. There are EMS providers who are hard-of-hearing or deaf. Consulting with an American with Disabilities Act (ADA) expert in these situations to determine any measures needed to assist the hard-of-hearing or deaf responder should be considered in order to make reasonable accommodations.

According to OSHA (1974), a study was conducted that found ambulance cab noise levels during siren use averaged 96 decibels (dBA) to 102.4 dBA, exceeding the Occupational Safety and Health Administration (OSHA) standard in use at the time. In a somewhat later study, Pepe, Jerger, Miller, and Jerger (1985) estimated the total number of hours of siren exposure for each of 192 male firefighters and, comparing those data with the results of hearing tests, concluded that (1) degree of hearing loss was positively correlated to duration of siren exposure, (2) the identified hearing loss could not be attributed to non-job-related exposure, and (3) the rate of hearing loss was 150 percent of that expected in age-matched, nonexposed men.

Almost 20 years later, Price and Goldsmith (1998) reinvestigated a group of Louisville EMTs and Paramedics. Based on comparisons between pre-employment baseline audiograms and follow-up audiograms as part of this study, the authors failed to find a significant correlation between the number of months between audiograms and pre-post age-adjusted hearing loss. (Note: There is an adjustment for hearing based on normal loss of hearing due to age. This study used information prior to this adjustment period.) Left ear hearing was reported to be somewhat more diminished than right-ear hearing, but still within overall normal limits. Overall, the authors concluded that for the group studied, there appeared to be no excessive loss of hearing acuity. The authors noted that the careers of the individuals tested partially or entirely spanned the era of General Services Administration KKK-1822 (Becker and Spicer, 2007) ambulance specifications requiring front-grill mount, rather than cab-roof mount, siren speakers.

Hearing loss in EMS providers must be taken seriously. Provisions must be provided in ambulance design and protection on the scene of an incident or other situation where the level of noise warrants protection. Currently there is a NFPA committee working to develop ambulance standards from the KKK standards published by the federal government.

BACK INJURIES

As discussed in Chapter 6, back injuries are very common for EMS personnel. Back injuries are typically the biggest category of workers' compensation claims and lost time injuries in the industry. The key to back injuries is prevention. This is really two-fold. First the EMS providers should stay physically active. They should be involved in a flexibility and strengthening program. Second, personnel should be trained to properly lift and carry patients and equipment. A lifting and moving program should be established to ensure that this takes place.

New patient-moving devices have been introduced into the industry to reduce injuries to personnel. Hydraulic stretchers are designed to reduce back injuries; however, there is concern about whether or not there is an increase in shoulder injuries as a result of the change in design. There is only anecdotal information on this to date, and additional research must be conducted to determine any significant injuries or reduction of injuries to personnel using hydraulic patient-moving devices. There have also been devices that have treads designed to move patients up and down stairs and inclines without the necessity for personnel to lift the patient. As the EMS safety officer, all of these devices should be taken into consideration.

CANCER

EMS personnel are subject to many different environments, including the exhaust from vehicles if the garage or bay area for vehicles is not properly ventilated. In many instances, personnel are not provided with the appropriate PPE for the environment. As a result they are subject to **carcinogens**: cancer-causing substances or agents. The carcinogens can be a result of working at the scene of a fire where breathing protection is needed, such as a self-contained breathing apparatus (SCBA). The inhalation of smoke is known to cause cancer from the toxins contained in the smoke. Hazmat scenes also increase the risk of exposure to carcinogenic environments. The importance of staging in a safe location and wearing the appropriate PPE in warm and hot zones is imperative to the protection of EMS personnel.

The World Trade Center collapse in September 2001 illustrates the potential of the harm to which EMS providers are subjected. The dust from the building collapse was known to contain asbestos. The incident of cancer has been illustrated since the event by personnel being diagnosed with various terminal diseases, including cancer, as a result of inhaling the dust at the incident scene.

There is limited research on the causes of cancer in EMS personnel. However, firefighters have been getting screened for many years, and the results of those studies indicate a high incidence of various cancers among firefighters, including thyroid, testicular, lung, and throat cancer. EMS personnel respond to the same incident scenes as fire personnel. Depending on the staging of the EMS unit and personnel, the environment remains the same. In addition, there has been some recognition of the increase of cancer in individuals who work the night shift.

EMS personnel should be screened for various cancers. An annual physical examination is the first step.

WELLNESS PROGRAMS

The most important part of any EMS organization is the personnel. Without healthy personnel, the EMS organization is in jeopardy. Thus, a number of areas should be considered when developing an EMS wellness program. EMS has not had a set of standards developed like the fire service has in with the NFPA standards and guidelines in place. NFPA 1500 (NFPA, 2007) and subsequent standards in the 1500 series deal with the health and wellness of firefighters. Many of these standards could be emulated for EMS personnel; however, it is imperative for EMS to begin to establish a set of nationally recognized standards for EMS agencies that are not fire based or are for fire-based EMS where personnel do not fall under the standards for firefighters' health and well-being.

EMS organizations should focus on five areas based on the NFPA 1500 (2007) standard. This will create a foundation for a wellness program. These are the five areas:

- Medical evaluations, including offer of employment or membership to volunteer organizations, annual and periodic
- Infection control
- **Employee assistance programs (EAP)**, including alcohol and substance abuse treatment
- Physical fitness program
- Emergency incident rehabilitation

ANNUAL MEDICAL EVALUATIONS

At best, EMS organizations will give a medical evaluation when they offer a position to someone. It should not matter whether the person is paid or a volunteer—everyone should receive a medical evaluation prior to starting the job. After the person is with the organization, a medical evaluation should be offered on an annual basis.

Standards such as NFPA 1582 (2007) differentiate when firefighters undergo certain medical testing. As we know, you can be subject to medical conditions regardless of your age. In fact, it is much better to find a medical condition early and begin treatment than to wait. Therefore, it is in the best interest of personnel to conduct annual medical examinations on all personnel. The type of testing may vary based on the recommendations of medical professionals.

There should be no discrimination between volunteer or paid personnel. They both do the same job and evaluated in the same manner. It should be stressed that the annual medical evaluation is intended to assist personnel in providing for their health, not as a means to eliminate a position or put someone out of work as paid or volunteer personnel. No discrimination should exist between volunteer or paid personnel. They both do the same job and should be evaluated in the same manner. The most important point from management's perspective is to have a plan and procedure in place that describe what happens when someone does not pass the medical evaluation. This should be documented and maintained in the personnel medical files.

A baseline medical exam for EMS personnel based on NFPA 1582 (2007) might include the following tests, examinations, and information:

- Basic medical examination by an appropriate licensed medical professional
- Electrocardiogram (ECG) with stress test
- Height
- Weight
- Blood pressure
- Heart rate
- Respiration
- Complete medical history of illnesses/injuries
- Cholesterol level
- Triglycerides
- Chest X-ray
- TB skin test
- Check for skin cancer
- Complete blood count
- Chemistry 23 blood test
- Hepatitis antibodies status
- Urinalysis
- Tetanus update
- PSA blood test for males
- Vision test
- Hearing test
- Current list of medications

In addition, a strength and fitness examination should be administered to test for the strength and flexibility of personnel by an individual qualified to administer such an evaluation. Currently there is no standard test for EMS personnel; however, NFPA 1582 (2007) can be used as a guideline for EMS personnel.

INFECTION CONTROL

Chapter 6 presented information on infection control procedures and the requirements for an exposure control plan. EMS personnel should be offered appropriate vaccinations at no cost. A post-exposure protocol should be in place if an exposure occurs. (Table 11-1).

Post-exposure exams should be offered when there is an exposure, whether it is a hazmat incident or infectious disease. You should

TABLE 11-1 ■ Recommended Vaccines for EMS Providers

Vaccine	Recommendations in Brief
Hepatitis B	Give 3-dose series (dose #1 now, #2 in 1 month, #3 approximately 5 months after #2). Give IM. Obtain anti-HBs serologic testing 1–2 months after dose #3.
Influenza	Give 1 dose of TIV or LAIV annually. Give TIV intramuscularly or LAIV intranasally.
Measles Mumps Rubella (MMR)	For health care personnel (HCP) born in 1957 or later without serologic evidence of immunity or prior vaccination, give 2 doses of MMR, 4 weeks apart. For HCP born prior to 1957, see below. Give subcutaneous.
Varicella	For HCP who have no serologic proof of immunity, prior vaccination, or history of varicella disease (chickenpox), give 2 doses of varicella vaccine, 4 weeks apart. Give SC.
Tetanus, diphtheria	Give all HCP a Td booster dose every 10 years, following the completion of the primary 3-dose series. Give 1-time dose of Tdap to all HCP younger than age 65 years with direct patient contact. Give intramuscularly (IM).

Source: Immunization Action Coalition. (2008). "Healthcare Personnel Vaccination Recommendations. #P2017." (See the organization website.)

establish a policy with guidelines for a post-exposure exam. It is important that the organization establish a relationship with a physician or medical center prior to an incident. The center should be able to understand the needs of the organization if a post-exposure exam is required. The time of the incident is not the time to establish the protocol for a post-exposure exam or educate the medical center on what you need.

EMPLOYEE ASSISTANCE PROGRAM

An employee assistance program (EAP) is used to help personnel who are experiencing personal problems (Figure 11.2). It is great to think that personnel check their issues at the door when they walk into the EMS station; however, this is not true. Providing an assistance program can help personnel get through tough situations. In addition, the program should include the family. Family issues contribute to the individual's well-being and must be considered.

The major components of an EAP are substance abuse program for alcoholism, tobacco use, and addiction to legal or illegal drugs; stress management; family relations; legal and financial concerns; and health promotion. Check with your health insurance provider about obtaining these services. In some instances, they are part of the package, in others a special program must be purchased. The EAP program is an alternative to CISD and CISM (discussed at the end of this chapter).

PHYSICAL FITNESS PROGRAM

Physical fitness programs can reduce the number of EMS personnel injuries and deaths, but must

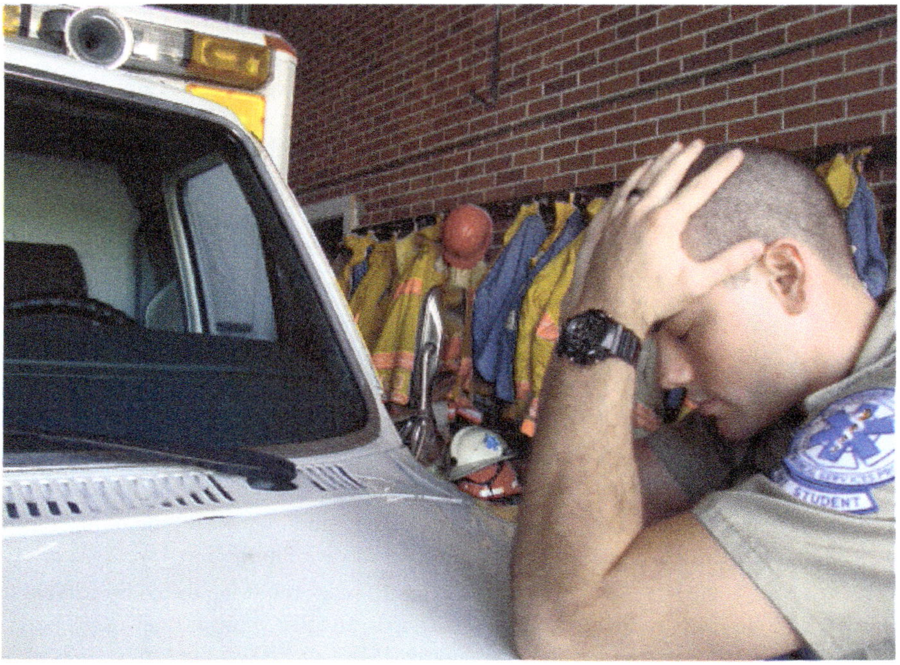

FIGURE 11.2 ■ An EAP can assist personnel in getting through tough times. *Courtesy of Jeffrey T. Lindsey, Ph.D.*

be developed to be comprehensive and aimed at improving overall personnel health.

The program must be designed for the provider. A qualified fitness trainer is an ideal person to work with in order to establish such a program. However, the cost of a fitness trainer may not be feasible.

> **Side Bar**
>
> **College and Universities**
>
> If you live near a college or university, check to see if it has a physical fitness program of any kind. Practically every college and university has some type of program. Many P.E. students must perform community service, and you may find someone who must do an internship and can assist you with your program for little or no cost.

A fitness program should include a medical screening, a fitness assessment, defined fitness standards, an exercise program, and nutrition education.

Medical Screening

Medical screening should begin before the person starts with the organization. A medical exam cannot be given prior to offering a person a position with the organization, paid or volunteer. The offer of employment or membership can be conditional upon meeting the medical requirements or physical fitness requirements of the position. If after the exam the person is not medically qualified to perform the duties of the position, then he should not be hired or allowed to volunteer for the position.

Personnel should receive an annual medical evaluation. This exam can determine if the person is able to do any physical fitness activities and to what level. If the organization does not provide medical screening, the provider must check with their medical doctor prior to beginning a fitness program.

Fitness Assessment

Once the medical exam is complete and the individual is deemed medically fit to participate in a physical fitness program, the next step would be to conduct a **fitness assessment** to determine the level the individual is at in their fitness. Four areas should be included in the fitness assessment: cardiovascular (aerobic), muscular strength, muscular endurance, and flexibility.

The tests can be conducted in various ways. It is recommended that an individual who is trained and certified in fitness assessments conduct the fitness assessment. Programs are available that focus on emergency responders and emergency service personnel getting a **peer fitness trainer** certification, including a course developed by the International Association of Fire Fighters. A fitness assessment should never be conducted by an inexperienced person or by someone who has not been trained or certified in the assessment process.

Fitness Standards

Currently there are no national fitness standards for EMS personnel, although some organizations have established their own levels of those standards. A **fitness standard** must contain three validity tests:

> **Content validity**. Test elements are similar or identical to those of the job being tested.
>
> **Criterion validity**. Uses statistical tests to predict job performance.
>
> **Construct validity**. Measures underlying theoretical concepts.

These tests are developed by experts in fitness standards who do not necessarily understand the job responsibilities of EMS personnel. Hence, they may not always measure the aspects of EMS performance correctly. You must be sure that the tests address the job duties and expectations of responders.

Exercise Program

Once the individual is cleared medically and has gone through a fitness assessment, it is time to start an **exercise program**. When you mention the word *exercise*, some people cringe. If the organization is truly committed to a fitness program, consider allocating time for personnel to exercise while on duty (Figure 11.3). There are many ways to be able to offer personnel a means to exercise. If the organization does not have a fitness center, consider speaking with the local YMCA/YWCA, gym, school, college, or any group that has a fitness center to either allow personnel to use the facilities for no cost or at reduced cost. In some instances, facility managers may ask that you provide CPR and first aid training in return for use of the fitness center.

The organization should continue to offer a personal trainer or peer fitness trainer to assist and monitor personnel. One thing you do not want to do is make the fitness program a punitive action program. The fitness program should be designed to help personnel, not to create an environment that makes personnel fearful of discipline.

In addition, personnel who are assigned to a unit in a system status deployment model should consider taking stretching breaks throughout the shift. Sitting in a vehicle is not a good practice and is similar to sitting for prolonged periods at a desk. Stretching exercises can improve circulation and keep personnel alert.

Nutrition Program

The last, but not least, component of the physical fitness program is **nutrition**. EMS personnel are not always able to eat properly, and in many instances fast food becomes the norm. Depending on the type of system, personnel may never be at a station during their shift. In addition, depending on the call volume, personnel may not have much time to eat.

Personnel should be educated on proper nutrition. Working with a dietician or nutritionist would be of great value to personnel. The best place to find someone versed in nutrition and diet would be at a local college or university. You should be able to find a professor or student who must do an internship to work with the personnel of the organization to create a nutrition program. You can also check with the dietician at local nursing homes, schools, hospitals, and colleges.

Personnel must know how to read labels and determine the nutritional value in the foods they select. In addition, they should be educated about choosing foods when eating out. Avoiding fast foods and convenience stores are important aspects of maintaining a healthy lifestyle. Eating in the ambulance also creates issues including the possibility of communicable diseases contaminating the food. Eating while the vehicle is moving causes distractions and is a safety issue. As the EMS safety officer, you should ensure that personnel are properly trained in nutrition and diet.

INCIDENT REHABILITATION

Incident rehabilitation must be considered at major incidents and training events. In addition, mass gatherings will require EMS personnel to establish a medical center similar to

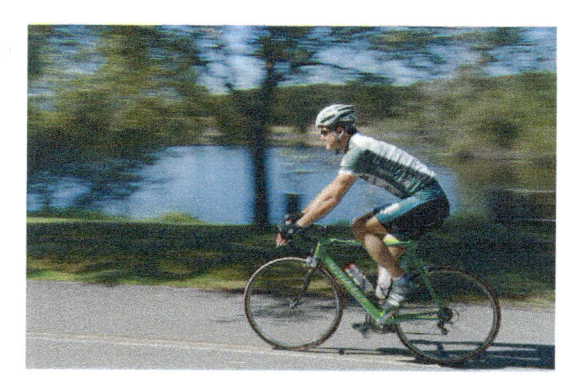

FIGURE 11.3 ■ An exercise program is an essential element of the fitness program.

a rehab station. EMS personnel must be cautious because they are called on in many instances to establish the rehab site. EMS personnel also should go through rehab in many cases, if for no other reason than to take a break from the continuous work that often occurs at these sites. Depending on the nature of the incident and the involvement of EMS personnel, a separate rehab area for them may need to be considered. Each individual has a role he plays at the scene of an incident.

Incident Commander

The incident commander must consider the circumstances of each incident and make adequate provisions early in the incident for the rest and rehabilitation of all personnel operating at the scene. These provisions must include medical evaluation, treatment, and monitoring; food and fluid replenishment; mental rest; and relief from extreme climatic conditions and the other environmental parameters of the incident. The rehabilitation also should include the provision of EMS and Basic Life Support (BLS) or higher. NFPA 1584 (2008) covers the necessary requirements for incident rehabilitation. All EMS personnel must be familiar with this standard.

Supervisors

All supervisors must maintain an awareness of the condition of each responder operating within a span of control and ensure that adequate steps are taken to provide for each responder's safety and health. The command structure is to be utilized to request relief and the reassignment of fatigued crews. This includes the crews working at rehab.

Personnel

During periods of hot weather, personnel should be encouraged to drink water and activity beverages such as sports drinks throughout the workday. During any emergency incident or training, all personnel should advise their supervisor when they believe that their level of fatigue or exposure to heat or cold is approaching a level that could affect themselves, their crew, or the operation in which they are involved. Personnel also should remain aware of the health and safety of other members of their crew.

Location

The location for the rehabilitation area is normally designated by the incident commander. If a specific location has not been designated, the rehab officer will need to select an appropriate location based on the site characteristics and designations.

Sites should include the following characteristics:

- Is a location that will provide physical rest by allowing the body to recuperate from the demands and hazards of the emergency operation or training evolution (Is far enough away from the scene that personnel may safely remove their turnout gear and SCBA and be afforded mental rest from the stress and pressure of the emergency operation or training evolution)
- Provides suitable protection from the prevailing environmental conditions; during hot weather, in a cool, shaded area; during cold weather, in a warm, dry area
- Enables personnel to be free of exhaust fumes from apparatus, vehicles, or equipment (including those involved in the rehabilitation sector/group operations)
- Is large enough to accommodate multiple crews, based on the size of the incident
- Is easily accessible by EMS units, including the transport units
- Allows prompt reentry back into the emergency operation upon complete recuperation

Rehabilitation Sector/Group Establishment

Rehabilitation should be considered by officers during the initial planning stages of an

NOAA's National Weather Service
Heat Index

Temperature (°F) →	80	82	84	86	88	90	92	94	96	98	100	102	104	106	118	110
Relative Humidity (%)																
40	80	81	83	85	88	91	94	97	101	105	109	114	119	124	130	136
45	80	82	84	87	89	93	96	100	104	109	114	119	124	130	137	
50	81	83	85	88	91	95	99	103	108	113	118	124	131	137		
55	81	84	86	89	93	97	101	106	112	117	124	130	137			
60	82	84	88	91	95	100	105	110	116	123	129	137				
65	82	85	89	93	98	103	108	114	121	128	136					
70	83	86	90	95	100	105	112	119	126	134						
75	84	88	92	97	103	109	116	124	132							
80	84	89	94	100	106	113	121	129								
85	85	90	96	102	110	117	126	135								
90	86	91	98	105	113	122	131									
95	86	93	100	108	117	127										
100	87	95	103	112	121	132										

Likelihood of Heat Disorders with Prolonged Exposure or Strenuous Activity

☐ Caution   ☐ Extreme Caution   ☐ Danger   ☐ External Danger

FIGURE 11.4 ■ Heat stress index chart. *Source: NOAA/National Weather Service.*

emergency response. However, the climatic or environmental conditions of the emergency scene should not be the sole justification for establishing a rehabilitation area. Any activity/incident that is large in size, long in duration, and/or labor intensive will rapidly deplete the energy and strength of personnel and therefore merits consideration for rehabilitation. Climatic or environmental conditions that indicate the need to establish a rehabilitation area are a **heat stress index** (Figure 11.4) above 90°F or a **windchill index** (Figure 11.5) below 10°F.

Hydration

A critical factor in the prevention of heat injury is the maintenance of water and electrolytes. Water must be replaced during exercise periods and while at emergency incidents. During heat stress, the individual should consume at least 1 quart of water per hour. Rehydration is important even during cold weather operations where, despite the outside temperature, heat stress may occur during strenuous activity when protective equipment is worn. Alcohol and caffeine beverages should be avoided before and during heat stress because both interfere with the body's water conservation mechanisms. Carbonated beverages should be avoided.

Nourishment

The organization that is overseeing the incident typically provides food at the scene of an extended incident when units are engaged for 3 or more hours. A cup of soup, broth, or stew is highly recommended because it is digested much faster than sandwiches and fast food products. In addition, foods such as apples, oranges, and bananas provide supplemental forms of energy replacement. Fatty and/or salty foods should be avoided.

Rest

The objective evaluation of an individual's fatigue level should be the criteria for rehab time. Rest must not be less than 10 minutes

NWS Windchill Chart

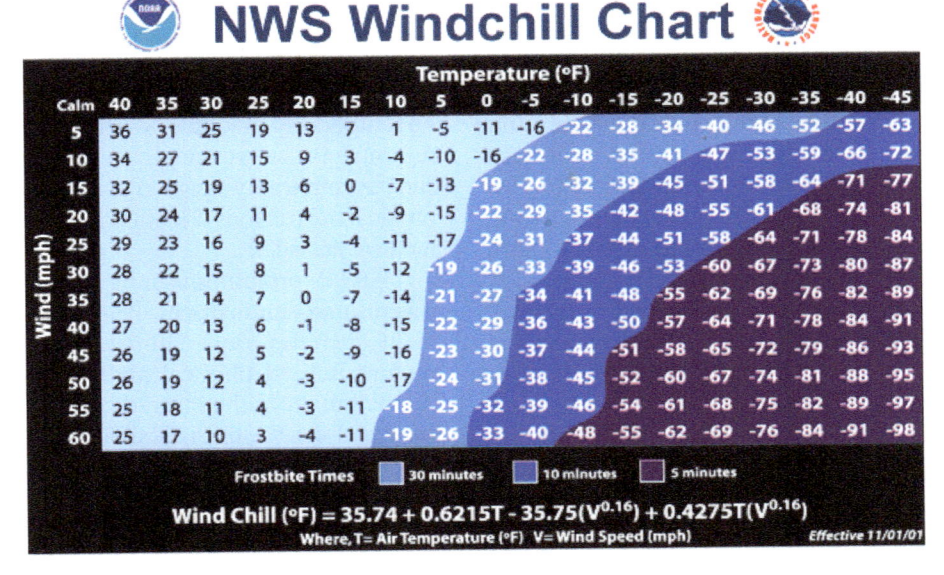

Wind (mph) \ Temp (°F)	40	35	30	25	20	15	10	5	0	-5	-10	-15	-20	-25	-30	-35	-40	-45
Calm	40	35	30	25	20	15	10	5	0	-5	-10	-15	-20	-25	-30	-35	-40	-45
5	36	31	25	19	13	7	1	-5	-11	-16	-22	-28	-34	-40	-46	-52	-57	-63
10	34	27	21	15	9	3	-4	-10	-16	-22	-28	-35	-41	-47	-53	-59	-66	-72
15	32	25	19	13	6	0	-7	-13	-19	-26	-32	-39	-45	-51	-58	-64	-71	-77
20	30	24	17	11	4	-2	-9	-15	-22	-29	-35	-42	-48	-55	-61	-68	-74	-81
25	29	23	16	9	3	-4	-11	-17	-24	-31	-37	-44	-51	-58	-64	-71	-78	-84
30	28	22	15	8	1	-5	-12	-19	-26	-33	-39	-46	-53	-60	-67	-73	-80	-87
35	28	21	14	7	0	-7	-14	-21	-27	-34	-41	-48	-55	-62	-69	-76	-82	-89
40	27	20	13	6	-1	-8	-15	-22	-29	-36	-43	-50	-57	-64	-71	-78	-84	-91
45	26	19	12	5	-2	-9	-16	-23	-30	-37	-44	-51	-58	-65	-72	-79	-86	-93
50	26	19	12	4	-3	-10	-17	-24	-31	-38	-45	-52	-60	-67	-74	-81	-88	-95
55	25	18	11	4	-3	-11	-18	-25	-32	-39	-46	-54	-61	-68	-75	-82	-89	-97
60	25	17	10	3	-4	-11	-19	-26	-33	-40	-48	-55	-62	-69	-76	-84	-91	-98

Frostbite Times: 30 minutes, 10 minutes, 5 minutes

$$\text{Wind Chill (°F)} = 35.74 + 0.6215T - 35.75(V^{0.16}) + 0.4275T(V^{0.16})$$

Where, T = Air Temperature (°F) V = Wind Speed (mph) Effective 11/01/01

FIGURE 11.5 ■ Windchill index chart. *Source: NOAA/National Weather Service.*

and may exceed an hour as determined by the rehab officer. Fresh crews, or crews released from the rehabilitation sector/group, are to be available in the staging area to ensure that fatigued responders are not required to return to duty before they are rested, evaluated, and released by the rehab officer.

Recovery

Personnel in the rehabilitation area should maintain a high level of hydration. Personnel should not be moved from a hot environment directly into an air conditioned area because the body's cooling system can shut down in response to the external cooling. An air conditioned environment is acceptable after a cool-down period at ambient temperature with sufficient air movement.

Certain drugs impair the body's ability to sweat and extreme caution must be exercised if the individual has taken antihistamines, such as Actifed or Benadryl, or has taken diuretics or stimulants.

Medical Evaluation

The EMS provider will typically be called on to provide and staff the rehab scene. It is best to give ALS-level care, but BLS-level care is acceptable. Personnel in rehab must evaluate vital signs, examine personnel, and determine proper disposition (return to duty, continued rehabilitation, or medical treatment and transport to medical facility). Continued rehabilitation should consist of additional monitoring of vital signs, providing rest, and providing fluids for rehydration. Medical treatment for personnel, whose signs and/or symptoms indicate potential problems, should be provided in accordance with local medical control procedures. EMS personnel must be assertive in an effort to find potential medical problems early.

All medical evaluations are to be recorded on standard forms along with the individual's name and complaints and must be signed, dated, and timed by the rehab officer or his designee.

Accountability

Personnel assigned to the rehabilitation sector/group must enter and exit the rehabilitation area as a crew. The crew designation, number of crew members, and times of entry to and exit from the rehabilitation area must be documented by the rehab officer or his designee on the check-in/out sheet. Crews are not to leave the rehabilitation area until authorized to do so by the rehab officer.

All personnel, including EMS personnel, should go through the rehab process when warranted. EMS personnel must take care of their own just as they take care of other responders on the scene of an incident or at a training event.

RETURN TO WORK

Injuries occur in EMS. However, many organizations do not have a standard return-to-work program in place. Essentially, when an individual is injured, there must be some way to know when he is medically able to come back to function in the capacity expected of him. A physician's note approving return to active duty may be all that an organization requires. Is this enough to state that the individual is capable of doing the job? In many cases the answer is a resounding "No." This is a result of the physician not necessarily knowing and understanding the job responsibilities of the EMS responder. The organization should have a document that outlines the responsibilities of the individual in order to perform the job. The evaluating physician must complete the document attesting to the fact that the individual is capable of performing the job functions.

A return-to-work program must be developed and implemented by all EMS organizations. An **early return-to-work (ERTW) program** provides short-term duties within a specified time frame for personnel who have been injured and cannot return to their time-of-injury duties. ERTW assumes that personnel are valuable assets. When an individual is injured, every attempt should be made to bring the individual back to full duty quickly. In many cases, the individual's existing position or work schedule can be temporarily modified. When injuries prevent returning to the individual's own job, other duties can be temporarily assigned to accommodate the physical restrictions identified by the treating medical provider.

ERTW programs usually are referred to as **transitional employment**. Transitional employment includes only short-term duties that require limited physical ability requirements, can be taught to the injured employee quickly, can be done within a flexible work schedule, and would minimize exposure of the injured worker to further injury and would not slow down recovery time. This can also be accomplished with a volunteer.

Light-duty positions are permanent reserved positions within an organization for personnel who are temporarily or permanently unable to return to their positions due to a disabling condition. This is not transitional employment.

Purpose of an ERTW Program

Studies show that when individuals remain off work for 6 months, only 50 percent return (American College of Occupational and Environmental Medicine, 2006). Only 10 percent return when off work for more than a year. With an early return-to-work commitment, organizations can encourage an increased quality of life for injured personnel. Individuals report that often ERTW increases their morale and they feel valued by their organization.

Workers' compensation payments also can be significantly reduced through an ERTW program. The wages paid an individual in transitional employment offset the payments made by the insurance company. Often the expenses for an industrial injury are less when the individual returns to work quickly.

Benefits of an ERTW Program

Returning injured personnel to work is a win-win proposition. An injured individual remains active and has a sense of value, and the organization retains a valuable and trained individual (American College of Occupational and Environmental Medicine, 2006):

Your organization receives some level of production. While the individual is at home, you are paying direct and indirect costs without receiving any productivity in return. An ERTW program gives the organization an opportunity to generate some productivity during the healing period.

Your organization can avoid replacement and training costs. While the individual is recovering, the work still must be completed. Returning the individual to work can minimize the costs associated with training and replacing that person.

Depending on the role of the individual injured, your organization may be able to identify workflow improvements and generate efficiencies while developing modified jobs. As you examine the injured person's position, you may find new and creative ways to bring the injured individual back to work. You may even discover efficiencies at the same time.

Your organization can significantly reduce compensation payments. Compensation costs, one of the most expensive components of workers' compensation, are dramatically reduced.

Medical costs go down. An injured individual in an ERTW program typically recovers more quickly and uses less medical care. This also can result in decreased premiums.

The loyalty of valuable personnel increases. Loyalty to your organization increases when you demonstrate a caring and concerned attitude.

A problem individual's opportunity to defraud the system decreases. With a mandatory ERTW program, you remove the incentive for filing fraudulent claims.

Your injured person remains in the work force and maintains social contact with fellow personnel. This helps the healing process. Experience shows injured individuals with ERTW options heal much quicker and return to full productive duty much earlier than those who do not have the same opportunity.

Components of an ERTW Program

The guidelines previously discussed are designed to help EMS supervisors develop an effective early return-to-work program. Because each organization is different, you can modify the components to fit your own work environment. As you develop your ERTW program, keep in mind the primary purpose is to transition the injured individual back to full, productive work. The following are the components of an ERTW Program.

Executive Support. You must have management support, from the chief down, for the program to be successful. If the individual's position has been temporarily filled while the individual is unable to work, your supervisors must determine where the individual will come from to hire the individual for transitional duties. This can be determined ahead of time or on a case-by-case basis.

Formalize Your Organization's Commitment. ERTW options must be provided to all personnel injured on the job, regardless of their productivity or performance. A formal statement outlining the organization's commitment to ERTW should be developed and provided to all personnel.

Assign Responsibility for Managing the Program. An individual or team should be assigned to coordinate and manage ERTW activities. A team could include a safety committee representative, a human resources expert knowledgeable in the ADA and the Family Medical Leave Act (FMLA), a supervisor, and a union representative if applicable. This team should meet to develop and formalize the program, and then meet weekly whenever a lost-time claim occurs. The injured individual and direct supervisor should be invited to develop customized transitional work. If the individual grants permission, it also would be appropriate to have staff members discuss ways to modify and assist the injured individual return to duty.

Develop Clear Guidelines for Reporting Injuries. Identify the person responsible for accepting notice of injuries and immediately notifying the workers' compensation insurance company. Train your personnel on the reporting procedures.

Establish a Target Return-to-Work Date. Send a return-to-work form and cover letter with the injured individual to give to the medical provider during the initial visit. Some organizations report a positive result when supervisors accompany the injured individual to the first visit and obtain a return-to-work release in person. You will need a copy of the individual's job description, including the physical requirements and working conditions, for the medical provider's review. If a release does not occur on the first visit, maintain contact with your individual and the workers' compensation insurance company claim adjuster on a weekly basis to establish an anticipated return-to-work date. Obtain the limitations or injured individual's abilities, anticipated target return-to-work dates, proposed length of restricted duty, and anticipated release to full duty.

If Possible, Modify Your Individual's Existing Job. Based on limitations described by the medical provider, focus first on modifying the individual's existing job. This may include reducing the number of hours worked in a shift and allowing time to visit the health care provider. Find meaningful, productive work for the individual and, if necessary, create temporary duties to accommodate the individual's limitations. Use existing procedures to establish the position. A "transitional worker" classification title is available. A letter with a list of duties for a specific amount of pay, with a specific hire date and end date, is sufficient documentation for classification purposes.

Determine an Appropriate Wage for the Temporary Work. If wages are decreased, the workers' compensation insurance company will pay the individual the difference between pre-injury wage and temporary wage, not to exceed the temporary total disability rate.

Follow Up with the Injured Individual. After the individual returns to work, maintain frequent contact to determine potential problems and the necessity for additional modifications. If necessary, make adjustments to accommodate the individual's needs.

Maintain Confidentiality. Remember that the individual's medical information must be kept confidential, unless the individual specifically grants permission for the supervisor to disclose information to personnel or anyone else who does not have access to confidential medical information. All information collected regarding medical examinations or inquiries must be treated as confidential records and collected and maintained on separate forms in separate files as required by the organization's recordkeeping policy. If your agency establishes a team, ask the individual to grant permission for the team members to have access to medical information and have a permission form signed before releasing any information to members of the team.

Remain Flexible. Remember, the goal is to return the injured individual to the original position at the time of injury. Complications commonly arise during this transition period. Do not give up. If problems occur, continue to modify to reach the desired outcome.

Complications

Poorly performing individuals, individuals facing termination due to a reduction in force, short-term individuals, substance-abusing individuals, or individuals nearing retirement age have the potential to complicate efforts to develop an effective ERTW program. They may refuse to take a modified job, or you may not have appropriate work available. Resolving problems requires effort and coordination. Remaining firm with your commitment to provide ERTW options is the most effective tool you have to combat complications.

Personnel Involved in ERTW

ERTW requires coordination among personnel managers, safety coordinators, workers' compensation insurance company adjusters, agency workers' compensation coordinator or team, union representatives, managed care organizations, referring physician, vocational rehabilitation counselor, and other medical providers.

Steps of an ERTW Program

When an individual is injured, the claim adjuster at the workers' compensation insurance company or managed care organization should be contacted. You should discuss options regarding placement of the injured individual into transitional duties.

If an injured individual qualifies for ERTW, your organization must provide to the attending medical provider a job description that includes the physical requirements. This will allow an accurate decision regarding the type of duties the injured individual is able to perform while in the ERTW program. Individuals must be evaluated on a case-by-case basis.

If possible, the agency should first modify the individual's current duties. This can be as simple as reducing the normal working hours until the individual can work full time. In some cases, a separate position may be temporarily created to allow the individual to perform meaningful work during the healing process. The medical provider can assess the temporary physical limitations of the individual and recommend the kinds of duties that may be performed safely. The agency has to determine what duties are available within the organization that would qualify for transitional duty. These duties may be identified and described on a periodic basis, or when the need arises to bring an individual back to duty.

Once the description of duties is approved, your organization must make an offer of employment or volunteer status to the injured individual. Transitional employment is temporary and must have a designated start and end date set at the time of return to work. The end date may be extended for another specific time if the individual needs additional time to recover, or the individual may be assigned to other transitional duties with specific start and end dates.

The individual then must notify the insurance claim adjuster of the offer. At that time, the claim adjuster will adjust the compensation benefits based on the number of hours offered per week and the wage. These amounts will equal the usual wage of the injured individual. This adjustment occurs whether the individual accepts the offer of employment or not, unless the temporary position requires relocation.

Finally, the organization must notify the claim adjuster when an injured individual accepts or refuses the offer. The claim adjuster will adjust the benefits promptly. It is possible for an injured individual to lose benefits if the individual refuses an offer equal to normal wages and hours. If an individual accepts transitional duty, the insurance company may underwrite the workers' compensation coverage until the injured individual can return to the time-of-injury job.

STRESS AND MENTAL HEALTH

The media is replete with accounts of the **stress** experienced by emergency providers. High work-stress burnout can be formally described as consisting of three components: emotional exhaustion that may lead to negative, cynical attitudes toward patients; deindividuation and depersonalization of patients; and a tendency for providers to evaluate themselves negatively when assessing their work with patients.

There are a number of studies of EMS personnel and stress. *The Feasibility for an EMS Workforce Safety and Health Surveillance System* (Becker and Spicer, 2007) contains an accumulation of these studies. Stress and tension are normal reactions to events that threaten us. Such threats can come from accidents, financial troubles, and problems on the job or with family. The way we deal with these pressures has a lot to do with mental, emotional, and physical health.

The Canadian Mental Health Association (n.d.) offers 18 tips for dealing with the stress and tension in your life:

1. Recognize your symptoms of stress.
2. Look at your lifestyle and see what can be changed—in your work situation, your family situation, or your schedule.
3. Use relaxation techniques: yoga, meditation, deep breathing, or massage.
4. Exercise. Physical activity is one of the most effective stress remedies around!
5. Time management. Do essential tasks and prioritize the others. Consider those who may be affected by your decisions, such as family and friends. Use a checklist so you will receive satisfaction as you check off each job as it is done.
6. Watch your diet. Alcohol, caffeine, sugar, fats, and tobacco all put a strain on your body's ability to cope with stress. A diet with a balance of fruits, vegetables, whole grains, and foods high in protein but low in fat will help create optimum health. Contact your local branch of the Heart and Stroke Foundation for further information about healthy eating.
7. Get enough rest and sleep.
8. Talk with others. Talk with friends, professional counselors, support groups, or relatives about what is bothering you.
9. Help others. Volunteer work can be an effective and satisfying stress reducer.
10. Get away for a while. Read a book, watch a movie, play a game, listen to music, or go on vacation. Leave yourself some time that is just for you.
11. Work off your anger. Get physically active, dig in the garden, start a project, get your spring-cleaning done.
12. Give in occasionally. Avoid quarrels whenever possible.
13. Tackle one thing at a time. Don't try to do too much at once.
14. Don't try to be perfect.
15. Ease up on criticism of others.
16. Don't be too competitive.
17. Make the first move to be friendly.
18. Have some fun! Laugh and be with people you enjoy.

Stress is a very real element of EMS, and it is important for EMS organizations to identify personnel who are having issues related to stress. They must be encouraged to seek professional help. It is important to remember that everyone is different and everyone handles matters in different ways. The worse thing is to force a method on an individual who may not want to deal with stress in a manner you suggest.

Critical incident stress management (CISM) has undergone scrutiny in the past few years. Some individuals strongly believe in CISM, yet others strongly dissent that CISM is not effective. Regardless, CISM has a purpose and must be used with the realms of its effectiveness. Personnel must seek professional assistance when dealing with stress as a result of a significant incident.

CHAPTER REVIEW

Summary

The most important asset of any organization is its personnel. This chapter has presented a number of areas of importance for establishing programs for the health and well-being of EMS personnel. EMS does not have any national standards, like the fire service does, to provide guidance in medical exams, fitness programs, or any other health and well-being activities. It is important for EMS organizations to establish those programs and utilize the resources available. It starts before the individual walks in the door. Once the individual is with the organization, the organization must do its part in helping personnel ensure their own health and well-being.

WHAT WOULD YOU DO? Reflection

You have prepared a plan to implement the physical fitness program. You have arranged for a company that specializes in medical screening for emergency service personnel to come to the station and perform a medical evaluation on all personnel.

You have spoken to your local university, which has a physical therapy program with a track in fitness. The program director has assigned a student to do an internship with the organization and conduct the fitness assessment. He has also agreed to monitor the progress of personnel and work with them during the next 4 months. You have solicited and selected two individuals who expressed interest in becoming certified as peer fitness trainers. In addition, the intern from the university will work with you and your personnel to establish a set of fitness standards. You have also been informed that management is committed to the program and will allow personnel to have 45 minutes of on-duty time to work out.

The last piece of the puzzle is nutrition. You have spoken to a friend who is a dietician and is more than willing to do classes for the crews. In addition, she will provide sample meals, and work with crews to learn how to prepare well-balanced meals for themselves. The leadership of the organization is pleased with the progress of the program and will be participating in the program to set the example for the rest of the organization.

Review Questions

1. Describe at least three high-risk factors for EMS personnel.
2. What are the five areas that EMS organizations should focus on to build a strong wellness program?
3. You are asked to create an annual medical evaluation for personnel. What would be your recommendation for this evaluation?
4. What vaccinations are recommended for EMS personnel?

5. What are the major components of an EAP program?
6. You have been asked to create a fitness program. Your first step is to provide the components you think would be best for the program. What components would you recommend?
7. You have created a physical ability testing course for your applicants. How would you validate the test?
8. You are assigned as the rehab sector leader for a major incident. The first task is to establish the rehab sector in an appropriate location. Discuss your thoughts on what you would look for to secure the best site.
9. One of your personnel was injured on the job. She cannot return to full duty, but you both agreed along with her physician that she can return to transitional duty on an early return-to-work program. What are the benefits of placing her on the ERTW program?
10. What tips does the Canada Mental Health Association recommend for dealing with stress?

References

American College of Occupational and Environmental Medicine. (2006, September). "Preventing Needless Work Disability by Helping People Stay Employed." *Journal of Emergency Medicine.* (See the organization website.)

Austin-Travis County EMS. (2009). "Austin-Travis EMS Physical Ability Testing." Austin, TX: Author. (See the organization website.)

Becker, L. R., and R. Spicer. (2007, May). *Feasibility for an EMS Workforce Safety and Health Surveillance System.* Washington, DC: National Highway Traffic Safety Administration.

Canadian Mental Health Association. (n.d.). "Coping with Stress: 18 Tips for Dealing with Stress and Tension." Ottawa, ON: Author. (See the organization website.)

Immunization Action Coalition. (2008). Healthcare Personnel Vaccination Recommendations. #P2017. (See the organization website.)

Montana Worker's Compensation Management Bureau. (n.d.). "Early Return to Work." (See the organization website.)

National Fire Protection Association (NFPA). (2007). "1500: Standard on Comprehensive Occupational Medical Program for Fire Departments, 2007 Edition." Quincy, MA: Author.

National Fire Protection Association (NFPA). (2007). "1582: Standard on Fire Department Occupational Safety and Health Program, 2007 Edition." Quincy, MA: Author.

National Fire Protection Association (NFPA). (2008). "1584: Standard on the Rehabilitation Process for Members During Emergency Operations and Training Exercises, 2008, Edition." Quincy, MA: Author.

Occupational Safety and Health Administration (OSHA). (1974). Occupational Safety and Health Act. *Federal Register 39*(37), 773–778.

Pepe, P., J. Jerger, R., Miller, and S. Jerger. (1985). "Accelerated Hearing Loss in Urban Emergency Medical Services Personnel." *Annals of Emergency Medicine 14*(5), 438–442.

Price, T., and J. Goldsmith. (1998). "Changes in Hearing Acuity in Ambulance Personnel." *Prehospital Emergency Care* **2**, 308–311.

U.S. Fire Administration (July 1992) (See the organization website for Emergency Incident Rehabilitation.)

Key Terms

carcinogens Cancer-causing substances or agents.

content validity A test of elements that are similar or identical to those of the job being tested.

criterion validity A test that uses statistical tests to predict job performance.

critical incident stress management (CISM) A method of managing stress after a critical incident including mass casualties, suicides, pediatric incidents, and other incidents that have an effect on personnel.

construct validity A method of measuring underlying theoretical concepts.

early return-to-work program A program that provides short-term duties within a specified time frame for personnel who have been injured and cannot return to their time-of-injury duties.

employee assistance programs (EAP) Programs used to help personnel who are experiencing personal problems.

exercise program Programs designed for personnel to do exercises in order to maintain good health.

fitness assessment An assessment conducted to determine the strength, flexibility, and endurance of personnel.

fitness standards The level of fitness expected of personnel to perform the job.

heat stress index A chart that dictates the heat index by combining the temperature and relative humidity; the feels-like temperature.

medical screening A medical evaluation that is conducted to determine if the person is able to participate in a physical fitness program.

nutrition A part of the fitness program that deals with what and the way one eats.

peer fitness trainer A certified individual who monitors and constructs a physical fitness program.

permissible noise level The maximum level of noise permissible by OSHA at 90dB for an 8-hour period.

physical ability testing (PAT) A test of applicants conducted to test whether or not they are physically able to perform the duties and requirements of the job.

physical fitness programs The programs used to help personnel remain physically fit to perform the duties of the task or job.

post-exposure exams The medical exam that is conducted if a provider is exposed to hazmat chemicals or infectious disease.

stress Emotional exhaustion that may lead to negative, cynical attitudes towards their patients; deindividuation and depersonalization of patients; and a tendency for providers to evaluate themselves negatively when assessing their work with patients.

transitional employee An individual allowed only short-term duties such as those with limited physical ability requirements, those that can be taught to the injured employee quickly, those that fit into a flexible work schedule, those that would minimize exposure of the injured worker to further injury, and those that would minimize the injured worker's exposure to further injury and would not slow down the recovery time.

windchill index The chart that gives the feels-like temperature after combining the actual temperature with wind speed.

APPENDIX I: Occupational Safety and Health Administration (OSHA)

OSHA can provide extensive help through a variety of programs, including assistance about safety and health programs, state plans, workplace consultations, Voluntary Protection Programs, strategic partnerships, training and education, and more. Whether you are an OSHA state or not (see below), these resources are available.

SAFETY AND HEALTH PROGRAM MANAGEMENT

Effective management of worker safety and health protection is a decisive factor in reducing the extent and severity of work-related injuries and illnesses and their related costs. In fact, an effective safety and health program forms the basis of good worker protection and can save time and money, about $4 for every dollar spent, and increase productivity.

To assist employers and employees in developing effective safety and health systems, on January 26, 1989, OSHA published recommended "Safety and Health Program Management Guidelines" (*Federal Register* 54(18), 3908–3916). These voluntary guidelines can be applied to EMS.

The guidelines identify four general elements that are critical to the development of a successful safety and health management program: management leadership and employee involvement, worksite analysis, hazard prevention and control, and safety and health training.

The guidelines recommend specific actions under each of these general elements to achieve an effective safety and health program. The *Federal Register* notice is available online at www.osha.gov.

STATE PLANS

State plans are OSHA-approved job safety and health programs operated by individual states or territories instead of federal OSHA. The Occupational Safety and Health Act of 1970 (OSH Act) encourages states to develop and operate their own job safety and health plans and permits state enforcement of OSHA standards if the state has an approved plan. Once OSHA approves a state plan, it funds 50 percent of the program's operating costs. State plans must provide standards and enforcement programs, as well as voluntary compliance activities that are at least as effective as those of federal OSHA.

There are 26 state plans: 23 cover both private and public (state and local government) employment, and three (Connecticut, New Jersey, and New York) cover only the public sector. For more information on state plans, visit OSHA's website at www.osha.gov.

CONSULTATION ASSISTANCE

In addition to helping employers identify and correct specific hazards, OSHA's consultation service provides free, on-site assistance in developing and implementing effective workplace safety and health management systems that emphasize the prevention of worker injuries and illnesses.

Comprehensive consultation assistance provided by OSHA includes a hazard survey of the worksite and an appraisal of all aspects of the employer's existing safety and health management system. In addition, the service offers assistance to employers in developing and implementing an effective safety and health management system. Employers also may receive training and education services, as well as limited assistance away from the worksite.

TRAINING

The OSHA Training Institute in Des Plaines, Illinois, provides basic and advanced training and education in safety and health for federal and state compliance officers, state consultants, other federal agency personnel, and private-sector employers, employees, and their representatives.

Institute courses cover diverse safety and health topics including electrical hazards, machine guarding, personal protective equipment, ventilation, and ergonomics. The facility includes classrooms, laboratories, a library, and an audiovisual unit. The laboratories contain various demonstrations and equipment, such as power presses, woodworking and welding shops, a complete industrial ventilation unit, and a sound demonstration laboratory. More than 57 courses dealing with subjects such as safety and health in the construction industry and methods of compliance with OSHA standards are available for personnel in the private sector.

In addition, OSHA's 73 area offices are full-service centers offering a variety of informational services such as personnel for speaking engagements, publications, audiovisual aids on workplace hazards, and technical advice.

FUNDING

OSHA awards grants through its Susan Harwood Training Grant Program to nonprofit organizations to provide safety and health training and education to employers and workers in the workplace. The grants focus on programs that will educate workers and employers in small business (fewer than 250 employees) and train workers and employers about new OSHA standards or high-risk activities or hazards. Grants are awarded for 1 year and may be renewed for an additional 12 months depending on whether the grantee has performed satisfactorily.

OSHA expects each organization awarded a grant to develop a training and/or education program that addresses a safety and health topic named by OSHA, to recruit workers and employers for the training, and to conduct the training. Grantees also are expected to follow up with people who have been trained to find out what changes were made to reduce the hazards in their workplaces as a result of the training.

Each year OSHA has a national competition that is announced in the *Federal Register* and on the Internet at www.osha.gov/Training/sharwood/sharwood.html. If you do not have access to the Internet, you can contact the OSHA Office of Training and Education, 1555 Times Drive, Des Plaines, IL 60018, (847) 297-4810, for more information.

OTHER RESOURCES

OSHA has a variety of materials and tools available on its website at www.osha.gov. These include eTools, Expert Advisors, Electronic Compliance Assistance Tools (e-CATs), Technical Links, regulations, directives, publications, videos, and other information for employers and employees. OSHA's software programs and compliance assistance tools guide participants through challenging safety and health issues and common problems to find the best solutions for their workplace. OSHA's comprehensive publications program includes more than a hundred titles to help understand OSHA requirements and programs.

OSHA's CD-ROM includes standards, interpretations, directives, and more and can be purchased from the U.S. Government Printing Office. To order, write to the Superintendent of Documents, U.S. Government Printing Office, Washington, DC 20402, or phone (202) 512-1800. Specify *OSHA Regulations, Documents and Technical Information on CD-ROM (ORDT)*, GPO Order No. S/N 729-013-00000-5.

OSHA PUBLICATIONS

A single free copy of the following materials can be obtained from the OSHA Area or Regional Office, or contact the OSHA Publications Office, U.S. Department of Labor, 200 Constitution Avenue NW, N-3101, Washington, DC 20210, or call (202) 693-1888, or fax (202) 693-2498.

- Access to Medical and Exposure Records—OSHA 3110
- All About OSHA—OSHA 2056 (Spanish version 3173)
- Control of Hazardous Energy (Lockout/Tagout)—OSHA 3120
- Emergency Exit Routes Quick Card—OSHA 3183
- Employee Workplace Rights—OSHA 3021 (Spanish version 3049)
- Employer Rights and Responsibilities Following an OSHA Inspection—OSHA 3000 (Spanish version 3195)
- Hand and Power Tools—OSHA 3080
- How to Plan for Workplace Emergencies and Evacuations—OSHA 3088
- It's the Law Poster—OSHA 3165 (Spanish version 3167)
- Job Hazard Analysis—OSHA 3071
- Model Plans & Programs for the OSHA Bloodborne Pathogens and Hazard Communications Standard—OSHA 3186
- Occupational Safety and Health Act—OSHA 2001
- OSHA Inspections—OSHA 2098
- Personal Protective Equipment—OSHA 3151

The following publications are available from the U.S. Government Printing Office (GPO), Superintendent of Documents, Washington, DC 20402, phone toll-free (866) 512-1800, fax (202) 512-2250. Include GPO Order Number and make checks payable to Superintendent of Documents. All prices are subject to change by GPO.

- Hazard Communication: A Compliance Kit—OSHA 3111, Order No. 029-016-00200-6
- Materials Handling and Storing—OSHA 2236, Order No. 029-016-00215-4
- Internet—An enormous amount of compliance assistance information that can be useful to the small business owner is available on OSHA's website: www.osha.gov/dcsp/compliance_assistance/index.html
  OSHA standards, interpretations, directives, and additional information are also available at www.osha.gov and www.osha.gov
- CD-ROM—A wide variety of OSHA materials, including standards, interpretations, directives, and more, can be purchased on CD-ROM from the U.S. Government Printing Office, Superintendent of Documents, phone toll-free (866) 512-1800

OSHA REGIONAL AND AREA OFFICES

OSHA REGIONAL OFFICES

Note: States and territories marked with an asterisk (*) operate their own OSHA-approved job safety and health programs (Connecticut, New Jersey and New York plans cover public employees only). States with approved programs must have a standard that is identical to, or at least as effective as, the federal standard.

Region I
(CT*, ME, MA, NH, RI, VT*)
JFK Federal Building, Room E340
Boston, MA 02203
(617) 565-9860

Region II
(NJ*, NY*, PR*, VI*)
201 Varick Street, Room 670
New York, NY 10014
(212) 337-2378

Region III
(DE, DC, MD*, PA*, VA*, WV)
The Curtis Center
170 S. Independence Mall West
Suite 740 West
Philadelphia, PA 19106-3309
(215) 861-4900

Region IV
(AL, FL, GA, KY*, MS, NC*, SC*, TN*)
Atlanta Federal Center
61 Forsyth Street SW, Room 6T50
Atlanta, GA 30303
(404) 562-2300

Region V
(IL, IN*, MI*, MN*, OH, WI)
230 South Dearborn Street
Room 3244
Chicago, IL 60604
(312) 353-2220

Region VI
(AR, LA, NM*, OK, TX)
525 Griffin Street, Room 602
Dallas, TX 75202
(214) 767-4731 or 4736, ext. 224

Region VII
(IA*, KS, MO, NE)
City Center Square
1100 Main Street, Suite 800
Kansas City, MO 64105
(816) 426-5861

Region VIII
(CO, MT, ND, SD, UT*, WY*)
1999 Broadway, Suite 1690
Denver, CO 80202-5716
(303) 844-1600

Region IX
(American Samoa, AZ*, CA*, HI, NV*, Northern Mariana Islands)
71 Stevenson Street, Room 420
San Francisco, CA 94105
(415) 975-4310

Region X
(AK*, ID, OR*, WA*)
1111 Third Avenue, Suite 715
Seattle, WA 98101-3212
(206) 553-5930

OSHA AREA OFFICES

Birmingham, AL: (205) 731-1534
Mobile, AL: (251) 441-6131
Anchorage, AK: (907) 271-5152
Little Rock, AR: (501) 324-6291/5818
Phoenix, AZ: (602) 640-2348
Sacramento, CA: (916) 566-7471
San Diego, CA: (619) 557-5909
Denver, CO: (303) 844-5285
Greenwood Village, CO: (303) 843-4500
Bridgeport, CT: (203) 579-5581
Hartford, CT: (860) 240-3152

Wilmington, DE: (302) 573-6518
Fort Lauderdale, FL: (954) 424-0242
Jacksonville, FL: (904) 232-2895
Tampa, FL: (813) 626-1177
Savannah, GA: (912) 652-4393
Smyrna, GA: (770) 984-8700
Tucker, GA: (770) 493-6644/6742/8419
Des Moines, IA: (515) 284-4794
Boise, ID: (208) 321-2960
Calumet City, IL: (708) 891-3800
Des Plaines, IL: (847) 803-4800
Fairview Heights, IL: (618) 632-8612
North Aurora, IL: (630) 896-8700
Peoria, IL: (309) 671-7033
Indianapolis, IN: (317) 226-7290
Wichita, KS: (316) 269-6644
Frankfort, KY: (502) 227-7024
Baton Rouge, LA: (225) 389-0474/0431
Braintree, MA: (617) 565-6924
Methuen, MA: (617) 565-8110
Springfield, MA: (413) 785-0123
Linthicum, MD: (410) 865-2055/2056
Bangor, ME: (207) 941-8177
Augusta, ME: (207) 622-8417
Portland, ME: (207) 780-3178
Lansing, MI: (517) 327-0904
Minneapolis, MN: (612) 664-5460
Kansas City, MO: (816) 483-9531
St. Louis, MO: (314) 425-4249
Jackson, MS: (601) 965-4606
Billings, MT: (406) 247-7494
Raleigh, NC: (919) 856-4770
Bismark, ND: (701) 250-4521
Omaha, NE: (402) 221-3182
Concord, NH: (603) 225-1629
Avenel, NJ: (732) 750-3270
Hasbrouck Heights, NJ: (201) 288-1700
Marlton, NJ: (856) 757-5181
Parsippany, NJ: (973) 263-1003
Carson City, NV: (775) 885-6963
Albany, NY: (518) 464-4338
Bayside, NY: (718) 279-9060
Bowmansville, NY: (716) 684-3891
New York, NY: (212) 337-2636
North Syracuse, NY: (315) 451-0808
Tarrytown, NY: (914) 524-7510
Westbury, NY: (516) 334-3344
Cincinnati, OH: (513) 841-4132
Cleveland, OH: (216) 522-3818
Columbus, OH: (614) 469-5582
Toledo, OH: (419) 259-7542
Oklahoma City, OK: (405) 278-9560
Portland, OR: (503) 326-2251
Allentown, PA: (610) 776-0592
Erie, PA: (814) 833-5758
Harrisburg, PA: (717) 782-3902
Philadelphia, PA: (215) 597-4955
Pittsburgh, PA: (412) 395-4903
Wilkes-Barre, PA: (570) 826-6538
Guaynabo, PR: (787) 277-1560
Providence, RI: (401) 528-4669
Columbia, SC: (803) 765-5904
Nashville, TN: (615) 781-5423
Austin, TX: (512) 916-5783/5788
Corpus Christi, TX: (361) 888-3420
Dallas, TX: (214) 320-2400/2558
El Paso, TX: (915) 534-6251
Fort Worth, TX: (817) 428-2470, 485-7647
Houston, TX, North office: (281) 591-2438/2787
Houston, TX, South office: (281) 286-0583
Lubbock, TX: (806) 472-7681/7685
Salt Lake City, UT: (801) 530-6901

Norfolk, VA: (757) 441-3820
Bellevue, WA: (206) 553-7520
Appleton, WI: (920) 734-4521
Eau Claire, WI: (715) 832-9019
Madison, WI: (608) 264-5388
Milwaukee, WI: (414) 297-3315
Charleston, WV: (304) 347-5937

OSHA-APPROVED SAFETY AND HEALTH PLANS

Alaska
Alaska Department of Labor and Workforce Development
Commissioner
(907) 465-2700
Fax: (907) 465-2784
Program Director
(907) 269-4904
Fax: (907) 269-4915

Arizona
Industrial Commission of Arizona
Director, ICA
(602) 542-4411
Fax: (602) 542-1614
Program Director
602) 542-5795
Fax: (602) 542-1614

California
California Department of Industrial Relations
Director
(415) 703-5050
Fax: (415) 703-5114
Chief (415) 703-5100
Fax: (415) 703-5114
Manager, Cal/OSHA Program Office
(415) 703-5177
Fax: (415) 703-5114

Connecticut
Connecticut Department of Labor
Commissioner
(860) 566-5123
Fax: (860) 566-1520
CT OSHA Director
(860) 566-4550
Fax: (860) 566-6916

Hawaii
Hawaii Department of Labor and Industrial Relations
Director
(808) 586-8844
Fax: (808) 586-9099
Administrator (808) 586-9116
Fax: (808) 586-9104

Indiana
Indiana Department of Labor
Commissioner
(317) 232-2378
Fax: (317) 233-3790
Deputy Commissioner
(317) 232-3325
Fax: (317) 233-3790

Iowa
Iowa Division of Labor
Commissioner
(515) 281-6432
Fax: (515) 281-4698
Administrator (515) 281-3469
Fax: (515) 281-7995

Kentucky
Kentucky Labor Cabinet
Secretary (502) 564-3070
Fax: (502) 564-5387
Federal/State Coordinator
(502) 564-3070, ext. 240
Fax: (502) 564-1682

Maryland
Maryland Division of Labor and Industry
Commissioner
(410) 767-2999
Fax: (410) 767-2300
Deputy Commissioner
(410) 767-2992
Fax: (410) 767-2003

Assistant Commissioner, MOSH
(410) 767-2215
Fax: (410) 767-2003

Michigan
Michigan Department of Consumer and
   Industry Services
Director
(517) 322-1814
Fax: (517) 322-1775

Minnesota
Minnesota Department of Labor and
   Industry
Commissioner
(651) 296-2342
Fax: (651) 282-5405
Assistant Commissioner
(651) 296-6529
Fax: (651) 282-5293
Administrative Director, OSHA Management
   Team
(651) 282-5772
Fax: (651) 297-2527

Nevada
Nevada Division of Industrial Relations
Administrator
(775) 687-3032
Fax: (775) 687-6305
Chief Administrative Officer
(702) 486-9044
Fax: (702) 990-0358
Las Vegas: (702) 687-5240

New Jersey
New Jersey Department of Labor
Commissioner
(609) 292-2975
Fax: (609) 633-9271
Assistant Commissioner
(609) 292-2313
Fax: (609) 292-1314
Program Director, PEOSH
(609) 292-3923
Fax: (609) 292-4409

New Mexico
New Mexico Environment Department
Secretary
(505) 827-2850
Fax: (505) 827-2836
Chief
(505) 827-4230
Fax: (505) 827-4422

New York
New York Department of Labor
Acting Commissioner
(518) 457-2741
Fax: (518) 457-6908
Division Director
(518) 457-3518
Fax: (518) 457-6908

North Carolina
North Carolina Department of Labor
Commissioner
(919) 807-2900
Fax: (919) 807-2855
Deputy Commissioner, OSH Director
(919) 807-2861
Fax: (919) 807-2855
OSH Assistant Director
(919) 807-2863
Fax: (919) 807-2856

Oregon
Oregon Occupational Safety and Health
   Division Administrator
(503) 378-3272
Fax: (503) 947-7461
Deputy Administrator for Policy
(503) 378-3272
Fax: (503) 947-7461
Deputy Administrator for Operations
(503) 378-3272
Fax: (503) 947-7461

Puerto Rico
Puerto Rico Department of Labor and
   Human Resources
Secretary
(787) 754-2119

Fax: (787) 753-9550
Assistant Secretary for Occupational Safety and Health
(787) 756-1100/1106, 754-2171
Fax: (787) 767-6051
Deputy Director for Occupational Safety and Health
(787) 756-1100/1106, 754-2188
Fax: (787) 767-6051

South Carolina
South Carolina Department of Labor, Licensing, and Regulation
Director
(803) 896-4300
Fax: (803) 896-4393
Program Director
(803) 734-9644
Fax: (803) 734-9772

Tennessee
Tennessee Department of Labor
Commissioner
(615) 741-2582
Fax: (615) 741-5078
Acting Program Director
(615) 741-2793
Fax: (615) 741-3325

Utah
Utah Labor Commission
Commissioner
(801) 530-6901
Fax: (801) 530-7906
Administrator
(801) 530-6898
Fax: (801) 530-6390

Vermont
Vermont Department of Labor and Industry
Commissioner
(802) 828-2288
Fax: (802) 828-2748
Project Manager
(802) 828-2765
Fax: (802) 828-2195

Virgin Islands
Virgin Islands Department of Labor
Acting Commissioner
(340) 773-1990
Fax: (340) 773-1858
Program Director
(340) 772-1315
Fax: (340) 772-4323

Virginia
Virginia Department of Labor and Industry
Commissioner
(804) 786-2377
Fax: (804) 371-6524
Director, Office of Legal Support
(804) 786-9873
Fax: (804) 786-8418

Washington
Washington Department of Labor and Industries
Director
(360) 902-4200
Fax: (360) 902-4202
Assistant Director
(360) 902-5495
Fax: (360) 902-5529
Program Manager, Federal-State Operations
(360) 902-5430
Fax: (360) 902-5529

Wyoming
Wyoming Department of Employment
Safety Administrator
(307) 777-7786
Fax: (307) 777-3646

OSHA CONSULTATION PROJECTS

Anchorage, AK: (907) 269-4957
Tuscaloosa, AL: (205) 348-3033
Little Rock, AR: (501) 682-4522
Phoenix, AZ: (602) 542-1695
Sacramento, CA: (916) 263-2856

Fort Collins, CO: (970) 491-6151
Wethersfield, CT: (860) 566-4550
Washington, DC: (202) 541-3727
Wilmington, DE: (302) 761-8219
Tampa, FL: (813) 974-9962
Atlanta, GA: (404) 894-2643
Tiyam, GU: 9-1-(671) 475-1101
Honolulu, HI: (808) 586-9100
Des Moines, IA: (515) 281-7629
Boise, ID: (208) 426-3283
Chicago, IL: (312) 814-2337
Indianapolis, IN: (317) 232-2688
Topeka, KS: (785) 296-2251
Frankfort, KY: (502) 564-6895
Baton Rouge, LA: (225) 342-9601
West Newton, MA: (617) 727-3982
Lansing, MI: (517) 322-1809
Laurel, MD: (410) 880-4970
Augusta, ME: (207) 624-6400
Saint Paul, MN: (651) 284-5060
Jefferson City, MO: (573) 751-3403
Pearl, MS: (601) 939-2047
Helena, MT: (406) 444-6418
Raleigh, NC: (919) 807-2905
Bismarck, ND: (701) 328-5188
Lincoln, NE: (402) 471-4717
Concord, NH: (603) 271-2024
Trenton, NJ: (609) 292-3923
Santa Fe, NM: (505) 827-4230
Albany, NY: (518) 457-2238
Henderson, NV: (702) 486-9140
Columbus, OH: (614) 644-2631
Oklahoma City, OK: (405) 528-1500
Salem, OR: (503) 378-3272
Indiana, PA: (724) 357-2396
Hato Rey, PR: (787) 754-2171
Providence, RI: (401) 222-2438
Columbia, SC: (803) 734-9614
Brookings, SD: (605) 688-4101
Nashville, TN: (615) 741-7036
Austin, TX: (512) 804-4640
Salt Lake City, UT: (801) 530-6901
Richmond, VA: (804) 786-6359
Christiansted St. Croix, VI: (809) 772-1315
Montpelier, VT: (802) 828-2765
Olympia, WA: (360) 902-5638
Madison, WI: (608) 266-9383
Waukesha, WI: (262) 523-3044
Charleston, WV: (304) 558-7890
Cheyenne, WY: (307) 777-7786

APPENDIX II Federal Resources

NATIONAL HIGHWAY TRAFFIC SAFETY ADMINISTRATION

The National Highway Traffic Safety Administration (NHTSA) mission statement is to "Save lives, prevent injuries and reduce economic costs due to road traffic crashes, through education, research, safety standards and enforcement activity." NHTSA is the home of EMS in the federal government. Over time, controversy has characterized the discussion of whether or not EMS should be regulated under this agency. As of this writing, EMS still falls under NHTSA. NHTSA and the National Association of Emergency Medical Technicians (NAEMT) offer a lot of valuable information at their websites: www.naemt.org and www.nhtsa.gov. You can access the EMS office at NHTSA at www.ems.gov.

NATIONAL INSTITUTE FOR OCCUPATIONAL SAFETY AND HEALTH

The National Institute for Occupational Safety and Health (NIOSH) is a research agency in the U.S. Department of Health and Human Services. NIOSH conducts research and makes recommendations to prevent work-related illness and injury. The NIOSH toll-free phone number is (800) 356-4674, and its website address is www.cdc.gov/niosh.

U.S. DEPARTMENT OF TRANSPORTATION MANUAL ON UNIFORM TRAFFIC CONTROL DEVICES

The *Manual on Uniform Traffic Control Devices* (MUTCD) defines the standards used by road managers nationwide to install and maintain traffic control devices on all streets and highways. The MUTCD is published by the Federal Highway Administration (FHWA) under 23 Code of Federal Regulations (CFR), Part 655, Subpart F. The electronic version of the MUTCD 2003 Edition with Revisions 1 and 2 incorporated is the most current edition on the MUTCD website and is the official FHWA publication. You can access it at http://mutcd.fh-wa.dot.gov/HTM/2003/part1/part1a.htm

U.S. FIRE ADMINISTRATION

The U.S. Fire Administration (USFA) is an entity of the Department of Homeland Security's Federal Emergency Management Agency. The mission of the USFA is to foster a solid foundation in prevention, preparedness, and response by providing national leadership to local fire and emergency services. EMS agencies are reluctant to utilize the USFA as it has the word *fire* in the title; however, practically all programs are available to EMS providers and have an implication to EMS. You can access additional information at www.usfa.fema.gov.

CENTERS FOR DISEASE CONTROL AND PREVENTION

The website of the Centers for Disease Control and Prevention (CDC) contains a wealth of information and, quite frankly, can be overwhelming. The CDC can provide information on virtually everything from any type of illness or disease to injury prevention. www.cdc.gov is the CDC's primary online communication channel. The CDC.gov site provides users with credible, reliable health information on many topics, including these:

- Data and Statistics
- Diseases and Conditions
- Emergencies and Disasters
- Environmental Health
- Healthy Living
- Injury, Violence, and Safety
- Life Stages and Populations
- Travelers' Health
- Workplace Safety and Health

The CDC is a must resource for safety officers. You can find the agency's information at www.cdc.gov.

APPENDIX III: Associations

AMERICAN SOCIETY OF SAFETY ENGINEERS

The American Society of Safety Engineers is a member organization. It represents safety professionals and provides a wealth of information. You can find additional information at www.asse.org.

AMERICAN INDUSTRIAL HYGIENE ASSOCIATION

The American Industrial Hygiene Association is a member organization. It represents industrial hygienists. You can find out more information at www.aiha.org.

NATIONAL FIRE PROTECTION ASSOCIATION

This is another organization that has *fire* in its name, yet it has so many resources applicable to EMS. The National Fire Protection Association (NFPA) creates consensus standards in fire protection. In addition, it has a number of standards applicable to EMS. In order to access the standards you must be a member and subscribe to the standards or purchase the individual standards. You can obtain the standards at a higher cost if you are not a member. To find out more, you can access www.nfpa.org.

NATIONAL ACADEMY OF EMERGENCY DISPATCH

The National Academy of Emergency Dispatch (NAED) is a nonprofit standard-setting organization promoting safe and effective emergency dispatch services worldwide. Comprised of three allied academies for medical, fire, and police dispatching, the NAED supports first responder-related research, unified protocol application, legislation for emergency call center regulation, and strengthening of the emergency dispatch community through education, certification, and accreditation. You can find more information at www.naemd.org.

NATIONAL ASSOCIATION OF EMTS

NAEMT is a member organization representing EMS personnel at all levels. The Health and Safety Committee assists the board of directors in advocating for a nationwide EMS work environment in which health and safety are top operational priorities. Responsibilities include the following:

- Monitor the EMS community on a regular basis for trends in health and safety issues, and bring to the attention of the board any issues that may warrant action by the association.

- Identify best practices in addressing EMS health and safety issues and share them with the institutions that employ EMS providers.
- Identify the education and training that should be provided to EMS employers to help them create and maintain healthy and safe EMS work environments.

You can learn more about the Health and Safety Committee at www.naemt.org/emshealthsafety/emshealthsafety_home.aspx.

NATIONAL SAFETY COUNCIL

The National Safety Council (NSC) has a broad range of information services available. If you have a local chapter of the NSC in your area, you can call or visit to see how you can use materials pertaining to your organization. You also can access the organization's website at www.nsc.org.

PUBLIC RISK MANAGEMENT ASSOCIATION

The Public Risk Management Association is really targeted toward those who are in the public sector. The association provides a wealth of information on risk management along with a variety of education programs. You can find more information at www.primacentral.org.

OTHER ASSOCIATIONS

The list of organizations in this appendix is by no means an exhaustive list of associations that the safety officer should be looking to join. Many other associations provide valuable services. The NAEMT health and safety committee is the most applicable association for EMS safety officers. The following associations are also potential resources:

Fire Department Safety Officer Association, www.fdsoa.org

Fire and Emergency Services Higher Education, www.usfa.dhs.gov/nfa/higher_ed

International Association of Fire Chiefs, www.iafc.org

National Association of EMS Educators www.naemse.org

APPENDIX IV Other Resources

■ WORKERS' COMPENSATION CARRIERS AND OTHER INSURANCE COMPANIES

Many workers' compensation carriers, as well as many liability and fire insurance companies, conduct periodic inspections and visits to evaluate safety and health hazards. Managers of small and medium-size businesses need to know what services are available from these sources. Contact your carrier and see what it has to offer.

■ UNIONS AND EMPLOYEE GROUPS

If your employees are organized, set up some communications, as you do in normal labor relations, to ensure coordinated action on hazards in your business. Safety and health constitute an area where advance planning will produce action on common goals. Many unions have safety and health expertise that they are willing to share.

■ YOUR LOCAL LIBRARY

Many local or university libraries contain information on specific safety and health subjects pertaining to your business. These materials are usually in reference rooms or technical subject areas. Ask your reference librarian what is available. The library may be able to obtain materials for you through interlibrary loan, purchase, and so on.

Glossary

acquired abilities The abilities by which each individual coordinates and handles a vehicle based on a number of driving characteristics that he has acquired from the time he began to drive.

action Something that is done by an actor. Actions may or may not be observable. An action may describe something that is done or not done. Failure to act should be thought of as an act in itself.

actor Person who conducts an act. An individual or object that directly influenced the flow of the sequence of events. An actor may participate in the process or merely observe the process. An actor initiates a change by performing or failing to perform an action.

administrative controls Control measures aimed at reducing exposures to hazards, generally by designing safe work practices, scheduling, and job enrichment; should be used in conjunction with, and not as a substitute for, more effective or reliable engineering controls.

adverse selection Occurs when the more claims an insurer pays out, the higher the premium has the potential to go.

analysis Separation of an intellectual or substantial whole into its parts for individual study.

ANSI/ISEA Standard 207-2006 The American National Standards Institute and the International Safety Equipment Association standards for high-visibility public safety vests.

backlight The process of illuminating the subject from the back.

bloodborne pathogens Bacteria, viruses, or other microorganisms that can cause disease in humans, including but not limited to hepatitis B virus (HBV) and human immunodeficiency virus (HIV).

buffer zone A neutral area around an area of danger that serves to prevent a safe environment.

carcinogens Cancer-causing substances or agents.

change process A strategy intended to help focus on process rather than on individual tasks.

Class III safety vest A type of PPE that is required to be worn by all public safety personnel while on the scene of a highway or roadway incident.

commercial lines Insurance policies that help to protect businesses against losses, including errors and omissions, theft, vehicle, and liability.

computer terminal hazards Dangers or safety risks associated with the use of computers in buildings and in vehicles.

concealment Hides a person's body from view, but does not offer any ballistic protection. Compare *cover*.

construct validity A method of measuring underlying theoretical concepts.

contaminated sharps Any object contaminated with blood or other potentially infectious material that can penetrate the skin, including but not limited to needles, scalpels, broken glass, broken capillary tubes, and exposed ends of dental wires.

content validity A test of elements that are similar or identical to those of the job being tested.

cover Hides a person's body from sight and at the same time offers some ballistic protection.

crisis maintenance Maintenance needed to be performed immediately; typically, the vehicle is placed out of service until completely repaired.

criterion validity A test that uses statistical tests to predict job performance.

critical incident stress management (CISM) A method of managing stress after a critical incident including mass casualties, suicides, pediatric incidents, and other incidents that have an effect on personnel.

culture of consequences An environment in which individuals are rewarded or recognized and held accountable for their actions.

decontamination The use of physical or chemical means to remove, inactivate, or destroy pathogens on a surface or item to the point where they are no longer capable of transmitting infectious particles and the surface or item is rendered safe for handling, use, or disposal.

direct costs Costs that are paid as a result of a loss—for example, workers' compensation claims, which cover medical costs and indemnity payments for an injured or ill member.

driver proficiency The demonstration of the ability to perform in all the varying components of driving emergency vehicles.

driver selection The process of choosing an individual to drive an emergency vehicle.

driver training A comprehensive program to teach an individual how to drive an emergency vehicle; the program should include both written and practical testing.

early return-to-work program A program that provides short-term duties within a specified time frame for personnel who have been injured and cannot return to their time-of-injury duties.

egress The pathway out of a building.

electrical equipment hazards Dangers or safety risks associated with office equipment, electrical components of a building, and electricity in general.

emergency vehicle technician (EVT) A person certified through a testing process who can mechanically work on emergency vehicles.

employee assistance programs (EAP) Programs used to help personnel who are experiencing personal problems.

EMS safety officer The person responsible for the safety, health, and well-being of the EMS provider.

engineering controls To the extent feasible, the work environment and the job itself should be designed (not necessarily by an engineer) to eliminate hazards or reduce exposure to hazards.

epidemiology The study of the causes, distribution, and control of disease in populations.

ergonomics The study of the relationship between people and their workplaces.

exercise program Programs designed for personnel to do exercises in order to maintain good health.

exit The place to leave a building.

expert power A concept that stems from the realization that individuals who are considered experts in their fields play the role of an internal consultant to the organization.

exposure An act of subjecting or an instance of being subjected to an action or an influence on a hazard.

exposure incident A specific eye, mouth, other mucous membrane, or nonintact skin contact with blood or other potentially infectious materials that results from the performance of an employee's duties.

fire hazards Dangers or safety risks of any kind that can result in a fire if left uncorrected.

fitness assessment An assessment conducted to determine the strength, flexibility, and endurance of personnel.

fitness standards The level of fitness expected of personnel to perform the job.

forecasting Predicting or estimating; in the fire service this refers to determining what a fire in a building will do.

full check inspection An evaluation of all vehicle systems that can be checked without special equipment or facilities.

goals Benchmarks that are established to affect a certain outcome.

handling and storage hazards Dangers or safety risks associated with the handling and storage of various materials, including medical supplies, cleaning supplies, and office supplies.

hazard The potential for harm. In practical terms, a hazard often is associated with a condition or activity that, if left uncontrolled, can result in an injury or illness.

hazard identification The process of identifying hazards or unsafe processes or conditions.

hazardous conditions Things and states that directly cause an accident.

heat stress index A chart that dictates the heat index by combining the temperature and relative humidity; the feels-like temperature.

hierarchy of controls Four general strategies for managing hazards: engineering controls, administrative controls, personal protective equipment (PPE), and interim measures.

housekeeping The task of keeping an area clean and free of clutter and debris, especially as it relates to dangers or safety risks.

housekeeping hazards Dangers of safety risks associated with crowding, lack of privacy, and slips, trips, and falls.

human aspects Factors that can promote a change in human activity to produce the safest possible emergency vehicle driver.

illumination hazards Dangers or safety risks associated with lighting in a building or environment in which personnel work.

incident action plan An oral or written plan that contains objectives reflecting the overall incident strategy and specific tactical actions and supporting information for the next operational period.

incident command system A standardized on-scene emergency management concept specifically designed to allow its users to adopt an integrated organizational structure equal to the complexity and demands of single or multiple incidents, without being hindered by jurisdictional boundaries.

incident safety officer An officer who ensures safety on the scene of an incident.

indirect costs Costs related to added administrative time, lower morale, increased absenteeism, and poorer internal and external customer relations.

insurance A social device in which a group of individuals transfer the potential cost of risk in order to combine experience, which permits mathematical prediction of losses and provides for payment of losses from funds contributed by all members who transferred risk.

interim measures Temporary uses of engineering or administrative controls.

job hazard analysis A technique that focuses on job tasks as a way to identify hazards before they occur, and focuses on the relationship among member, task, tools, and work environment.

job transfer When a member is placed into another position because of an illness or injury that prevents him from performing his normal functions. In many organizations this is referred to "light duty."

liability loss exposure A set of circumstances that presents the possibility that one must spend time and money for the investigation, negotiation, settlement, defense, and/or payment of a claim or suit that arises out of a real or alleged failure to fulfill an obligation or duty imposed by law.

loss consequences The financial result of a peril that has caused property to be lost, damaged, or destroyed.

loss control A function of management that occurs after an incident.

loss exposure Any condition or situation that presents a possibility of financial loss, whether or not an actual loss ever occurs.

Manual on Uniform Traffic Control Devices for Streets and Highways (MUTCD) A document published by the Federal Highway Administration that addresses virtually every component of highway safety, including the national standard for all traffic control devices installed on any street, highway, or bicycle trail open to public travel.

material evidence Items valuable to an accident investigation, such as tools, equipment, and people.

medical plan A plan that provides information on incident medical aid stations, transportation services, hospitals, and medical emergency procedures.

medical screening A medical evaluation that is conducted to determine if the person is able to participate in a physical fitness program.

noise hazards Dangers or safety risks associated with noise in the work environment, such as the ambulance siren or machines in vehicle maintenance bays.

nutrition A part of the fitness program that deals with what and the way one eats.

objectives The means by which a goal is obtained, by establishing plans that support the completion of the goal.

Occupational Safety and Health Administration (OSHA) The federal agency that oversees the safety of all occupations in the United States.

office furniture hazards Dangers or safety risks associated with various types of office furniture, including desks, chairs, and filing cabinets, such as using a chair instead of a ladder to reach.

office machinery/tools hazards Dangers or safety risks associated with various office machinery and tools, which include photocopiers, paper cutters, staplers.

OSHA 300 log A record of injury and illnesses from an on-the-job occurrence.

peer fitness trainer A certified individual who monitors and constructs a physical fitness program.

peril The cause that might lead to loss, damage, or destruction of property.

permissible noise level The maximum level of noise permissible by OSHA at 90dB for an 8-hour period.

personal lines Insurance policies that help to protect an individual's home, auto, and life.

personal protective equipment (PPE) Equipment such as eye and hearing protection, gloves, and respiratory filters used in conjunction with administrative controls to limit exposure to a hazard in the workplace.

personnel records Those files that document the member's training, performance, and other demographic information.

physical ability testing (PAT) A test of applicants conducted to test whether or not they are physically able to perform the duties and requirements of the job.

physical fitness programs The programs used to help personnel remain physically fit to perform the duties of the task or job.

physical layout The actual arrangement of an office or room of a building and its contents.

position power A concept that stems from the realization that a person can be in a position to have influence on a decision maker.

post-exposure exams The medical exam that is conducted if a provider is exposed to hazmat chemicals or infectious disease.

preventive maintenance Maintenance that focuses on preventing the most likely vehicle malfunctions by replacing parts or making adjustments before a failure occurs.

probability The chances that, given an exposure to a hazard, an accident will result.

property Item subject to loss, damage, or destruction.

pure risk Refers to only two possible outcomes: financial loss or no financial loss.

quick check inspection An evaluation of all those vehicle systems that should be checked most often.

recordkeeping The process of documenting and maintaining documents.

reduced profile Making yourself less visible and less of a target in a dangerous or potentially dangerous environment.

relative risk Risks that are judged by specific undesirable events along a broad scale of undesirability.

restricted work Occurs when a member can still function in his role, but has restrictions.

retroreflective material Material made using tiny glass beads that reflect light directly back toward its source, from a much wider angle than reflective material.

retroreflectorized Reflects light or other radiation back to its source.

risk The possibility of meeting danger or suffering harm or loss; exposure to harm or loss.

risk avoidance The complete elimination of a particular risk in order to prevent an undesirable event from occurring.

risk management Activities that involve the comparison and/or evaluation of risks; the development of methods that will effect change in the probability or consequence of an act. Encompasses all management activities directed at the prevention, reduction, or elimination of the pure risks of providing emergency medical services.

risk manager Typically, personnel with responsibility for handling relations with outside agencies such as insurance companies.

risk retention Accomplished by testing, planning, training, and enforcement of safety and risk management-related issues.

risk transfer A means of mitigating risk potential.

routine maintenance Maintenance performed as needed; does not usually affect the performance of the vehicle.

safety Being free from risk, injury, or danger.

safety committee Personnel and management coming together on a regular basis to identify and solve everyday safety-and-health problems.

safety culture A combination of an organization's attitudes, behaviors, beliefs, values, ways of doing things, and other shared characteristics about safety.

safety program A program made up of the practical concerns of putting together the elements necessary to create a safe environment for personnel and patients.

scheduled maintenance Maintenance performed at regular intervals, usually based on manufacturer's recommendations; planned times at which parts of a vehicle require attention.

self-inspection An essential activity if you are to know where probable hazards exist and whether they are under control.

severity The degree of harshness or seriousness of an incident.

speculative risk A type of risk in which there may be a financial loss, no financial loss, or financial gain.

strategic map An overview of an organization's strategies.

stress Emotional exhaustion that may lead to negative, cynical attitudes towards their patients; deindividuation and depersonalization of patients; and a tendency for providers to evaluate themselves negatively when assessing their work with patients.

system weaknesses Underlying inadequate or missing programs, plans, policies, processes, and procedures that contributed to an accident.

transitional employee An individual allowed only short-term duties such as those with limited physical ability requirements, those that can be taught to the injured employee quickly, those that fit into a flexible work schedule, those that would minimize exposure of the injured worker to further injury, and those that would minimize the injured worker's exposure to further injury and would not slow down the recovery time.

unit log (ICS 214) A type of log used to record details of unit activity, including strike team activity. These logs provide the basic reference from which to extract information for inclusion in any after-action report.

unsafe behaviors Actions taken/not taken that contributed to the accident.

vehicle characteristics The capabilities and limitations of a vehicle, such as speed, road conditions, auxiliary braking systems, and weight transfer.

vehicle maintenance areas Areas of a facility where vehicle maintenance is conducted.

ventilation hazards Dangers or safety risks associated with air quality and air flow, including the exhaust from vehicles parked inside of stations.

windchill index The chart that gives the feels-like temperature after combining the actual temperature with wind speed.

worksite analysis A variety of worksite examinations that identify not only existing hazards, but also conditions and operations with a potential for hazards.

Index

A

acceptance, of risk, 102
accident investigations, 78, 217–250
   accident process, analysis, 229–232
   accident scene (*see* accident(s), scene)
   analysis, 234–236 (*see also* analysis, accident)
   causation theories, 229–232
      accident-proneness theory, 232
      domino theory, 230–231
      Haddon's energy transfer theory, 231
      multiple-cause theory, 232
      pure-chance theory, 232
      single-event theory, 232
   developing recommendations, 236–241
      effective, 236
      hierarchy of controls, 236–237 (*see also* hierarchy of controls)
      implementation-and-design root causes, 247
      primary surface causes, 246
      secondary surface causes, 246–247
      system improvements, 237–241 (*see also* system(s), improvements)
   documentation methods, 224–229
      documents reviewing, 227
      initial statements, 224–225
      interviews, conducting (*see* interviews, conducting)
      photo taking, 225–226
      sketches, 226
      videotaping scene, 226
   effective planning, 222–223
   implications, 222
   investigative techniques, 220–221
   investigator, 220
      kit, 224, 225
   near misses, 219–220
   overview, 218–219
   process initiation, 223–224 (*see also* accident(s), scene)
   purpose, 221–222
   report writing (*see* report writing, accident)
   safety engineers, role, 236
   sequence of events, determining, 232–233
   surface and root causes, determining, 233–236
      management perceptions, 234
   training, 220
accident-proneness theory, 232
accident(s). *see also* accident investigations
   computer terminal hazards, 200, 209–210
   defined, 219
   disabling, types, 200–201
   electrical hazards, 200, 206, 208–209
   exits and egress hazards, 200, 201–202, 203
   fire hazards, 200, 202, 204
   handling and storage hazards, 200, 202–204
   illumination hazards, 200, 210
   investigation (*see* accident investigations)
   noise hazards, 200, 210–211
   office furniture hazards, 200, 204–205
   office machinery and tool hazards, 200, 207, 209
   process analysis, 229–232
   reports, 261 (*see also* report writing, accident)
   scene
      documenting, 224
      securing, 224
      sketching, 226
      videotaping, 226
   street and roadway (*see* street and roadway incidents)
   summary, 247
   ventilation hazards, 200, 210
accountability
   incident rehabilitation, 284
   safety program, 25
      charge backs, 25
      safety activities, 25
      safety goals, 25
accreditation agencies, EMS safety, 2–3
   CAAS, 2
   CAMTS, 2–3
   CFAI, 3
acquired abilities, in driver training, 112–115
   defensive driving, 113–114
   driving knowledge and performance, 114
   licensing, 115
   new drivers, 112–113
   operator qualifications, 114–115
   participation, 115
action, defined, 219, 233
action plan, 57–58
actor, defined, 219, 233
ADA. *see* American with Disabilities Act (ADA)
administrative controls, 49–50
Advanced Hazmat Life Support (AHLS), 177
Advanced Safety Operations and Management (R154), 11
advanced warning sign, 148–149
adverse selection, 42
age, firefighters, 109, 111

Index

air operations, 177–180
  background, 178
  FAA (*see* Federal Aviation Administration (FAA))
  landing zone (*see* landing zone (LZ))
alcohol abuse, recordkeeping and, 118
ambulance(s)
  crashes (*see* crash injury and fatalities)
  office safety and health hazards and, 205
  safety, Levick on, 112
American Automobile Association Foundation for Traffic Safety, 124
American Industrial Hygiene Association, 304
American Society of Safety Engineers, 304
American with Disabilities Act (ADA), 274
analysis, accident, 221
  cause, 234–236
    event, 234
    injury, 234
    special-cause, 234
    systems (*see* system(s), analysis)
  process, 229–232
  purpose, 221
annual medical evaluations, 276–277
ANSI/ISEA Standard 207–2006, 149
antihistamines, 273
antilock braking systems (ABS), 116
antiseptic hand cleanser, 156
assessment, risk, 88
Association of Public-Safety Communications Officials (APCO), 151
attachment, report and, 247
attitude, driver selection and, 111–112
Austin-Travis County EMS, 272

Automotive Service Excellence (ASE) organization, 126
awareness training, 29

B

back injuries, 275
backlight, 172
Basic Life Support (BLS), 281
behavior-based safety, 238
bloodborne pathogens, 155
Bloodborne Standard 1910.1030, OSHA, 155, 156, 157, 158, 159, 160
body armor, tactical EMS and, 175–176
brazen/show-off, 112
buffer zone, 147
building
  age of, 153
  construction, 153
building fires, 151–154. *see also* fires
  forecasting tools, 152–154
    access for crews, 153
    age of building, 153
    attributes of smoke (*see* smoke, attributes of)
    construction type, 153
    egress for crews, 153
    features, 152–153
    functioning at, 154
bulletproof vests, 175–176
Bureau of Labor Statistics, 8, 46

C

CAAS. *see* Commission on Accreditation of Ambulance Services (CAAS)
CAMTS. *see* Commission on Accreditation of Medical Transport Systems (CAMTS)
Canadian Mental Health Association, 288, 292
cancer, 275–276
carcinogens, 275
CDC. *see* Centers for Disease Control and Prevention (CDC)

Census of Fatal Occupational Injuries (CFOI), 6
Centers for Disease Control and Prevention (CDC), 292, 303
CFAI. *see* Commission on Fire Accreditation International (CFAI)
CFOI. *see* Census of Fatal Occupational Injuries (CFOI)
chairs, office furniture hazards, 205
change analysis, 56
change process, 25
changing tires, 212
charge backs, 25
CISM. *see* critical incident stress management (CISM)
clandestine drug labs, 173–174
  actions, 173
  EMS concerns, 173–174
  hazards, 173
  types, 173
Class III safety vest, 147
clothing, gangs and, 172
Code of Federal Regulations (CFR), 144
comic attitude, 112
commercial lines, 38
Commission on Accreditation of Ambulance Services (CAAS), 2, 8
Commission on Accreditation of Medical Transport Systems (CAMTS), 2–3, 8
Commission on Fire Accreditation International (CFAI), 3, 8
commitment, management, 71–72
committee, safety. *see* safety committee
community risk management, 89. *see also* risk management process
comprehensive surveys, 56
compressed gases, 212–213
computer terminal hazards, 200, 209–210
concealment, in violent situations, 174

cones, traffic
  street and roadway incidents and, 146, 147, 148–149
confidentiality
  infectious disease, recordkeeping, 257
consensus standards, 102–103
construct validity, 279
contact tactics, tactical EMS and, 175
contaminated needles/sharps, 156–157, 158
content validity, 279
Contra Costa EMS, 4
controlled flight into terrain (CFIT), 178
cost-benefit analysis, 239–241
  risk management, 94, 97
cover
  tactics, tactical EMS and, 175
  in violent situations, 174
crash injury and fatalities, 107–109
  human factors, 108–109
  research, 107–108
crime scenes, EMS at, 176
crisis maintenance, 136
criterion validity, 279
critical incident stress management (CISM), 288
culture of consequences, 65

D

decontamination, 158
defensive driving, training for, 113–114
Deming, W. Edwards, 64
demographic information, in accident report forms, 245
desks, office furniture hazards, 205
direct costs, 22
disaster medical assistance team (DMAT), 12
distraction, in violence, 175
DMAT. *see* disaster medical assistance team (DMAT)
documentation
  accident scene, 224
  activities, recordkeeping, 253
  initial statements, 224–225
  methods, accident investigations, 224–229
  reviewing, documents, 227
domestic violence, 174
domino theory, 230–231
driver, safety and, 109–125
  proficiency, 119–125
    continuing physical and mental fitness, 125
    recertification, 119, 122
    shift work, 122–125
  responsibility for
    vehicle maintenance, 136
    vehicle repairs (*see* repairs, vehicle)
  selection, 110–112
    human aspects in (*see* human aspects)
  training, 112–119
    acquired abilities (*see* acquired abilities)
    courses, 118–119
    programs, 120–122
    recordkeeping, 116–118
    vehicle characteristics, 115–116
Driving Assessment 2009, 141–142
driving records, in selection, 110
driving under influence (DUI) convictions, 110
Drug Enforcement Administration, 173
drug labs, clandestine. *see* clandestine drug labs
duplicate resources, risk management, 92
duty transfer. *see* restricted work

E

EAP. *see* employee assistance programs (EAP)
early return-to-work (ERTW) program, 284
  benefits, 285
  complications, 287
  components, 285–287
  personnel involved, 287
  purpose of, 284
  steps, 287–288
electrical hazards, 200, 206, 208–209
emergency medical technicians (EMTs), 6
emergency personnel
  access, in fire building, 153
  egress, in fire building, 153
  functions, in street and roadway incidents, 147
  violence to (*see* violent situations, EMS personnel in)
emergency service organizations (ESOs), 150
Emergency Vehicle Safety Initiative, 141
emergency vehicles (EVs)
  characteristics, 115–116
  components and features, 116
  driver training programs, 120–122
  lighting, 149–151
  markings, 151
  safe parking, street and roadway incidents and, 145–146
  special driver training, 116
  technicians (*see* emergency vehicle technicians (EVTs))
  types, driver training and, 116
Emergency Vehicle Technician Certification Program, 142
emergency vehicle technicians (EVTs)
  ambulance certifications, 126
  Certification Commission, 126
employee assistance programs (EAP), 276, 278
Employee Polygraph Protection Act, 196
EMSARN, 250
EMSCloseCalls.com, 219, 220
EMS Event Reporting, 4
EMS organizational risk management, 89
EMS provider health and wellness. *see also* physical fitness programs
  back injuries, 275
  cancer, 275–276
  ERTW program (*see* early return-to-work (ERTW) program)
  hearing loss, 274–275

Index

history of illness, 272–273
medications, 273–274
overview, 271
physical fitness, lack of, 272
pre-employment physical ability testing, lack of, 272
risk factors, 272–276
tobacco, use of, 274
vaccines, 277
wellness programs (*see* wellness programs)
EMS Risk Management Resource Guide, 87
EMS safety. *see also* safety program, developing; safety program management
accreditation agencies, 2–3
high-risk profession, 3–5
risk managers and, 3
EMS safety officer, 3, 9–17. *see also* incident safety officer
duties and responsibilities, 14–16
effective, characteristics of, 16–17
incidents, respond to, 14–15
knowledge of duties, 14
minimum requirements, 15–16
OSHA and, 13, 16
role model, 14
role of, 12–13
EMTs. *see* emergency medical technicians (EMTs)
engineering controls, 49, 237
infectious disease and, 156–157
epidemiology, 160
Equal Employment Opportunity Commissions standards (EEOC), 166
equipment maintenance, recordkeeping, 265–267
equipment maintenance logs, 267
work requests, 267
ergonomics, 165
ERTW. *see* early return-to-work (ERTW) program
evaluation
medical, incident rehabilitation, 283
safety program management, 25

evasive tactics, in violence, 175
event analysis, 234
EVTs. *see* emergency vehicle technicians (EVTs)
exercise program, 280
exits and egress hazards, 200, 201–202, 203
expert power, 72
exposure, loss, 39, 88, 90–91, 94, 95
avoidance, 91
insurance, safety program, 39–41
separation of, 91
exposure control plan, infectious disease, 155–160
exposure determination, 156
Hepatitis B vaccination, 158–159
immunizations, 159–160
methods of compliance, 156–158
engineering and work practice controls, 156–157
housekeeping, 158
PPE, 157–158
regulated waste, 158
post-exposure evaluation and follow-up, 158–159
exposure incident, 159
exposure records, 256
eye protection, 211

F

FAA. *see* Federal Aviation Administration (FAA)
failure mode and effect analysis, 76
Fair Labor Standards Act, 192
Family and Medical Leave Act, 189, 193
FARS. *see* Fatality Analysis Reporting System (FARS)
Fatality Analysis Reporting System (FARS), 6, 107, 108, 141
fault tree analysis, 76
FDRs. *see* flight data recorders (FDRs)
The Feasibility for an EMS Workforce Safety and Health Surveillance System, 288
Federal Aviation Administration (FAA), 178

FDRs, 179
helicopter safety, 179
NVGs, 179
oversight, 178–180
TAWS, 179
weather, 178–179
Federal Bureau of Labor Statistics (BLS), 254
Federal Food Drug and Cosmetic (FFD&C) Act, 165
Federal Highway Administration (FHWA), 144
federal resources, 302–303
CDC, 303
MUTCD, 302
NIOSH, 302
USFA, 302–303
feedback system, safety program, 29
file cabinets, office furniture hazards, 205
financial aspects, safety program, 34–35
findings section, of accident report form, 245–246
design root cause, 246
implementation root cause, 246
primary surface, 245
secondary surface, 245–246
Fire and Emergency Services Higher Education, 305
The Fire and EMS Department Safety Officer, 10
Fire Department Safety Officer Association, 18, 305
FirefighterCloseCalls.com, 219, 220
firefighters, age limit for, 109, 111
fireground, EMS safety officer and, 15
fires
building (*see* building fires)
hazards, 200, 202, 204
wildland, 154–155
fitness
assessment, 279
mental, driver proficiency and, 125
standards, 279
flammables, in vehicle maintenance areas, 212, 213

flight data recorders (FDRs)
  FAA and, 179
flowchart, risk management, 90
Food & Drug Administration
  (FDA), 165
form, job hazard analysis, 33. *see
  also* report forms, accident
formal observation process,
  hazard identification, 77
full check vehicle inspection, 135
funding, risk management, 97

G

gangs, street, 172
General Accounting Office
  (GAO), 178
gloves, 157–158

H

Haddon's energy transfer
  theory, 231
handling and storage hazards,
  200, 202–204
hazard and operability study
  (HAZOP), 76
hazard-control strategies. *see*
  hierarchy of controls
hazardous conditions, 218, 223,
  233, 235
  categories of, 235
hazardous equipment, 79–80
hazardous materials, 79
Hazardous Waste Operations
  and Emergency Response
  (HAZWOPER), 177
hazard(s), 29–34
  analysis, 74–76
    HAZOP, 76
  classifications, 76
  defined, 29
  identification and control, 48,
    74–82
    accident/incident
      investigations, 78
    hazard analysis, 74–76
    hazard classifications, 76
    hazardous equipment, 79–80
    hazardous materials, 79

injury and illness trend
  analysis, 78–79
medical programs, 80
member reports of hazards, 78
preventive maintenance
  systems, 80–82
principles of, 76
processes, 76–78
safety-and-health training,
  80–82
systems to track hazard
  corrections, 80
JHA (*see* job hazard analysis
  (JHA))
workplace hazards, identifying,
  31–33
hazmat scenes, 176–177
HAZOP. *see* hazard and
  operability study (HAZOP)
Health and Safety Officer
  (F730), 11
Health Insurance Portability and
  Accountability (HIPAA)
  Act, 257
health officer, 3
hearing loss, 274–275
heat stress index, 282
Heinrich, W. H., 230
Helicopter Emergency Medical
  Service (HEMS), 178
helicopter safety, FAA and,
  179, 180
Hepatitis B vaccination, 158–159
HFACS, Inc., 250
hierarchy of controls, 48–49,
  236–237
  engineering controls, 237
  management controls, 237
  PPE, 237
Highway Incident Safety
  for Emergency
  Responders, 184
highways. *see also* street and
  roadway incidents
  limited access, operations, 147
  safety, in violent situations,
    169–171
  and street operations
    EMS safety officer and, 15

HIPAA. *see* Health Insurance
  Portability and
  Accountability
  (HIPAA) Act
housekeeping, 187
  hazards, 200
  infectious disease and, 158
  vehicle maintenance areas, 212
human aspects, in driver
  selection, 110–112
  attitude, 111–112
  driving records, 110
  judgment, 111
  knowledge, 111
  personal appearance and
    hygiene, 112
  physical fitness, 110–111
hydration, incident
  rehabilitation, 282
hygiene, in driver selection, 112

I

IAFF. *see* International Association
  of Fire Fighters (IAFF)
IAP. *see* incident action plan (IAP)
ICS. *see* incident command
  system (ICS)
illumination hazards, 200, 210.
  see also hazard(s)
immunizations, 159–160
implementation cost, risk
  management, 97
incident action plan (IAP), 12, 15
incident command system (ICS),
  11, 14
incident investigation. *see* accident
  investigations
incident rehabilitation, 280–284
  accountability, 284
  hydration, 282
  incident commander, 281
  location, 281
  medical evaluation, 283
  nourishment, 282
  recovery, 283
  rehabilitation sector/group
    establishment, 281–282
  rest, 282–283
  supervisors, 281

Index

incident safety officer, role of, 11–12
Incident Safety Officer (F729), 11
indirect costs, 22
infection control, 277–278
infectious diseases
  recordkeeping and, 256–258
    confidentiality, 257
    medical records, 257
    sharps injury log, 258
    training records, 257
    transfer of records, 257–258
  scene operations and, 155–161
    exposure control plan (*see* exposure control plan)
    information and training, 160–161
initial statements, documenting, 224–225
injury/illness
  analysis, 234
  prevention, 165–166
  records, 253–254
  reports, 254–256
    exposure records and others, 256
    lost workdays, defining, 255, 256
    restricted work/job transfer, 255, 256
Injury/Illness Prevention Program (IIP), 135
inspections, vehicle, 131
  full check, 135
  importance of maintaining records, 131
  methodology, 131
  negligence related to, 135
  quick check, 132–135
  schedule, 131–132
  systematic, 131
  types, 132–135
instinctive reactions, 112
insurance, 35–43
  benefits, 41
  companies, 306
  drawbacks, 41–42
  equipment and service disruption, 43

history of, 35–38
injury/damages/death in organization, 42
injury/damages/death to civilians, 42–43
long-term effects, 43
loss exposure, 39–41
present scenario, 38–39
risk management, 92, 95–97
insureds, 38
insurers, 38
interim measures, 51–52
International Association of Fire Chiefs, 305
International Association of Fire Chiefs EMS Section, 219
International Association of Fire Fighters (IAFF), 292
interviews, conducting, 227–229
  effective techniques, 228–229
  preparation for, 227–228
investigation, accident. *see* accident investigations
investigator, accident, 220
  kit, 224, 225
Isaacs, Andrew (A.J.), 117

J

James, Leon, Dr., 108
JHA. *see* job hazard analysis (JHA)
job hazard analysis (JHA), 29–31, 74–75. *see also* hazard(s)
  form, 33
  prevention, 33–34
  workplace hazards, identifying, 31–33
job transfer, 255, 256
Journal of Emergency Medical Services, 185
judgment, driver selection and, 111

K

knowledge, driver selection and, 111

L

ladders, office safety and health hazards and, 205–206, 207
laid back, 112

landing zone (LZ)
  coordinator responsibilities, 180
  criteria, 180
  marking, 180
leadership in safety and health, 22–23, 24–25
legal responsibility, 101–102
Levick, Nadine, Dr., 112
liability loss exposure, 39
licensing, driver training and, 115
lifting devices, in vehicle maintenance areas, 212
lifting dynamics, 166
lighting in street and roadway incidents, 149–151
limited access highways, operations, 147
load limits, tire maintenance, 128–129
local library, 306
long-term effects
  insurance, safety program, 43
loss consequences, 39
loss control
  risk management process, 98–100
    customer service, 99–100
    finance, 99
    leadership and supervision, 100
  vs. risk management, 5–6
loss exposure, 39. *see also* exposure, loss
lost workdays, defined, 255, 256

M

management commitment, 71–72
management controls, 237
Manual on Uniform Traffic Control Devices (MUTCD), 302
  for streets and highways, 144–145
masks, 158
material evidence, 223
material safety data sheets (MSDS), 189
medical device reporting (MDR), 165
medical evaluation, incident rehabilitation, 283
Medical Plan, 15

318 Index

medical programs, 80
medical records
   infectious disease, record-keeping, 257
medical screening, 279
medications, 273–274
Medtec Ambulance Inc., 117
meetings, planning
   EMS safety officer and, 15, 16
mental fitness, driver proficiency and, 125. *see also* fitness
mobile data computers (MDC), 210
Morgan Stanley, 202
multiple-cause theory, 232
MUTCD. *see* Manual on Uniform Traffic Control Devices (MUTCD)
Mycobacterium tuberculosis, 258

N

NAEMSP. *see* National Association of EMS Physicians (NAEMSP)
NAEMT. *see* National Association of Emergency Medical Technicians (NAEMT)
National Academies of Emergency Dispatch (NAEMD), 151
National Association of Emergency Medical Technicians (NAEMT), 291–292, 304–305
National Association of EMS Educators, 305
National Association of EMS Physicians (NAEMSP), 105
National Electronic Injury Surveillance System (NEISS), 6
National Fire Fighter Near-Miss Reporting System, 250
National Fire Protection Association (NFPA), 102, 260–261, 268, 276, 304
National Highway Traffic Safety Administration (NHTSA), 6

National Institute for Occupational Safety and Health (NIOSH), 117, 145, 206, 302
National Institute of Automotive Service Excellence, 142
National Patient Safety Foundation (NPSF), 249
National Safety Council (NSC), 239–241, 305
National Sleep Foundation (NSF), 124
near misses, 219–220
NEISS. *see* National Electronic Injury Surveillance System (NEISS)
NFPA. *see* National Fire Protection Association (NFPA)
NFPA 471, 177
NFPA 472, 177
NFPA 473, 177
NFPA 1500, 10
NFPA 1521, 10
NHTSA. *see* National Highway Traffic Safety Administration (NHTSA)
night vision goggles (NVGs)
   FAA and, 179
NIOSH. *see* National Institute for Occupational Safety and Health (NIOSH)
noise hazards, 200, 210–211
nourishment, incident rehabilitation, 282
NSC. *see* National Safety Council (NSC)
nutrition program, 280
NVGs. *see* night vision goggles (NVGs)

O

Occupational Safety and Health Administration (OSHA), 13, 16, 49, 53, 135, 155, 156, 157, 158, 159, 160, 269, 274, 293–301
   approved safety and health plans, 298–300

   consultation assistance, 294
   consultation projects, 300–301
   exposure records and others, 256
   funding, 294
   infectious diseases and, 256–258
   OSHA 300-A, 254
   OSHA 301 form, 254, 255
   OSHA 300 log, 254, 255
   OSHA Sections 1904.29, 254–255
   OSHA Sections 1904.35, 254
   OSHA Sections 1904.40, 254
   privacy issues, 258
   publications, 295
   recording and reporting injury/illness, 253–254
   regional and area offices, 296–298
   respiratory protection program, 259
   restricted work/job transfer and, 256
   safety and health program management, 293
   state plans, 293–294
   training, 294
   record, 260–261
   tuberculosis cases, 258–259
office safety and health hazards. *see also* station, office, and facility safety
   ambulances, 205
   computer terminal hazards, 200, 209–210
   disabling accidents, types, 200–201
   electrical hazards, 200, 206, 208–209
   exits and egress hazards, 200, 201–202, 203
   fire hazards, 200, 202, 204
   handling and storage hazards, 200, 202–204
   illumination hazards, 200, 210
   ladders, 205–206, 207
   machinery and tool hazards, 200, 207, 209
      paper cutters, 209
      pencils, pens, scissors, 209
      photocopying machines, 207
      staplers, 209

noise hazards, 200, 210–211
office furniture hazards, 200, 204–205
  chairs, 205
  desks, 205
  file cabinets, 205
ventilation hazards, 200, 210
organization, safety-and-health culture, 21. *see also* job hazard analysis (JHA)
OSHA. *see* Occupational Safety and Health Administration (OSHA)
OSHA 29 CFR 1910.120, 177
OSHA 300 log, 254, 255
other potentially infectious material (OPIM), 256–257
Out of the Crisis, 64

P

paper cutters, hazards, 209
participation, in driver training, 115
PAT. *see* physical ability testing (PAT)
patient drops, causes of, 162–163
patient handling, 161–166
  causes of patient drops
    improper balance/strength, 162–163
    improper use of equipment, 162
    improper maintenance, 164–165
    equipment failure/malfunction, 164–165
    provider haste, 165
  injury prevention, 165–166
  proper lifting dynamics, 166
patient safety, 4
peer fitness trainer, 279
PEL. *see* permissible exposure limit (PEL)
pencils, pens, scissors hazards, 209
Pennsylvania Emergency Health Services Council (2004), 87
performance measurement, safety program, 29
peril, 39
permissible exposure limit (PEL), 274

personal appearance, in driver selection, 112
personal lines, 38
personal protective equipment (PPE), 14, 51
  hazard-control strategies, 237
  infectious disease and, 157–158
  in street and roadway incidents, 149
personnel records, 110, 116–118
photocopy machine hazards, 207
photographs, 225–226
physical ability testing (PAT), 272
physical fitness. *see also* fitness
  driving, 110–111, 125
  lack of, 272
physical fitness programs, 278–280. *see also* wellness programs
  exercise program, 280
  fitness assessment, 279
  fitness standards, 279
  medical screening, 279
  nutrition program, 280
physical layout, 200
planning, accident investigation, 222–223
position power, 72
post-exposure exams, 277–278
postings, EMS facility and, 189
PPE. *see* personal protective equipment (PPE)
predicted effect, risk management, 96
pre-employment physical ability testing, 272
preserving evidence, 176
pressure, tire, 128–129
  checking, 129–130
preventive maintenance, 136
  systems, 80–82
primary surface causes, recommendations, 246
proactive recommendations, 238–239
probability, risk, 88, 94, 95
property, 39
protective clothing, 147, 211
provider haste, 165
provision of authority, safety program, 24–25

Public Risk Management Association, 305
pure-chance theory, 232
pure risk, 95

Q

quick check vehicle inspection, 132–135

R

Radio Technical Commission for Aeronautics (RTCA), 179
recertification, driver, 119, 122
recommendations, accident investigations and, 236–241
recordkeeping, 251–269
  accident reports, 261
  benefits, 261–262
  checklist, 267
  defined, 252
  documenting activities, 253
  driver training and, 116–118
    suspected drug and/or alcohol abuse, 118
    training records, 117–118
  equipment maintenance, 265–267
  infectious diseases (*see* infectious diseases, recordkeeping and)
  injury/illness records, 253–254
  injury reports (*see* injury/illness, reports)
  overview, 252–253
  privacy issues, 258
  respirator fit testing, 259
  safety and health, 253
  safety audits, 261
  safety meetings, 262, 263, 264
  training, 260–261
  tuberculosis cases, 258–259
  vehicle maintenance, 262–263, 265
Recordkeeping Forms and Recording Criteria, 254
reduced profile, 147
reflective vests, 149
regulated waste, 158

Index

rehabilitation sector/group establishment, 281–282
relative risk, 88
repairs, vehicle
  driver's responsibilities, 137–138
    driving vehicle with problems safely, 138
    making repairs, 137
    malfunctions during run, 137
    repairs during run, 138
report forms, accident, 241–246
  demographic information, 245
  description of accident, 245
  findings (*see* findings section)
reporting policy, 101
report writing, accident
  accident summary, 247
  attachment, 247
  recommendations, 246–247
  report forms (*see* report forms, accident)
  review and follow-up actions, 247
Rescorla, Rick, 202
residences, violent situations and, 171–172
respirator fit testing, record-keeping, 259
rest, incident rehabilitation, 282–283
restricted work, 255, 256
retention, risk management, 92, 94
retroreflective material, 149
retroreflectorized cones, 148
reviewing, documents, 227. *see also* documentation
reward participation, safety program, 29
risk
  assessment, 88
  avoidance, 98
  defined, 88
  managers, 3, 89–90
  retention, 97
  transfer, 97
risk management process, 86–103
  alternative risk management techniques, 91–94
  assessment, 88
  community risk management, 89
  control categories, 97
  defined, 88–89
  duplicate resources, 92
  EMS organizational risk management, 89
  exposure avoidance, 91
  flowchart, 90
  goals and objectives, 90
  insurance, 92, 95–97
  loss control, 98–100
  loss exposures, identifying and analyzing, 90–91
  monitoring, 98
  retention, 92, 94
  risk avoidance, 98
  risk manager, 89–90
  system, 90
  vs. loss control, 5–6
routine maintenance, 136

S

Sachs, Gordon, 10
Safe Medical Devices Act (SMDA), 165
safe parking, of EVs, 145–146
safe practices, 50–51
safe procedures, 50
safety, 6. *see also* EMS safety
  activities, 25
  audits, 261
  committee (*see* safety committee)
  culture, 48, 61–62
    building, 62–63
    management processes, 63
  engineers, role, 236
  goals, 25
  inspections, 77–78, 100–101
  meetings, 73–74, 262, 263, 264
  officer, 3 (*see also* EMS safety officer)
  prevention and (*see* safety and prevention)
  program (*see* safety program, developing)
safety-and-health culture, organization and, 21
safety-and-health policy, 23
safety and prevention
  acceptance of risk, 102
  consensus standards, 102–103
  legal responsibility, 101–102
  safety inspections, 100–101
  SOP, 100
safety committee, 48, 63–74, 101
  benefits, 66–67, 68–69
  costs *vs.* benefits, 66–67
  expert power, 72
  involvement, 67
  lack of interest, 70–71
  management commitment, 71–72
  minimum requirements, 73
  operations, 73
  position power, 72
  purpose, 64–65
  roles and responsibilities, 63–64
  safety meetings, 73–74
  starting, 65–66
  training, 72–73
  written plan, 68–69
safety program, developing, 47–83
  action plan, 57–58
  administrative controls, 49–50
  change analysis, 56
  comprehensive surveys, 56
  current situation, information on, 53–55
  designating responsibility, 52–53
  engineering controls, 49
  hazard identification (*see* hazard(s), identification and control)
  hierarchy of controls, 48–49
  interim measures, 51–52
  OSHA and, 49, 53
  PPE, 51
  safety committee (*see* safety committee)
  safety culture, 48, 61–63
  self-inspection, 58–61
  trend analysis, 56–57
  worksite analysis, 51, 55–57
safety program management, 19–44
  accountability, 25
  areas of improvement, 21–22
  assignment of responsibility, 24
  financial aspects, 34–35
  hazards, 29–34

Index

insurance concerns, 35–43
leadership in safety and health, 22–23
overview, 20–21
program evaluation, 25
provision of authority, 24–25
safety-and-health policy, 23
strategic map, 25–29
system components, overview of, 22
SCBA. *see* self-contained breathing apparatus (SCBA)
scene lighting, in street and roadway incidents, 149–151
scene operations, 143–185
   air operations (*see* air operations)
   building fires (*see* building fires)
   hazmat scenes, 176–177
   infectious disease and (*see* infectious diseases, scene operations and)
   overview, 144
   patient handling (*see* patient handling)
   street and roadway scenes (*see* street and roadway incidents)
   violent situations (*see* violent situations)
   wildland fire, 154–155
schedule, inspection, 131–132
scheduled maintenance, 136
scheduling and job enrichment strategies, 51
The Science Daily, 3, 4, 8
secondary surface causes, recommendations, 246–247
self-assessments and benchmarking, safety program, 28
self-contained breathing apparatus (SCBA), 275
self-inspection, 58, 187–188
   scope, 58, 61, 188–189
severity, risk, 88, 94
sharps injury log, 258
shift work, driver proficiency and, 122–125
simple cost-benefit analysis, 239–241

single-engine air tankers (SEATs), 154
single-event theory, 232
sketches, 226
sleep loss, driver proficiency and, 122–125
smoke, attributes of
   color, 154
   pressure, 154
   thickness, 154
   volume, 154
Solomon, Stephen , Dr., 150
SOP. *see* standard operating procedures (SOP)
special-cause analysis, 234
special operations, EMS safety officer and, 15
speculative risk, 95
St. Louis Fire Department, 151
standard operating procedures (SOP), 100
stapler hazards, 209
station, office, and facility safety, 186–216
   changing tires, 212
   checklist for general safety, 198–200
   compressed gases, 212–213
   maintaining healthy office environment, 189–211
   overview, 187
   safety and health hazards (*see* office safety and health hazards)
   towing, 212
   vehicle maintenance areas (*see* vehicle maintenance, areas)
   workplace, organising (*see* workplace, organising)
stimulants, 273
strategic map, safety program, 25–29
   awareness training, 29
   communicate results, 29
   conduct self-assessments and benchmarking, 28
   continue building buy-in on larger scale, 26–27
   develop policies, 28

   measurement and-feedback system, 29
   obtain top management buy-in, 26
   organization, alignment, 28
   performance measurement, 29
   process changes, 29
   provide ongoing support, 29
   reward participation, 29
   roles and responsibilities, 28
   steering committee, 28
   system of accountability, 28
   training, 28
   trust, 27
street and roadway incidents, 144–151
   challenge, 145
   command and control, 146–147
   emergency vehicle markings, 151
   limited access highway operations, 147
   MUTCD for, 144–145
   personnel functions, 147
   PPE, 149
   safety, 145–146
   scene lighting, 149–151
   traffic cones, 146, 147, 148–149
stress and mental health, 288
substance abuse, recordkeeping and, 118
Sunstar EMS, 265
Superfund Amendments and Reauthorization Act (SARA), 177
Supplemental Type Certificates (STCs), 179
system(s)
   of accountability, safety program, 28
   analysis, 234–235
      design, 235
      implementation, 235
   improvements, accident investigation, 237–241
      behavior-based safety, 238
      proactive recommendations, 238–239
      simple cost-benefit analysis, 239–241
   weaknesses, 221, 233

T

tactical EMS, in violent situations, 175–176
  body armor, 175–176
  contact and cover tactics, 175
TAWS. *see* terrain awareness warning systems (TAWS)
techniques, risk management process, 91–94
  implementing, 95–98
  selecting, 94–95
temperature grades, tire maintenance, 128
terrain awareness warning systems (TAWS)
  FAA and, 179
Thomco Insurance, 250
time, risk management, 96–97
tires, vehicle maintenance, 127–130
  load limits, 128–129
  pressure, 128–129
    checking, 129–130
  temperature grade, 128
  traction grade, 127
  tread-wear grade, 127
tobacco, use of, 274
towing, 212
traction grade, vehicle maintenance, 127
traffic cones, street and roadway incidents and, 146, 147, 148–149
traffic psychology, 108
training
  accident investigation, 220
  program, for infectious diseases, 160–161
  for recordkeeping, 260–261
  records, 117–118, 257, 260–261
  safety program, 28
transitional employment, 284
tread wear, vehicle maintenance, 127
trend analysis, 56–57
trust, safety program, 27

tuberculosis (TB) cases, recordkeeping, 258–259

U

Uniformed Services Employment and Reemployment Rights Act (USERRA), 194
uniforms, EMS personnel, 169
unions and employee groups, 306
Unit Log (ICS Form 214), 16
unsafe behaviors, 218, 233, 236
"upstream measures," 21
U.S. Department of Labor, 216
U.S. Fire Administration (USFA), 109, 302–303
U.S. National Highway Traffic Safety Administration (NHTSA), 124
USFA. *see* U.S. Fire Administration (USFA)

V

vaccination
  EMS providers, 277
  Hepatitis B, 158–159
vehicle characteristics, 115–116
vehicle driving and fleet maintenance, 106–142. *see also* emergency vehicles (EVs)
  crash injury and fatalities, 107–109
  maintenance, 125–138
    comprehensive programs (*see* vehicle maintenance, programs)
    EVTs, 126–127
    inspections (*see* inspections, vehicle)
    refusing to drive unsafe vehicle, 135
    support equipment, 131
    tires (*see* tires, vehicle maintenance)
  overview, 107
  safe driver (*see* driver, safety and)
vehicle maintenance
  areas, 211–212

  eye protection and protective clothing, 211
  flammables, 212, 213
  housekeeping, 212
  lifting devices, 212
  work clothing, 211–212
  programs, 135–138
    driver responsibility, 136
    driver responsibility for vehicle repairs (*see* repairs, vehicle)
    preventive maintenance, 136
    vehicle maintenance logs, 136–137
    work requests, 136
  recordkeeping, 262–263, 265
    vehicle maintenance logs, 265
    work requests, 263, 265
ventilation hazards, 200, 210
VFIS, 120–122, 133, 249–250
videotaping, accident scene, 226
violent situations, 167–176
  clandestine drug labs (*see* clandestine drug labs)
  cover and concealment, 174
  distraction and evasive tactics, 175
  domestic violence, 174
  EMS at crime scenes, 176
    preserving evidence, 176
  EMS personnel in, 167–169
    on scene, 167
    in workplace, 167–169
  groups and situations, 172–173
    gang characteristics, 172
    safety issues, 172–173
  highway safety, 169–171
    approaching vehicle, 170–171
    scene observation, 170
  residences, 171–172
  tactical EMS (*see* tactical EMS)
  uniforms, 169
visual flight rules (VFR), 179

Voluntary Protection Programs (VPP), 22, 23
VPP. *see* Voluntary Protection Programs (VPP)

W
weather, FAA and, 178–179
wellness programs. *see also* EMS provider health and wellness
   annual medical evaluations, 276–277
   EAP, 278
   incident rehabilitation, 280–284
   infection control, 277–278
   physical fitness program (*see* physical fitness programs)
   return to work, 284–288 (*see also* early return-to-work (ERTW) program)
   stress and mental health, 288
West, Kathy, 158
White, Jim, 117
wildland fire operations, 154–155
windchill index, 282
Winter Park ambulance safety design, 117
work clothing, in vehicle maintenance areas, 211–212
workers' compensation carriers, 306
workplace, organising, 187–189
   required postings, 189
   self-inspection scope, 188–189
workplace hazards, identifying, 31–33. *see also* job hazard analysis (JHA)
work practice controls, infectious disease and, 156–157
work requests
   equipment maintenance, 267
   vehicle maintenance, 136, 263, 265
worksite analysis, 51, 55–57